THE AUSTRALIAN Women's Weekly

Taking charge of
# DIABETES

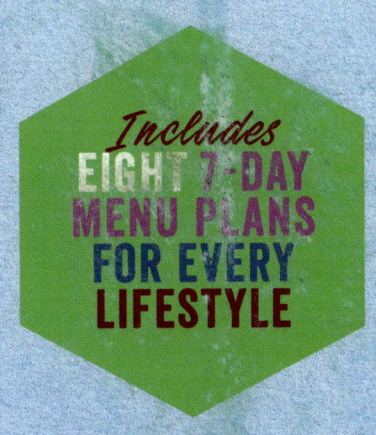

Includes
EIGHT 7-DAY
MENU PLANS
FOR EVERY
LIFESTYLE

BAUER
MEDIA GROUP

**PUBLISHED IN 2018 BY BAUER MEDIA BOOKS, AUSTRALIA.
BAUER MEDIA BOOKS IS A DIVISION OF BAUER MEDIA PTY LTD.**

## BAUER MEDIA BOOKS

**Publisher**
Jo Runciman

**Associate publisher**
Sally Eagle

**Editorial & food director**
Sophia Young

**Editorial director-at-large**
Pamela Clark

**Creative director**
Hannah Blackmore

**Managing editor**
Stephanie Kistner

**Senior designers**
Gayna Murphy, Jeannel Cunanan

**Editor**
Wendy Bryant

**Food editor**
Alexandra Elliott

**Operations manager**
David Scotto

**Photographer**
James Moffatt

**Stylists**
Olivia Blackmore, Kate Brown

**Photochefs**
Rebecca Clancy, Amal Webster

**Recipe developers**
Carly-Sophia Taylor, Nadia Fonoff, Rebecca Clancy,
Elizabeth Fiducia, Sarah Murphy, Angela Devlin,
Jane Howard, Tessa Immens, Kathy Knudsen,
Jordanna Levin

**Printed in China**
by Leo Paper Products Ltd

A catalogue record for this book is available
from the National Library of Australia.
**ISBN:** 978-1-92569-459-8

© Bauer Media Pty Limited 2018
ABN 18 053 273 546

This publication is copyright. No part of it
may be reproduced or transmitted in any form
without the written permission of the publisher.

**Published by Bauer Media Books**,
a division of Bauer Media Pty Ltd,
54 Park St, Sydney; GPO Box 4088,
Sydney, NSW 2001, Australia
Ph +61 2 9282 8618; Fax +61 2 9126 3702
www.awwcookbooks.com.au

**Order books**
phone 136 116 (within Australia)
**or order online at**
www.awwcookbooks.com.au
**Send recipe enquiries to**
recipeenquiries@bauer-media.com.au

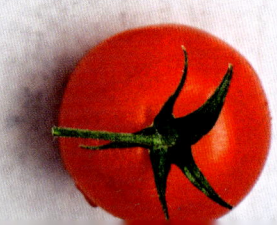

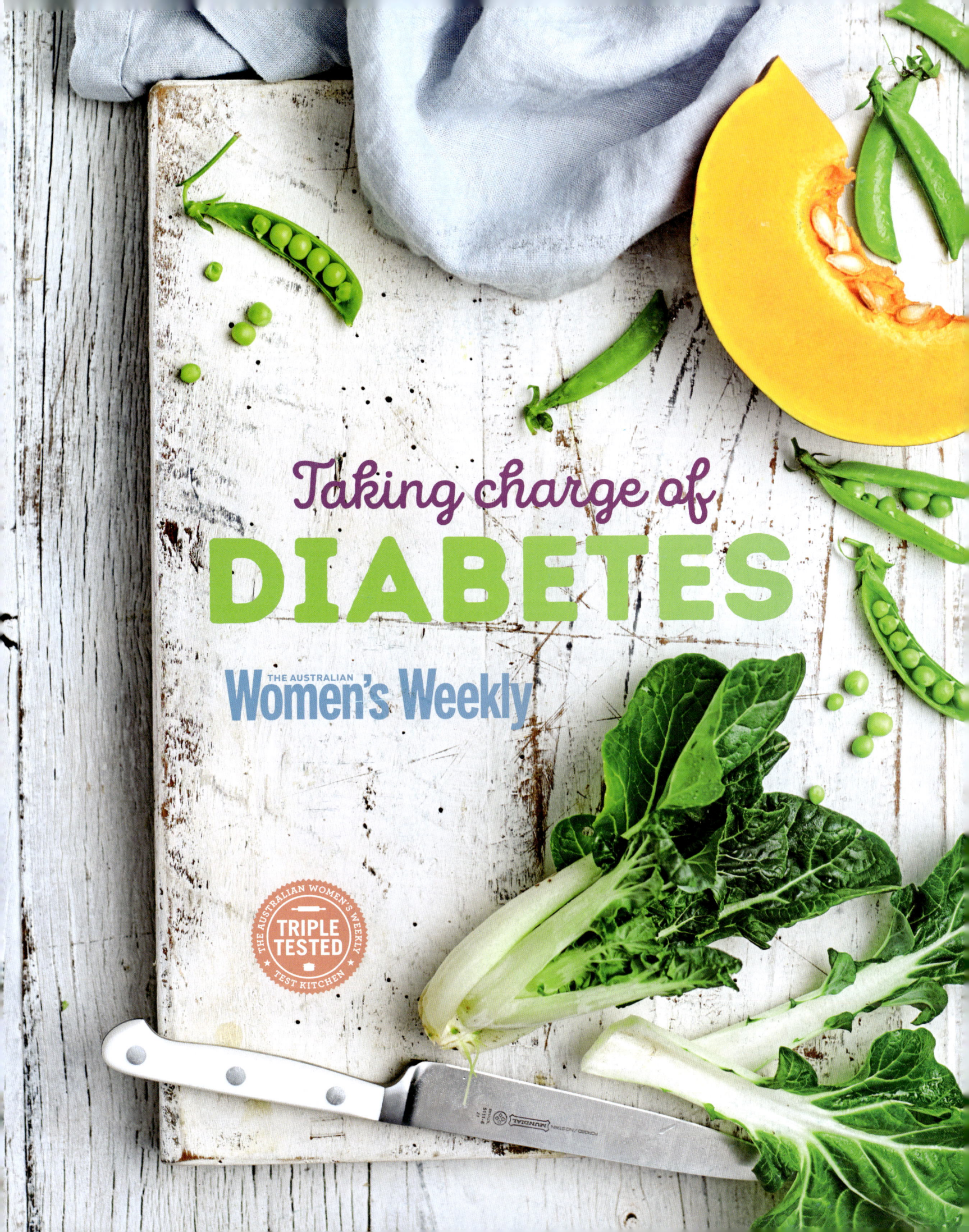

Taking charge of
DIABETES

THE AUSTRALIAN Women's Weekly

TRIPLE TESTED
THE AUSTRALIAN WOMEN'S WEEKLY
TEST KITCHEN

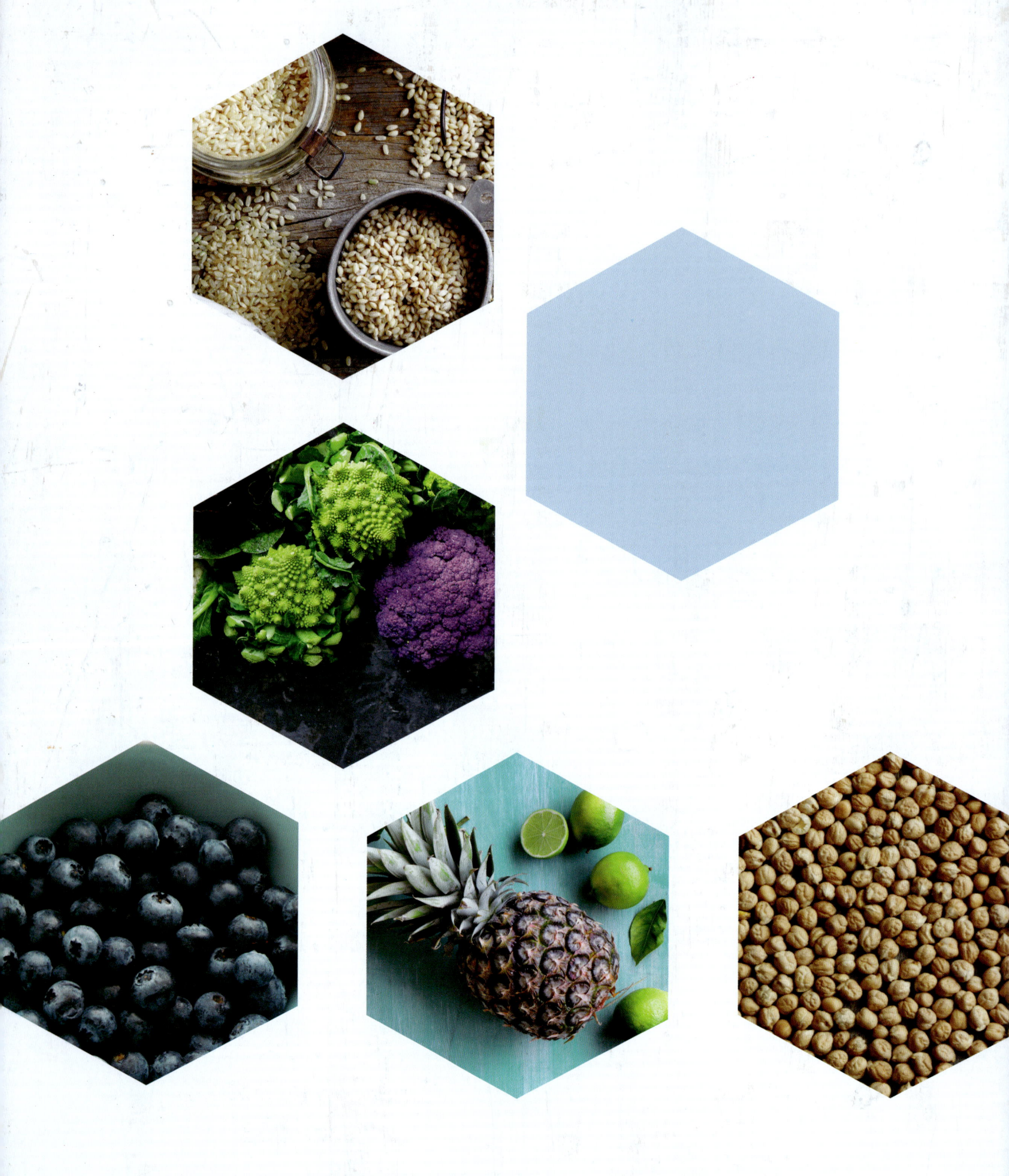

# CONTENTS

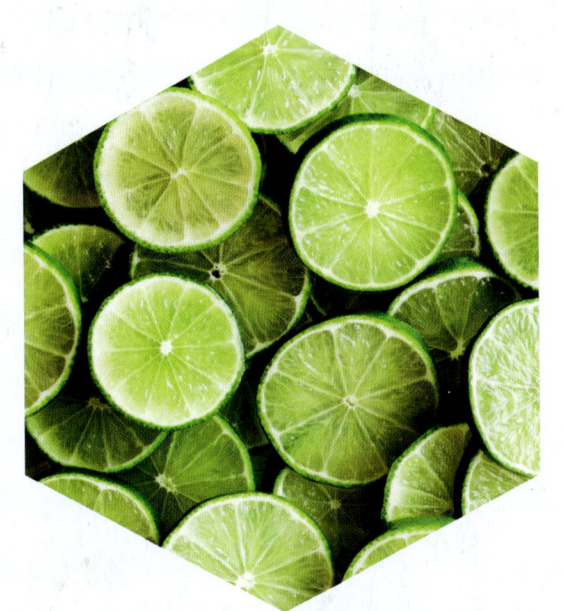

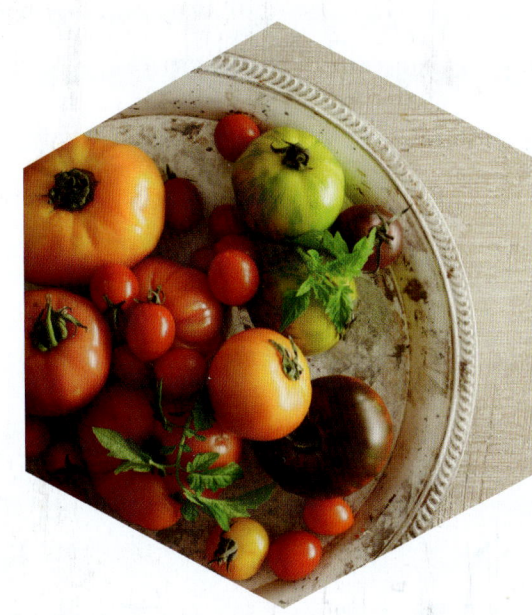

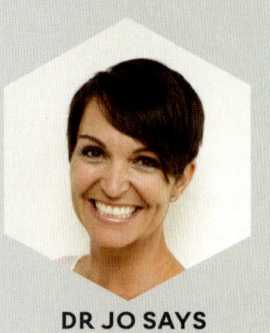

**DR JO SAYS**
As a PhD qualified nutrition scientist & dietitian, Dr Jo has spent over 20 years translating science into everyday diet and lifestyle advice. She is an author, TV presenter and founder of a lifestyle change program, *Get Lean*.

# Get yourself
# INTO
# SHAPE

In Australia, someone develops diabetes every five minutes. That's 280 Australians every day, and type 2 diabetes is our fastest growing chronic condition. There are around 1.2 million Australians diagnosed with diabetes (of all types), but of great concern is the estimated 500,000 more people who simply don't know they have it as they are yet to be diagnosed.

If your doctor says you have pre-diabetes, a condition in which your blood glucose levels are higher than normal but not yet at the level where diabetes is diagnosed, you may be able to turn the situation around and prevent the progression to type 2 diabetes. Pre-diabetes affects some 2 million Australians, and so tackling the condition at this early stage has huge potential to reduce the number of people developing diabetes in the future.

Whether you want to reduce your risk of diabetes, or you have pre-diabetes and want to turn that ship around, or you have a diabetes diagnosis and want to optimally manage the condition to avoid complications and maintain good health, this book is for you.

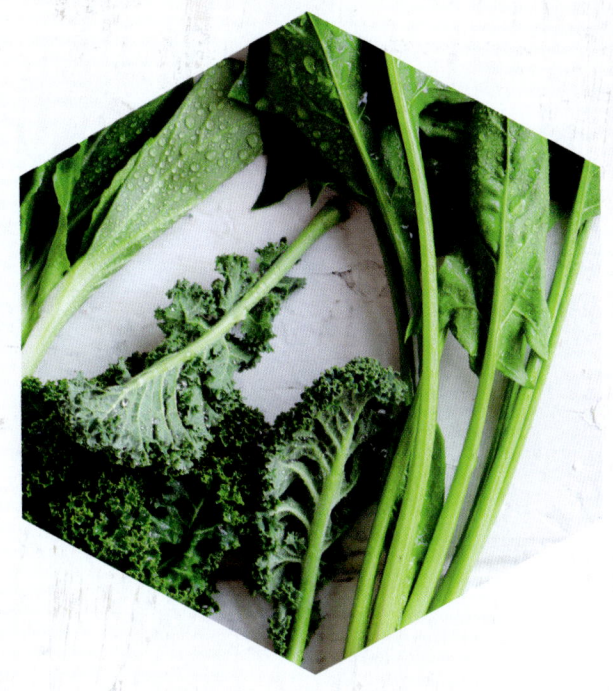
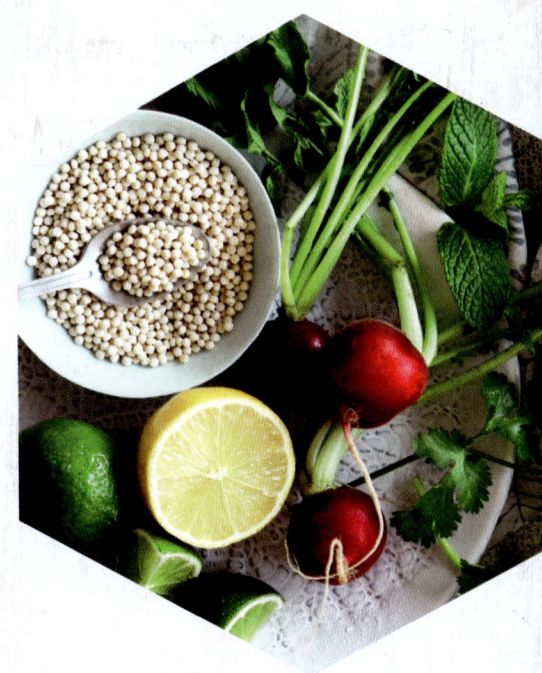

**DISCLAIMER**

The following information provides basic guidelines to healthy eating for people with diabetes. Please check with your doctor, dietitian or diabetes educator as to the suitability of this information for your diabetes management. Unless indicated otherwise, all serving portions, including accompaniments, are of equal size.

Type 2 diabetes can often be managed entirely by a healthy diet and lifestyle. Although medications and/or insulin may become necessary to reduce the risk of complications, remember that no matter the stage of diabetes, your diet and lifestyle choices remain crucial to managing the condition and are under your control.

## TYPES OF DIABETES

There are three types of diabetes, and it's important to understand the differences.

**Type 1 diabetes** is an auto-immune condition where the body's immune system attacks the cells in the pancreas that produce insulin. The onset can be very sudden and, with no insulin being produced, the body cannot get glucose out of the bloodstream to utilise as fuel.

The symptoms include excessive thirst, passing more urine, weight loss despite an increased appetite, blurred vision, headaches, mood swings and feeling incredibly lethargic, poor wound healing and/or skin infections. This type of diabetes accounts for about 10–15% of all diabetes cases, and most often occurs in those under 30 years of age, but can occur later.

Although there is a genetic link to the risk of developing type 1 diabetes, no one knows exactly what triggers it. But, importantly, it is not related to diet or lifestyle choices. Nevertheless, following a healthy diet and lifestyle is important in the management of the condition.

**Type 2 diabetes** is quite different. It tends to occur more gradually, developing over months and years. There is a genetic link, so if you have a close family member with type 2 diabetes, or come from a particular ethnic background, you are at a higher risk. However, this form of diabetes is also associated with diet and lifestyle. View this as good news: that means you have some control over the condition and can act now to improve your health and wellbeing, both today and in the long term. Following a healthy diet, maintaining a healthy weight and being more active every day are cornerstones to reducing the risk of and managing type 2 diabetes.

In type 2 diabetes, body cells becomes resistant to insulin and the pancreas pumps out more and more insulin to keep blood glucose levels under control. Eventually these cells may become exhausted and fail to produce enough insulin. So, in type 2 diabetes you may have defective insulin or insufficient insulin, and one frequently progresses to the other.

In the early days of type 2 diabetes, the condition can often be managed entirely through positive diet and lifestyle choices. However, as the condition progresses, medications and/or insulin may be necessary to reduce the risk of complications. It's important that you follow the advice of your doctor, but do remember that no matter the stage of diabetes, your diet and lifestyle choices remain vital, and are under your control.

**Gestational diabetes** is a type of diabetes that occurs during pregnancy and usually disappears after the baby is born. A mother who has had gestation diabetes is, however, at an increased risk of developing type 2 diabetes later in life. It is essential, therefore, that she takes action to reduce this risk as much as possible.

Losing any weight gained during the pregnancy (and more if overweight prior to pregnancy), within a realistic timeframe, following a healthy diet and living an active lifestyle, will all reduce the risk of developing type 2 diabetes later in life. Managing gestational diabetes can be done with healthy eating, regular exercise and ensuring appropriate weight gain. Some women may, however, find that insulin injections are required.

## MANAGING BLOOD GLUCOSE LEVELS

For all diabetes types, the key priority is to help the body manage blood glucose levels. During fasting, normal blood glucose levels in people without diabetes are between 3.9 and 5.5 mmol/L, and the goal for those with diabetes is for fasting levels to be in the range of 4–6 mmol/L.

**Hypoglycaemia, or hypo**, is when blood glucose levels drop too low. Symptoms include sweating, dizziness, confusion and trembling, and, if not corrected, you may pass out. A 'hypo' requires immediate treatment.

**Hyperglycaemia, or hyper**, is when blood glucose levels get too high. Symptoms include an increase in appetite, thirst and urination. If not corrected, over time 'hypers' can lead to heart, kidney and eye damage and limb amputation.

Long term blood glucose control is measured by glycated haemoglobin, or HbA1c. Glucose in the bloodstream can attach to haemoglobin (a protein in your red blood cells that carries oxygen around the body) to form 'glycated haemoglobin'. The amount of HbA1c is a good indicator of your blood glucose control over the previous 2–3 months. The more glucose there is, the higher the levels of HbA1c.

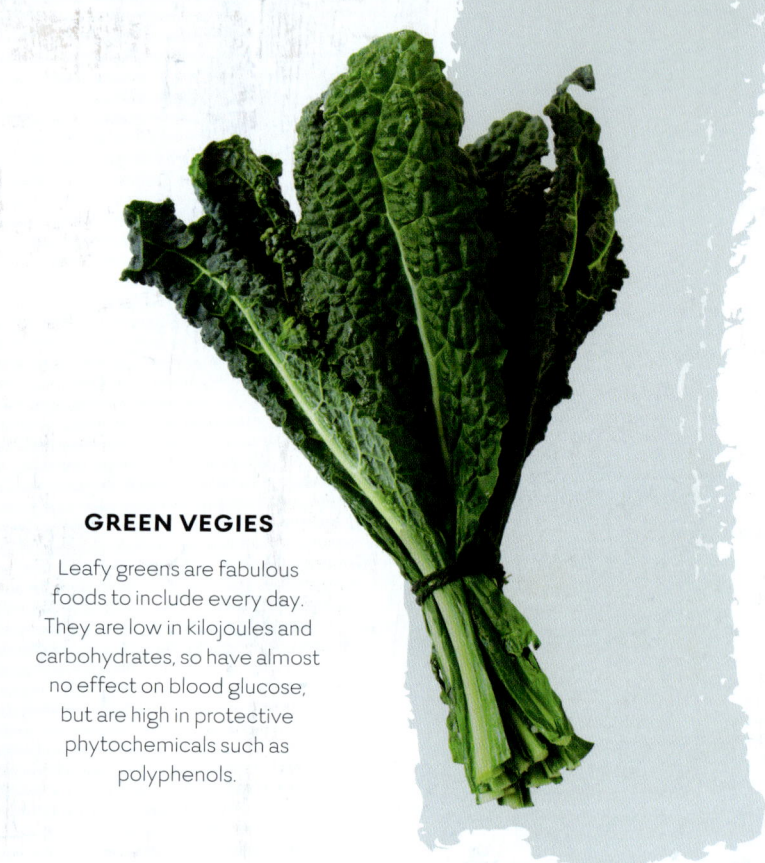

**GREEN VEGIES**

Leafy greens are fabulous foods to include every day. They are low in kilojoules and carbohydrates, so have almost no effect on blood glucose, but are high in protective phytochemicals such as polyphenols.

This measure is important as the higher your HbA1c, the greater the risk of complications. The target to aim for in most people is an HbA1c of 7% or less. If you're getting results higher than this, you don't have your blood glucose levels under control. Talk to your doctor, Credentialled Diabetes Educator or dietitian for further advice and help.

## BLOOD GLUCOSE SPIKES AFTER EATING

It's not just fasting levels of blood glucose that are important. Recent research has emphasised that the spike in blood glucose after eating (i.e. how high your blood glucose goes) and how quickly it returns to the normal healthy range is crucial for reducing the risk of complications.

High blood glucose spikes and levels that stay higher than normal for more than two hours are incredibly damaging to blood vessels around the body, including those in and around the heart, as well as the smaller vessels in the eyes, kidneys and extremities including the hands and feet.

It's therefore a good idea to test your blood glucose level 2 hours after eating. As a general guide, if the result is less than 7.8 mmol/L you're in the normal range, but if it's above 10 mmol/L you are in the potentially damaging zone. The more often this happens the greater the potential for damage.

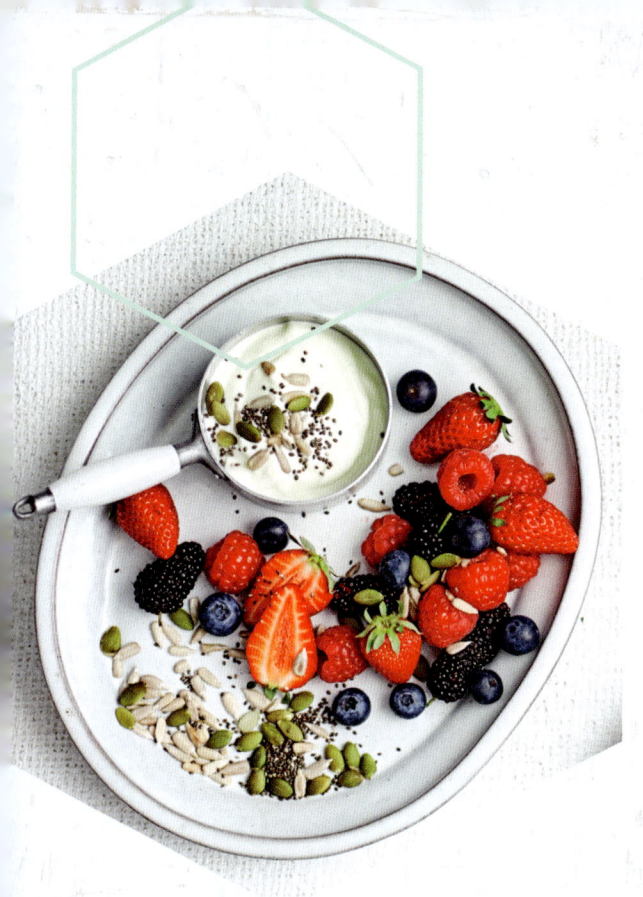

# THE OPTIMAL DIET FOR MANAGING DIABETES

A healthy diet for people living with diabetes is really the same as for those without the condition. You do, however, need to pay closer attention to the impact of your food choices on your blood glucose levels.

When you eat foods that contain carbohydrates, present in foods as starch or sugars, these are broken down in the small intestine and absorbed into the blood stream, resulting in a rise in blood glucose levels. Lots of factors can affect how quickly this happens. Firstly, the more carbohydrate in the meal, the larger the blood glucose rise will be. Secondly, several factors affect how quickly the food or meal is broken down to release the glucose.

Whole plant foods contain a mixture of carbohydrates, some we can break down (starch and sugars) and some we can't. The latter are broadly termed 'fibre'. Some of these fibres are soluble, and within the gut they form a kind of gel that slows down the attack of digestive enzymes. This, in turn, slows down the digestion and absorption of glucose from the digestible carbohydrates present.

The fibre eventually passes into the colon where it has a further benefit by fuelling the growth of the resident gut bugs, favouring a healthy balance of bacterial groups. This process is key not only for good gut health, but appears to be involved in the management of blood glucose, blood cholesterol and insulin sensitivity.

Almost all whole plant foods contain a mixture of digestible carbohydrates and fibre, while most junk and highly-processed foods are made from refined flours and added sugars where the fibre has been discarded, leaving only rapidly digestible carbohydrates. This is highly detrimental to the control of blood glucose and the maintenance of a healthy balanced microbiota. The knock-on effects for health and wellbeing are potentially huge.

## GREEK NATURAL YOGHURT

Yoghurt may have several health benefits, and recent research has shown that people who eat yoghurt regularly have a lower risk of developing diabetes or becoming overweight. No one understands why, but it may be the live 'good' bacteria present, the high calcium content or the types of protein. Yoghurt also has a low GI, making it a great choice. However, opt for unsweetened varieties, and add your own fruit if you wish.

## DR JO SAYS

Controlling your blood glucose levels is best managed by careful selection of the types of carbohydrate-containing foods you eat and by controlling your portion size. In general, whole plant foods that are minimally processed fit the bill, including wholegrains, legumes and some starchy vegetables eaten with their skin.

## TIPS ABOUT DIABETES

### LOSE WEIGHT AND AVOID WEIGHT GAIN
Carrying too much body fat tends to increase insulin resistance and the risk of developing diabetes. If you're overweight and diagnosed with diabetes, losing even 5% of your body weight can help to manage the condition and lower your risk of complications.

### ADOPT A HEALTHY EATING PATTERN
What you eat has a major effect on weight control, diabetes management and general health and wellbeing. Forget the latest diet fads, and focus on cutting out ultra-processed foods and drinks, including junk food and sweetened drinks. Enjoy a menu based on minimally-processed whole foods such as vegies, fruit, nuts, seeds, legumes, wholegrains, seafood, lean meats, dairy foods and extra virgin olive oil.

### LIVE A HEALTHY ACTIVE LIFESTYLE
Being active daily and limiting time spent on sedentary behaviours is key to managing and preventing diabetes. When you move, muscles are stimulated to take up glucose from the blood, helping you to control blood levels, while being regularly active improves insulin sensitivity. Over the long term, regular exercise plays an important role in weight control.

# GLYCAEMIC INDEX (GI) AND GLYCAEMIC LOAD (GL)

The glycaemic index (GI) is a measure of how quickly a carbohydrate–containing food raises blood glucose levels. It is a ranking system where foods are compared to the same amount of carbohydrate consumed as pure glucose dissolved in water.

Glucose is the reference, so therefore has a value of 100, and all other foods are ranked as a percentage of this. In other words, if a food has a GI of 50 it has half the blood glucose response of drinking the same amount of carbohydrate as pure glucose.

While there are individual variations in our responses to foods, GI research has shown that the ranking of foods is remarkably consistent. In other words, all of us will have a smaller blood glucose response to a low GI food, such as chickpeas, compared to a high GI food, such as white jasmine rice, even if our individual results vary from each other.

Think of the GI as a measure of the quality of the carbohydrate, but the quantity is also key. Eating a large portion of a low GI food, such as pasta, can have a bigger effect on your blood glucose than eating a small portion of a high GI food, such as white bread. This is where the Glycaemic Load (GL) comes in.

The GL is a more accurate measure of the absolute effect of the food on blood glucose levels. It is calculated by multiplying the grams of carbohydrate present in the serve of food by the GI.

GL = quantity (grams of carbohydrate) x quality (the GI).

Diets with a low glycaemic load are strongly supported by the scientific evidence to be beneficial in improving blood glucose control in people living with diabetes. They are now recommended by most diabetes foundations and organisations around the world including the International Diabetes Federation.

It may, at first, seem complicated to have to think about GI and GL, but be reassured that the absolute numbers don't matter. If you understand the concept then you can easily put it into practise.

The advantage of the GI is that the category doesn't change, whereas the GL does in relation to the portion size. This means that if you opt for mostly low GI foods and keep your portion size under control, you'll end up with a low GL diet.

The recipes in this book are all designed to utilise mostly low GI foods and keep the overall carbohydrate levels to no more than 50g in main meals and 25g in snacks, desserts and drinks. This will help you to achieve a low GL diet that is ideal for the management of diabetes.

## CHICKPEAS

Chickpeas are terrific to include as they have both a low GI and a low GL per typical serve. They are rich sources of several types of fibre, including those that specifically fuel healthy fermentation in the colon by the resident gut bacteria, and provide plant protein and a raft of vitamins and minerals including folate, magnesium, zinc and iron.

### DR JO SAYS

Think about both the quality and the quantity of carbohydrate in your diet. The GI is a useful tool for assessing the quality, but do remember a low GI does not always indicate a healthy food. Ice-cream, for example, may have a low GI, but clearly this is not an everyday food!

## WHY NOT JUST FOLLOW A LOW CARB DIET?

Low carb diets are not currently recommended for people living with diabetes for several reasons. Low carb also tends to mean low fibre, and it's very hard to meet the recommended fibre levels and the array of different fibres required for good gut health without plant foods that contain significant amounts of carbohydrate. Fibres are types of carbohydrate, after all.

If carbs are low, then fat and/or protein intake must be high. A high protein intake may place undue stress on your kidneys, particularly if you are unaware of any kidney damage from poorly managed blood glucose control. A high protein or a high fat diet may also have further damaging effects on gut health, particularly combined with low fibre, via changes to the gut microbiota.

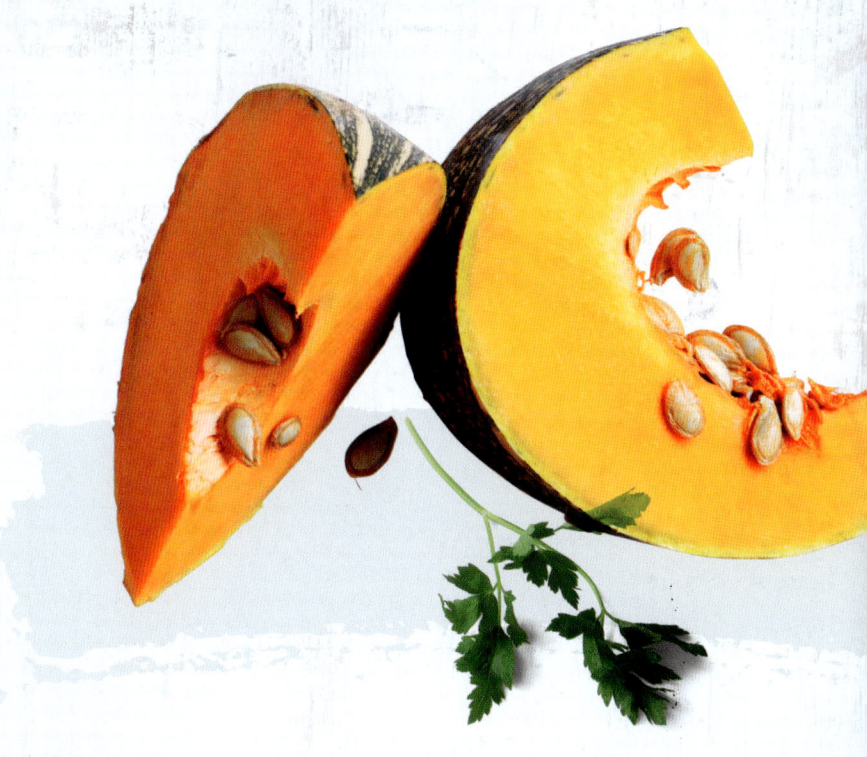

We all need some carbs, they provide our body with the energy it needs to function daily. And, depending on whether we are growing teenagers, athletes, manual labourers or sedentary workers, we all need different amounts. It's the type of carbs we eat that's the issue. Smart carbs are minimally processed and closer to their natural state, and these are the carbs we should choose.

### GRAINS, NUTS + SEEDS

The low-fat era is long gone, and nutrition research clearly shows the benefits of including foods containing good fats like nuts, seeds and wholegrains in the diet. These are rich in healthy unsaturated fats, fibres, nutrients and beneficial plant chemicals such as antioxidants.

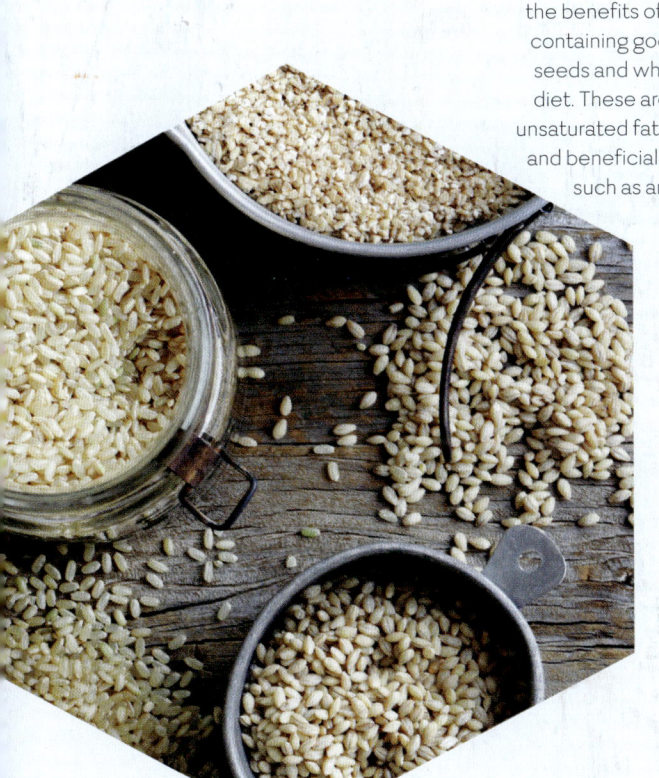

Early evidence also suggests that high protein/high fat diets may accelerate the aging process, particularly if followed in mid to later life, increasing the risk of other chronic diseases and an ultimately shortened life span.

There is interesting and valid research looking at the effects of diets high in good fats (rather than just any fats) and low in carbs, but the truth is that we simply don't know the long-term effects of these on the health of those living with diabetes.

And, don't forget, good carbs are also important providers of different types of fibre, as well as minerals, vitamins and numerous beneficial plant compounds, such as antioxidants, all of which are necessary to keep our bodies in good health.

Unless further substantial and convincing evidence comes to light, it is most prudent to follow the type of diet known to be beneficial, not just for diabetes management, but for long-term health and wellbeing. That is a diet based on plenty of fibre-rich plant foods with a balance of good carbs, protein and healthy fats.

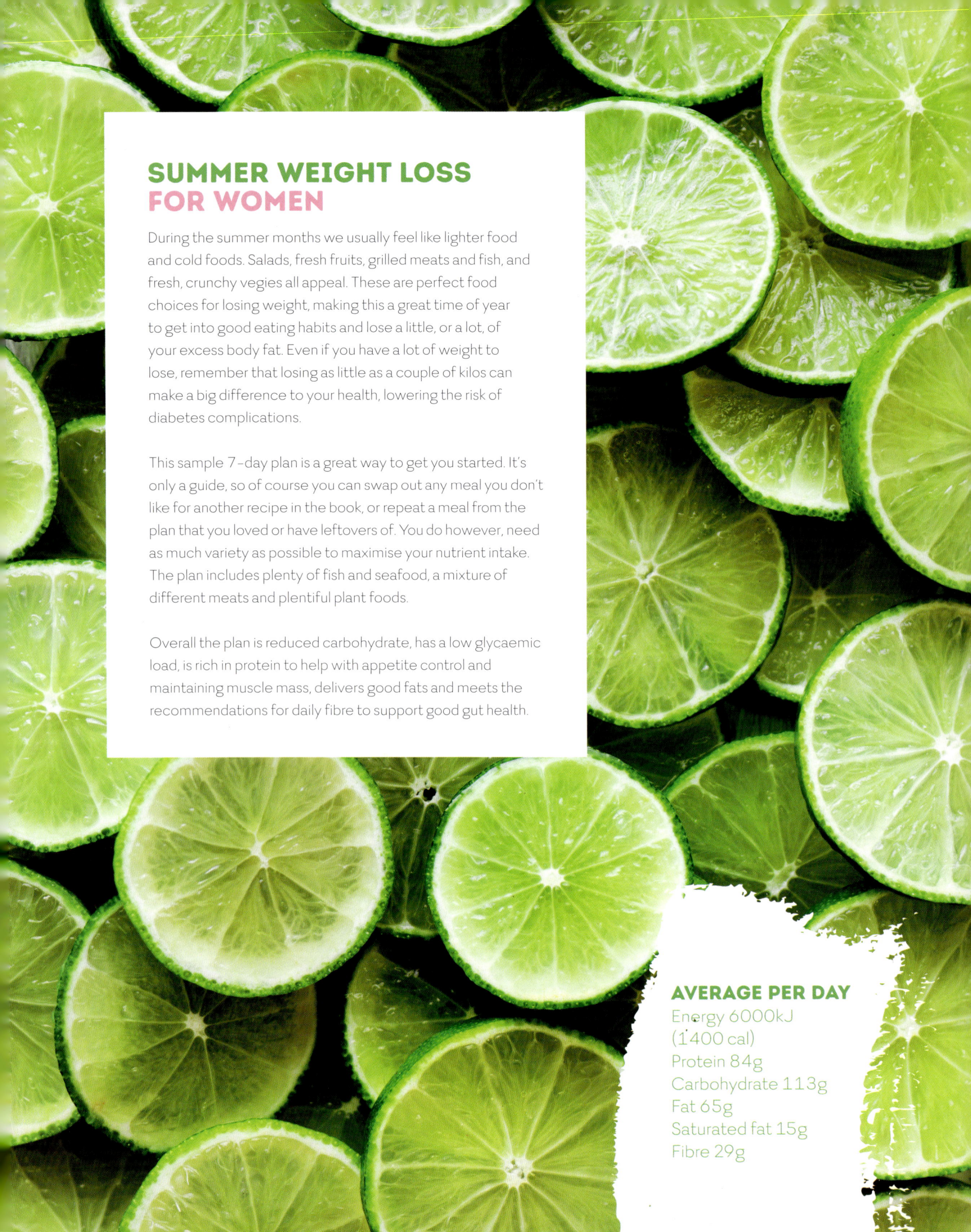

# SUMMER WEIGHT LOSS FOR WOMEN

During the summer months we usually feel like lighter food and cold foods. Salads, fresh fruits, grilled meats and fish, and fresh, crunchy vegies all appeal. These are perfect food choices for losing weight, making this a great time of year to get into good eating habits and lose a little, or a lot, of your excess body fat. Even if you have a lot of weight to lose, remember that losing as little as a couple of kilos can make a big difference to your health, lowering the risk of diabetes complications.

This sample 7-day plan is a great way to get you started. It's only a guide, so of course you can swap out any meal you don't like for another recipe in the book, or repeat a meal from the plan that you loved or have leftovers of. You do however, need as much variety as possible to maximise your nutrient intake. The plan includes plenty of fish and seafood, a mixture of different meats and plentiful plant foods.

Overall the plan is reduced carbohydrate, has a low glycaemic load, is rich in protein to help with appetite control and maintaining muscle mass, delivers good fats and meets the recommendations for daily fibre to support good gut health.

## AVERAGE PER DAY

Energy 6000kJ
(1400 cal)
Protein 84g
Carbohydrate 113g
Fat 65g
Saturated fat 15g
Fibre 29g

# 7-DAY MENU PLANNER

| DAY | BREAKFAST | SNACK | LUNCH | SNACK | DINNER |
|---|---|---|---|---|---|
| 1 | Lentil omelette with braised capsicum & watercress (page 71) | 1 apple | Spicy chicken, lettuce & avocado wrap (page 89) | 30g almonds | Teriyaki salmon with edamame & cucumber rice salad (page 169) |
| 2 | ½ cup natural muesli (with no dried fruit) with ½ cup low-fat milk, ¼ cup blueberries, 4 sliced strawberries & 2 tb greek yoghurt | 4 brazil nuts + 2 dried apricots | Sesame chicken & barley salad (page 81) | 1 carrot & 1 stick celery cut into batons served with 2 tb hummus (see page 29) | Cumin-spiced steak with white bean hummus (page 162) |
| 3 | Breakfast smoothie (page 63) | 1 stick celery spread with 1 tb natural peanut butter | Spicy chicken, lettuce & avocado wrap (page 89) | 1 orange | Prawn & zucchini 'noodle' pad thai (page 153) |
| 4 | Passionfruit & strawberry trifle (page 62) | 1 macadamia & fig bliss ball (page 28) | Zucchini, spinach & sweet potato frittata (page 120) | 1 cup mixed berries with ½ cup natural greek yoghurt | Fennel-rubbed pork with fennel & apple slaw (page 161) <br><br> 2 x 10g squares dark chocolate |
| 5 | Yoghurt, chia & apple oat bircher (page 42) | 1 carrot cut into batons with 2 tb hummus (see page 29) | Avocado, trout & fennel tzatziki open sandwich (page 107) | 1 macadamia & fig bliss ball (page 28) | Lamb kofta with broccoli barley salad (page 183) |
| 6 | Big mushrooms with fetta & spinach (page 34) | ½ cup blueberries + 10 almonds | Roasted root vegetable & rice salad with spiced yoghurt (page 93) | 2 x 10g squares dark chocolate | Sardines with roast broccoli and almond 'gremolata' (page 146) + ½ cup greek yoghurt with 6 sliced strawberries (see page 31) |
| 7 | Baked berry german pancake (page 72) | 30g cashews | Mediterranean beef salad (page 78) | Green smoothie (see page 30) | Braised chicken with mushrooms & artichokes (page 187) + Grilled mango cheeks with lime drizzle (page 233) |

NOTE: While you need to pay attention to your blood sugar levels, especially if taking insulin, the snacks are optional. If you're not hungry, and your blood sugar levels are ok, you can skip the snacks.

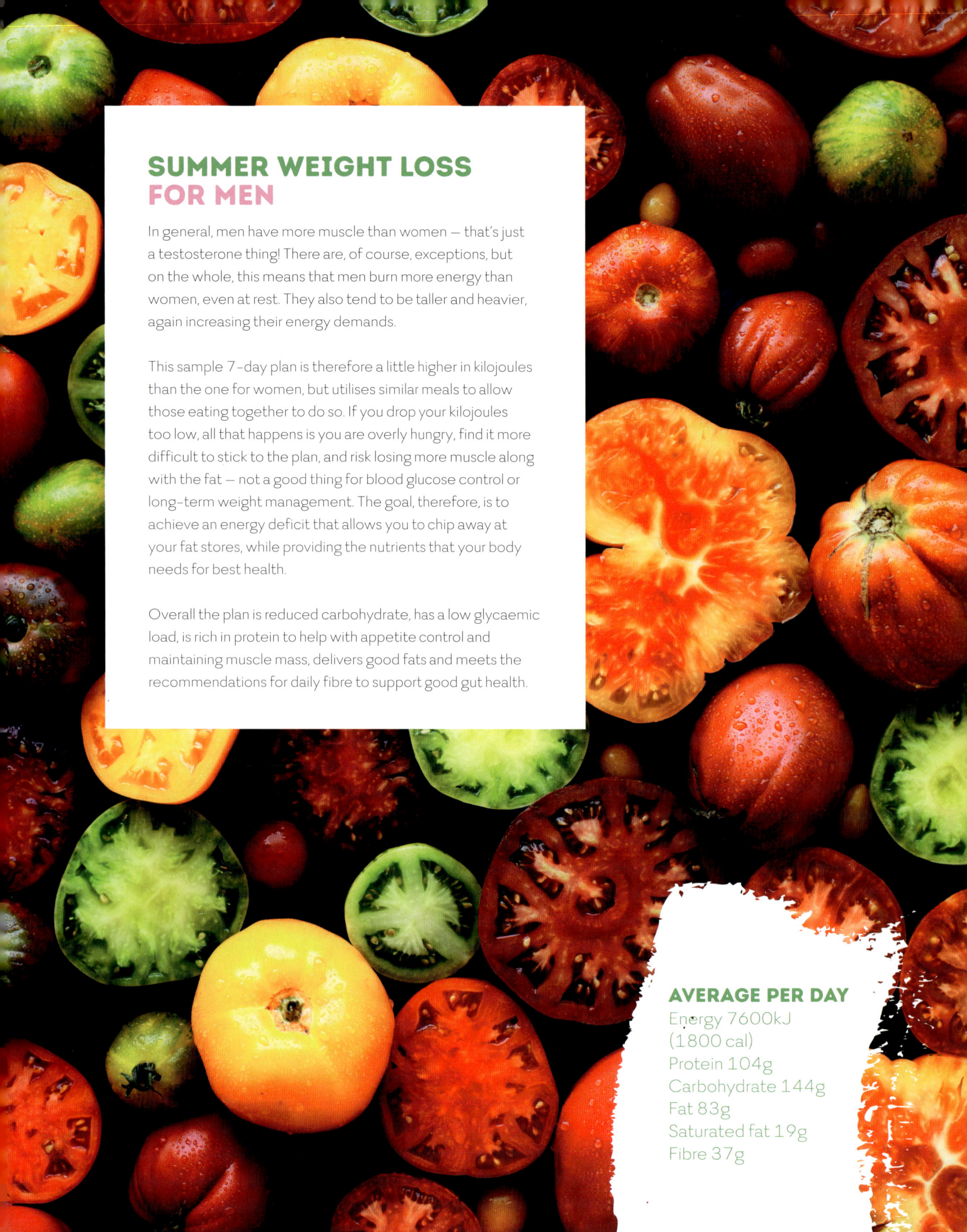

# SUMMER WEIGHT LOSS
## FOR MEN

In general, men have more muscle than women — that's just a testosterone thing! There are, of course, exceptions, but on the whole, this means that men burn more energy than women, even at rest. They also tend to be taller and heavier, again increasing their energy demands.

This sample 7-day plan is therefore a little higher in kilojoules than the one for women, but utilises similar meals to allow those eating together to do so. If you drop your kilojoules too low, all that happens is you are overly hungry, find it more difficult to stick to the plan, and risk losing more muscle along with the fat — not a good thing for blood glucose control or long-term weight management. The goal, therefore, is to achieve an energy deficit that allows you to chip away at your fat stores, while providing the nutrients that your body needs for best health.

Overall the plan is reduced carbohydrate, has a low glycaemic load, is rich in protein to help with appetite control and maintaining muscle mass, delivers good fats and meets the recommendations for daily fibre to support good gut health.

### AVERAGE PER DAY
Energy 7600kJ
(1800 cal)
Protein 104g
Carbohydrate 144g
Fat 83g
Saturated fat 19g
Fibre 37g

# 7-DAY MENU PLANNER

| DAY | BREAKFAST | SNACK | LUNCH | SNACK | DINNER |
|---|---|---|---|---|---|
| 1 | Lentil omelette with braised capsicum & watercress (page 71) + 1 slice wholegrain toast with ¼ avocado & 1 sliced tomato | 1 apple | Spicy chicken, lettuce & avocado wrap (page 89) + 1 orange | 50g almonds | Teriyaki salmon with edamame & cucumber rice salad (page 169) |
| 2 | ½ cup natural muesli (with no dried fruit) with ½ cup low-fat milk, ¼ cup blueberries, 4 sliced strawberries & 2 tb greek yoghurt | 50g brazil nuts | Sesame chicken & barley salad (page 81) + 1 apple | 1 carrot & 1 stick celery cut into batons served with 2 tb hummus (see page 29) | 1½ serves Cumin-spiced steak with white bean hummus (page 162) |
| 3 | Breakfast smoothie (page 63) + 1 slice wholegrain toast with ¼ avocado & 1 sliced tomato | 2 sticks celery spread with 2 tb natural peanut butter | 1½ serves Spicy chicken, lettuce & avocado wraps (page 89) | 1 orange | Prawn & zucchini 'noodle' pad thai (page 153) |
| 4 | 1½ serves Passionfruit & strawberry trifle (page 62) | 2 macadamia & fig bliss balls (page 28) | Zucchini, spinach & sweet potato frittata (page 120) + 1 slice wholegrain sourdough | 1 cup mixed berries with ½ cup natural greek yoghurt | 1½ serves Fennel-rubbed pork with fennel & apple slaw (page 161) 3 x 10g squares dark chocolate |
| 5 | 1½ serves Yoghurt, chia & apple oat bircher (page 42) | 1 carrot, cut into batons, with 2 tb hummus (see page 29) | Avocado, trout & fennel tzatziki open sandwich (page 107) | 2 macadamia & fig bliss balls (page 28) | 1½ serves Lamb kofta, with broccoli barley salad (page 183) |
| 6 | Big mushrooms with fetta & spinach (page 34) + 1 extra slice soy and linseed toast | ½ cup blueberries + 30g almonds | Roasted root vegetable & rice salad with spiced yoghurt (page 93) | 2 x 10g squares dark chocolate | 1½ serves Sardines with roast broccoli & almond 'gremolata' (page 146) + ½ cup greek yoghurt with 6 sliced strawberries (see page 31) |
| 7 | 1½ serves Baked berry german pancake (page 72) | 50g cashews | Mediterranean beef salad (page 78) + 1 slice wholegrain bread | Green smoothie (see page 30) | Braised chicken with mushrooms & artichokes (page 187) + Grilled mango cheeks with lime drizzle (page 233) |

NOTE: While you need to pay attention to your blood sugar levels, especially if taking insulin, the snacks are optional. If you're not hungry, and your blood sugar levels are ok, you can skip the snacks.

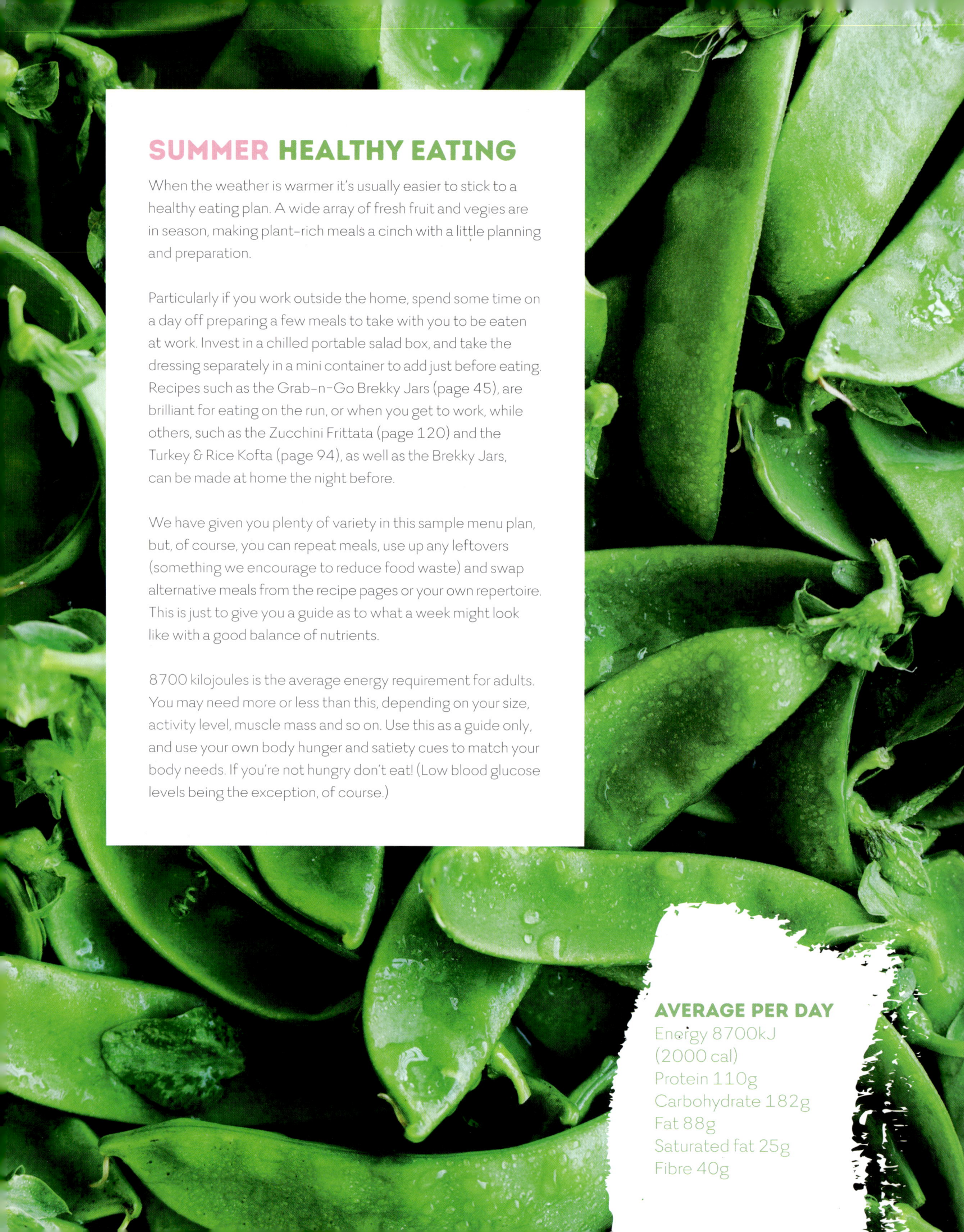

# SUMMER HEALTHY EATING

When the weather is warmer it's usually easier to stick to a healthy eating plan. A wide array of fresh fruit and vegies are in season, making plant-rich meals a cinch with a little planning and preparation.

Particularly if you work outside the home, spend some time on a day off preparing a few meals to take with you to be eaten at work. Invest in a chilled portable salad box, and take the dressing separately in a mini container to add just before eating. Recipes such as the Grab-n-Go Brekky Jars (page 45), are brilliant for eating on the run, or when you get to work, while others, such as the Zucchini Frittata (page 120) and the Turkey & Rice Kofta (page 94), as well as the Brekky Jars, can be made at home the night before.

We have given you plenty of variety in this sample menu plan, but, of course, you can repeat meals, use up any leftovers (something we encourage to reduce food waste) and swap alternative meals from the recipe pages or your own repertoire. This is just to give you a guide as to what a week might look like with a good balance of nutrients.

8700 kilojoules is the average energy requirement for adults. You may need more or less than this, depending on your size, activity level, muscle mass and so on. Use this as a guide only, and use your own body hunger and satiety cues to match your body needs. If you're not hungry don't eat! (Low blood glucose levels being the exception, of course.)

**AVERAGE PER DAY**
Energy 8700kJ
(2000 cal)
Protein 110g
Carbohydrate 182g
Fat 88g
Saturated fat 25g
Fibre 40g

# 7-DAY MENU PLANNER

| DAY | BREAKFAST | SNACK | LUNCH | SNACK | DINNER |
|---|---|---|---|---|---|
| 1 | Grab-n-Go brekky jar (page 45) (make the day before) | 30g almonds + 1 orange & 1 banana | Sesame chicken & barley salad (page 81) | 2 macadamia & fig bliss balls (page 28) | Lamb leg steaks with quinoa tabbouleh (page 176) + 3 x 10g squares dark chocolate |
| 2 | Spring vegetable & mint soufflé omelette (page 75) + 1 slice wholegrain toast with ¼ avocado | 30g brazil nuts + ½ cup blueberries | Pumpernickel with smoky tomato liptauer (page 86) + 1 apple | 2 wholegrain sandwich-size crackers topped with 40g (2 slices) cheddar cheese & 1 sliced tomato (see page 29) | Fish & quinoa salad with green hummus (page 165) + Yoghurt mango jellies (page 222) |
| 3 | ½ cup muesli with milk, 3 tb greek yoghurt, ½ cup mixed berries & pulp from 2 passionfruit | 2 wholegrain sandwich-sized crackers with ¼ avocado & 1 sliced tomato (see page 29) | Turkey & rice kofta with beetroot hummus (page 94) | 2 macadamia & fig bliss balls (page 28) + 1 orange | Tandoori chicken with roast chickpea salad (page 195) + 200g greek yoghurt with ½ cup raspberries |
| 4 | Asparagus, egg & white bean smash (page 50) | 1 apple + 30g mixed nuts & seeds | Zucchini, spinach & sweet potato frittata (page 120) + 2 slices wholegrain sourdough spread with 1 tb avocado | 1 carrot & 1 stick celery cut into batons with ¼ cup hummus (see page 29) | Cumin-spiced steak with white bean hummus (page 162) + Grilled mango cheeks with lime drizzle (page 233) |
| 5 | Green smoothie (see page 30) + 2 slices wholegrain sourdough toast with ¼ avocado, 40g cheddar cheese & 1 sliced tomato | 2 macadamia & fig bliss balls (page 28) | Ginger beef & quinoa salad (page 105) + 1 apple | 200g greek yoghurt with 1 cup mixed fresh fruit salad sprinkled with 1 tb chia seeds (see page 31) | Fast pipi & squid paella (page 138) + 3 x 10g squares dark chocolate |
| 6 | Open croque madame (page 46) | 200g greek yoghurt with ½ mango, ¼ cup blueberries & 1 tb sunflower seeds | Salmon & freekeh 'nasi goreng' (page 101) | 2 wholegrain sandwich-size crackers topped with ½ cup cottage cheese & ¼ sliced cucumber (see page 29) + 1 banana | Harissa chicken with barley & chickpea salad (page 158) + Yoghurt mango jellies (page 222) |
| 7 | Cauliflower dhal with poached egg (page 49) | 40g (2 slices) cheddar cheese + 1 apple | Open pork burgers with mustard yoghurt (page 111) + 200g greek yoghurt & 1 cup mixed fresh fruit salad | Guacamole (see page 132) with crudité (e.g. ½ carrot, 1 stick celery & ¼ sliced cucumber) | Spicy roast salmon burrito bowls (page 142) + Buttermilk panna cotta with strawberry salad (page 206) |

NOTE: While you need to pay attention to your blood sugar levels, especially if taking insulin, the snacks are optional. If you're not hungry, and your blood sugar levels are ok, you can skip the snacks.

# GLUTEN-FREE WEIGHT LOSS

It's estimated that up to 10% of people with type 1 diabetes also have coeliac disease. Both are auto-immune diseases and they share some of the same genetic characteristics. Coeliac disease is not associated with type 2 diabetes, but, of course, can occur.

There are also those who may have an intolerance to gluten. This is an important distinction as those with diagnosed coeliac disease must follow a strictly gluten-free diet for life, while those with a suspected intolerance need not be so strict. For them, lowering their intake of gluten to their threshold level will usually alleviate any symptoms.

For those with diabetes and coeliac disease, extra care must be taken to manage both conditions. Unfortunately, many commercially available gluten-free products have high GI values, making them inadvisable for blood glucose control. This is because they are usually made with refined potato and rice flours, which are quick to digest, and break down the starch into glucose for easy and rapid absorption into the bloodstream. These products are best avoided.

Thankfully you can successfully plan a healthy menu to both avoid gluten and manage your blood glucose levels. The basics are the same — to follow a plant-rich diet with a low glycaemic load — you just need to opt for gluten-free wholegrains, legumes and starchy vegies in place of the gluten containing grains, wheat, barley, rye and oats*.

The following is a gluten-free menu plan geared towards weight loss. If you're at a healthy weight, you can increase the portion sizes or add in a little extra food to meet your needs. Larger people, men, those who are very active and anyone with higher energy demands, may need to do the same. See this as your basic menu, and adapt accordingly to suit your needs.

*Oats do not contain gluten but a very similar protein. It seems that while some with coeliac disease can consume oats without problem, not all can. Oats may also be contaminated with other grains. The recommendation in Australia, therefore, is for those with coeliac disease to avoid oats. If you have a gluten intolerance, you may well be able to include oats in your menu plan. Speak with a dietitian for individual advice.

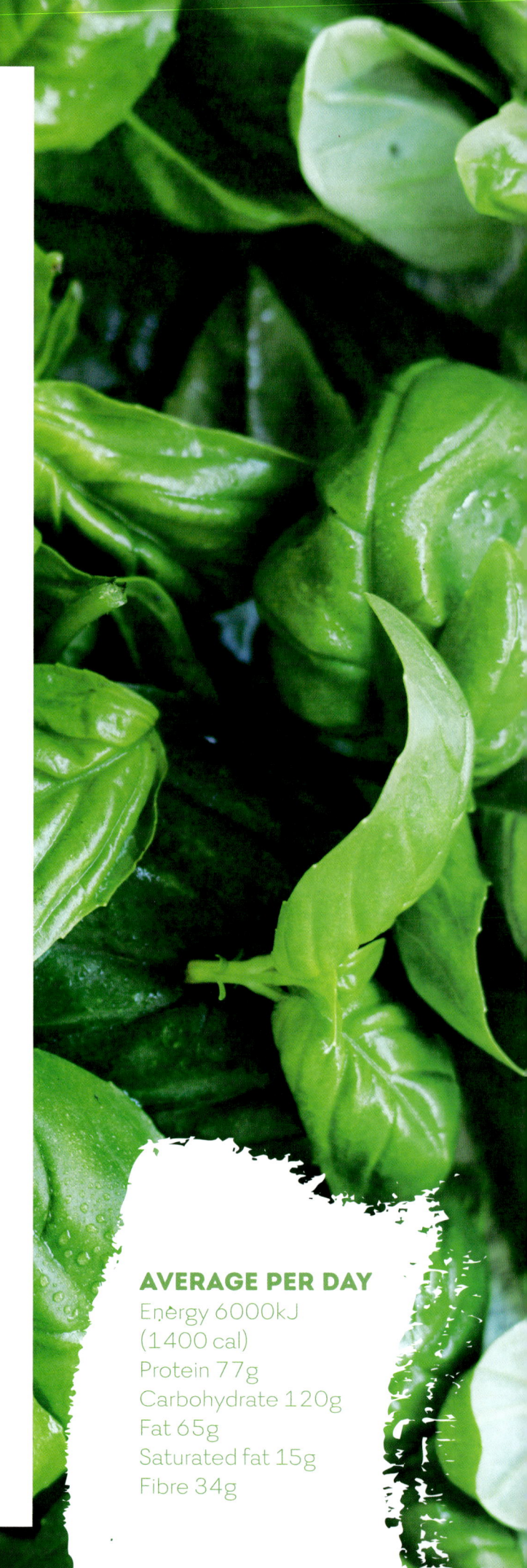

**AVERAGE PER DAY**
Energy 6000kJ
(1400 cal)
Protein 77g
Carbohydrate 120g
Fat 65g
Saturated fat 15g
Fibre 34g

# 7-DAY MENU PLANNER

| DAY | BREAKFAST | SNACK | LUNCH | SNACK | DINNER |
|---|---|---|---|---|---|
| 1 | Rose, cardamom & pistachio quinoa porridge (page 64) | 30g almonds + 2 prunes | Spiced cauliflower soup with chickpea croûtons (page 128) | Green smoothie (see page 30) | Cumin-spiced steak with white bean hummus (page 162) + Baked rice pudding with raspberries (page 217) |
| 2 | Creamy polenta porridge with roasted rhubarb & sweet dukkah (page 58) | 30g brazil nuts | Grilled beef, pear, rocket & avocado salad (page 127) | 2 x 10g squares dark chocolate | Spicy roast salmon burrito bowls (page 142) |
| 3 | Muesli 'soldiers' with yoghurt dipping sauce (page 54) | 30g mixed nuts & seeds | Rawslaw with poached chicken (page 108) | 1 pear | Fast pipi & squid paella (page 138) |
| 4 | Muesli 'soldiers' with yoghurt dipping sauce (use leftovers from the previous day) (page 54) | 30g walnuts | Spiced cauliflower soup with chickpea croûtons (page 128) | 1 cup low-fat milk heated with 2 tsp pure cocoa powder | Fast lamb curry with sticky chickpea & cauliflower rice (page 149) |
| 5 | Spring vegetable & mint soufflé omelettes (page 75) + 1 slice high-fibre gluten-free bread, toasted | 1 apple | Prawn & broccoli fried 'rice' (page 116) | 1 apple & pepita bliss ball (page 28) | Herb-roasted pork with sweet potato & turnip fries (be sure to use gluten-free dijon mustard) (page 141) |
| 6 | Baked pumpkin, tomato & egg skillet (page 38) | ½ cup greek yoghurt with ¼ cup blueberries | Mediterranean beef salad (page 78) | 30g almonds | Spinach & paneer curry (page 191) |
| 7 | Cinnamon crumpets with autumn fruit (page 37) | 30g cashews | Zucchini, spinach & sweet potato frittata (page 120) | 1 carrot cut into batons with 2 tb hummus (see page 29) | Sardines with roast broccoli and almond 'gremolata' (page 146) + Buttermilk panna cotta with strawberry salad (page 206) |

NOTE: While you need to pay attention to your blood sugar levels, especially if taking insulin, the snacks are optional. If you're not hungry, and your blood sugar levels are ok, you can skip the snacks.

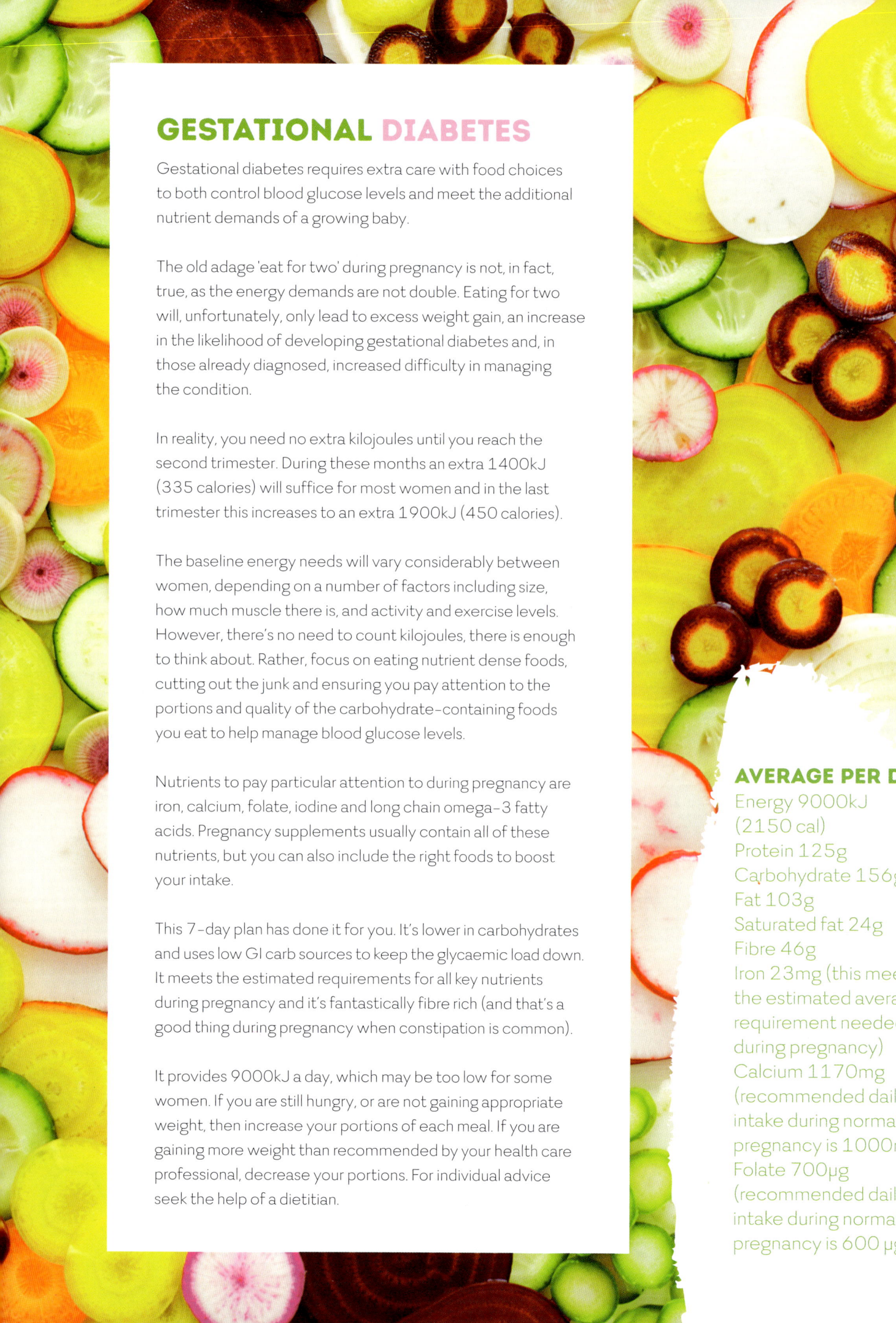

# GESTATIONAL DIABETES

Gestational diabetes requires extra care with food choices to both control blood glucose levels and meet the additional nutrient demands of a growing baby.

The old adage 'eat for two' during pregnancy is not, in fact, true, as the energy demands are not double. Eating for two will, unfortunately, only lead to excess weight gain, an increase in the likelihood of developing gestational diabetes and, in those already diagnosed, increased difficulty in managing the condition.

In reality, you need no extra kilojoules until you reach the second trimester. During these months an extra 1400kJ (335 calories) will suffice for most women and in the last trimester this increases to an extra 1900kJ (450 calories).

The baseline energy needs will vary considerably between women, depending on a number of factors including size, how much muscle there is, and activity and exercise levels. However, there's no need to count kilojoules, there is enough to think about. Rather, focus on eating nutrient dense foods, cutting out the junk and ensuring you pay attention to the portions and quality of the carbohydrate–containing foods you eat to help manage blood glucose levels.

Nutrients to pay particular attention to during pregnancy are iron, calcium, folate, iodine and long chain omega–3 fatty acids. Pregnancy supplements usually contain all of these nutrients, but you can also include the right foods to boost your intake.

This 7–day plan has done it for you. It's lower in carbohydrates and uses low GI carb sources to keep the glycaemic load down. It meets the estimated requirements for all key nutrients during pregnancy and it's fantastically fibre rich (and that's a good thing during pregnancy when constipation is common).

It provides 9000kJ a day, which may be too low for some women. If you are still hungry, or are not gaining appropriate weight, then increase your portions of each meal. If you are gaining more weight than recommended by your health care professional, decrease your portions. For individual advice seek the help of a dietitian.

## AVERAGE PER DAY

Energy 9000kJ (2150 cal)
Protein 125g
Carbohydrate 156g
Fat 103g
Saturated fat 24g
Fibre 46g
Iron 23mg (this meets the estimated average requirement needed during pregnancy)
Calcium 1170mg (recommended daily intake during normal pregnancy is 1000mg)
Folate 700µg (recommended daily intake during normal pregnancy is 600 µg)

# 7-DAY MENU PLANNER

| DAY | BREAKFAST | SNACK | LUNCH | SNACK | DINNER |
|---|---|---|---|---|---|
| 1 | ¾ cup fortified wholegrain breakfast cereal, ¼ cup blueberries, 4 sliced strawberries, 2 tb greek yoghurt & ½ cup milk | 2 slices wholegrain toast spread with 2 tb almond or cashew butter | Salmon & freekeh 'nasi goreng' (page 101) | 200g greek yoghurt & ½ cup raspberries, 1 tb pepitas & 1 tsp chia seeds (see page 31) | Pot-roasted beef with mushrooms & thyme (page 175) + 2 extra 100g slices beef |
| 2 | 2 serves Big mushrooms with fetta & spinach (page 34) + 1 extra slice soy and linseed toast | 50g cashews + 1 apple | Mediterranean beef salad (using 150g leftover roast beef from last night) (page 78) | 200g greek yoghurt with pulp from 2 passionfruit | Sardines with roast broccoli and almond 'gremolata' (page 146) + Fruits of the forest cookie 'pizza' (page 209) |
| 3 | ½ cup muesli with ½ cup milk, 4 sliced strawberries & ¼ cup blueberries | 2 hard-boiled eggs (see page 31) | Turkey & rice kofta with beetroot hummus (page 94) | 2 wholegrain crispbreads topped with 40g (2 slices) cheddar cheese, 1 sliced tomato & 6 slices cucumber (see page 29) | 1½ serves Lamb & pumpkin shepherd's pie (page 150) + 2 cups garden salad dressed with 2 tsp extra virgin olive oil & 1 tsp vinegar + 2 apple & pepita bliss balls (page 28) |
| 4 | Lentil omelette with braised capsicum & watercress (page 71) | 1 carrot & 1 stick celery cut into batons with ¼ cup hummus (see page 29) | Rawslaw with poached chicken (page 108) | Green smoothie (see page 30) | 2 serves Steak & cannellini bean bubble-n-squeak (page 188) + 2 apple & pepita bliss balls (page 28) |
| 5 | Yoghurt chia & apple oat bircher (page 42) | 2 slices wholegrain toast spread with 2 tb almond or cashew butter | Black bean chilli with guacamole & 'corn chips' (page 132) | 1 pear + 40g (2 slices) cheddar cheese | Baked fish with cauliflower crumble (page 157) + 200g greek yoghurt with ½ cup raspberries, 1 tb pepitas & 1 tsp chia seeds (see page 31) |
| 6 | Spring vegetable & mint soufflé omelette (page 75) + 1 slice wholegrain toast | 1 banana + 30g almonds | Curried lentil soup with roast pumpkin seeds (page 85) | Green smoothie (see page 30) | Tandoori chicken with roast chickpea salad (page 195) + Ginger-poached rhubarb almond fillo tart (page 202) |
| 7 | Breakfast smoothie (page 63) + 2 slices wholegrain toast spread with 2 tb almond butter | 2 dried figs + 25g pepitas | Grilled beef, pear, rocket & avocado salad (page 127) + 1 orange | 2 apple & pepita bliss balls (page 28) | Pasta with salmon & minty pea pesto (page 172) + 2 cups garden salad dressed with 2 tsp extra virgin olive oil & 1 tsp vinegar |

NOTE: While you need to pay attention to your blood sugar levels, especially if taking insulin, the snacks are optional. If you're not hungry, and your blood sugar levels are ok, you can skip the snacks.

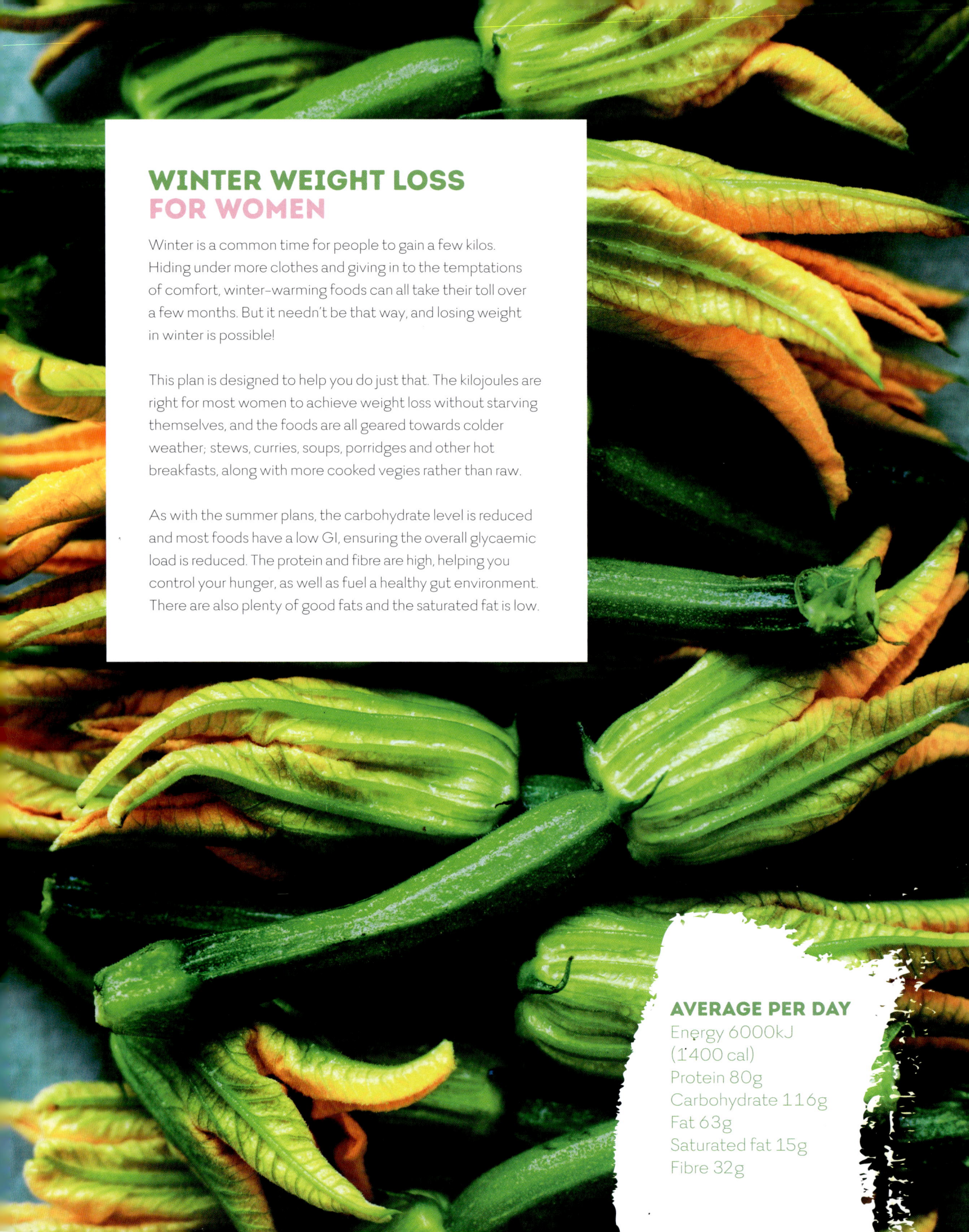

# WINTER WEIGHT LOSS
## FOR WOMEN

Winter is a common time for people to gain a few kilos. Hiding under more clothes and giving in to the temptations of comfort, winter-warming foods can all take their toll over a few months. But it needn't be that way, and losing weight in winter is possible!

This plan is designed to help you do just that. The kilojoules are right for most women to achieve weight loss without starving themselves, and the foods are all geared towards colder weather; stews, curries, soups, porridges and other hot breakfasts, along with more cooked vegies rather than raw.

As with the summer plans, the carbohydrate level is reduced and most foods have a low GI, ensuring the overall glycaemic load is reduced. The protein and fibre are high, helping you control your hunger, as well as fuel a healthy gut environment. There are also plenty of good fats and the saturated fat is low.

**AVERAGE PER DAY**
Energy 6000kJ
(1400 cal)
Protein 80g
Carbohydrate 116g
Fat 63g
Saturated fat 15g
Fibre 32g

# 7-DAY MENU PLANNER

| DAY | BREAKFAST | SNACK | LUNCH | SNACK | DINNER |
|---|---|---|---|---|---|
| 1 | Creamy polenta porridge with roasted rhubarb & sweet dukkah (page 58) | 1 macadamia & fig bliss ball (page 28) | Curried lentil soup with roast pumpkin seeds (page 85) | 30g mixed nuts | Sichuan beef noodles with creamy sesame dressing (page 166) |
| 2 | Turkish-style scrambled eggs (page 67) | 1 apple | Miso chicken noodle soup (page 90) | 30g almonds | Baked fish with cauliflower crumble (page 157) |
| 3 | Big mushrooms with fetta & spinach (page 34) | ½ cup red grapes + 10 cashews | Tuna pasta with pesto & tomatoes (page 131) | 1 macadamia & fig bliss ball (page 28) | Fast lamb curry with sticky chickpea & cauliflower rice (page 149) |
| 4 | Cauliflower dhal with poached egg (page 49) | 1 macadamia & fig bliss ball (page 28) | Creamy broccoli soup with crispy quinoa (page 115) | 1 pear with 20g (1 slice) cheddar cheese | Coq au vin with endive salad (page 192) |
| 5 | Rose, cardamom & pistachio quinoa porridge (page 64) | 1 apple | Curried lentil soup with roasted pumpkin seeds (page 85) (or, leftover broccoli soup from yesterday's lunch, if you prefer) | ½ cup greek yoghurt + 1 orange | Mustard-roasted lamb, roast cauliflower & minted greens (page 154) |
| 6 | Polenta, corn & sausage pancakes (page 41) | 1 slice wholemeal toast topped with 1 tb natural peanut butter & ½ banana sliced | Spanakopita quesadillas (page 112) | 30g mixed nuts & seeds | Pasta with salmon & minty pea pesto (page 172) |
| 7 | Turkish-style scrambled eggs (page 67) | 1 apple | Creamy seafood soup (page 123) | 1 stick celery, cut into batons, with 2 tb cottage cheese (see page 29) | Herb-roasted pork with sweet potato & turnip fries (page 141) + Ginger-poached rhubarb almond fillo tart (page 202) |

NOTE: While you need to pay attention to your blood sugar levels, especially if taking insulin, the snacks are optional. If you're not hungry, and your blood sugar levels are ok, you can skip the snacks.

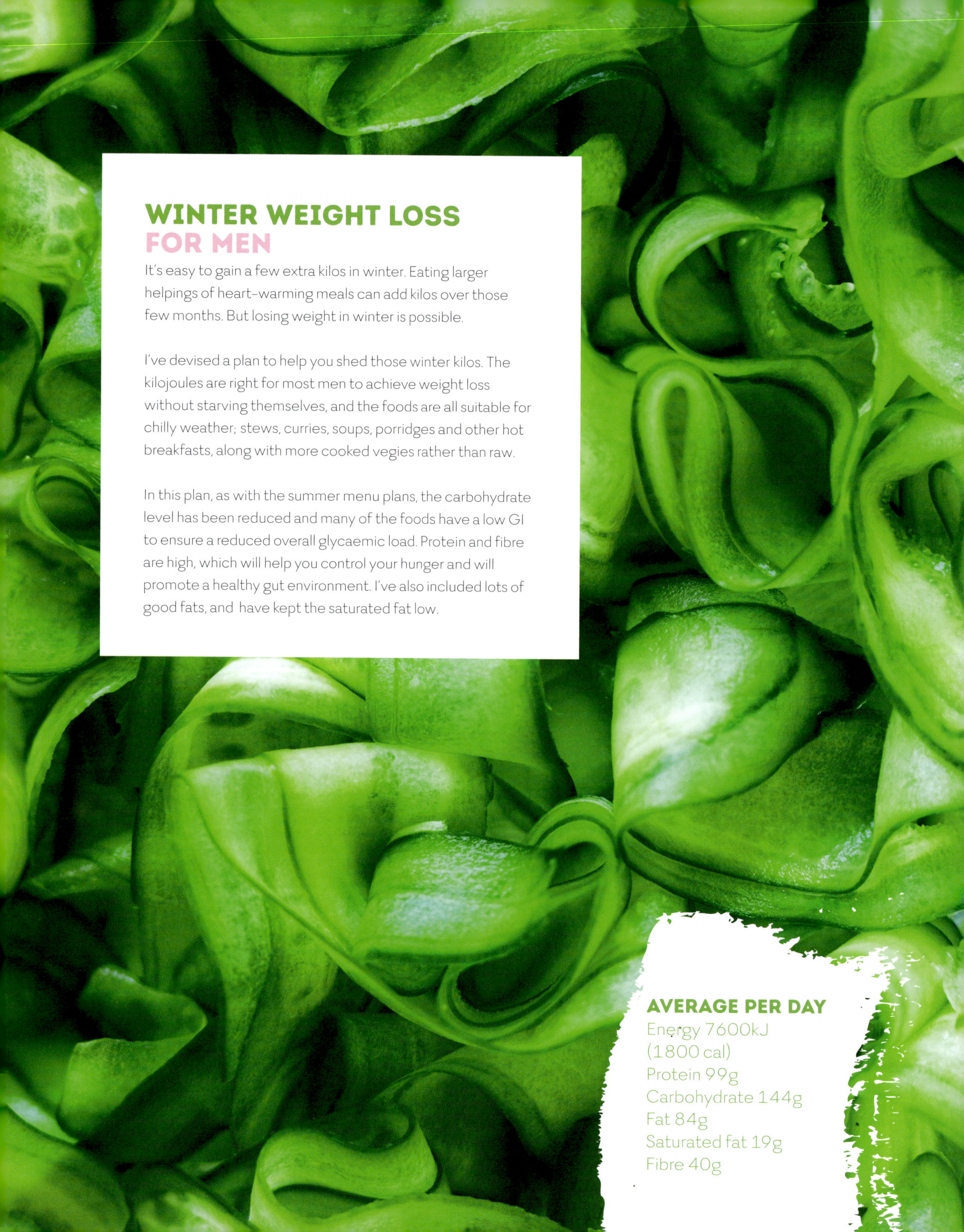

# WINTER WEIGHT LOSS
## FOR MEN

It's easy to gain a few extra kilos in winter. Eating larger helpings of heart–warming meals can add kilos over those few months. But losing weight in winter is possible.

I've devised a plan to help you shed those winter kilos. The kilojoules are right for most men to achieve weight loss without starving themselves, and the foods are all suitable for chilly weather; stews, curries, soups, porridges and other hot breakfasts, along with more cooked vegies rather than raw.

In this plan, as with the summer menu plans, the carbohydrate level has been reduced and many of the foods have a low GI to ensure a reduced overall glycaemic load. Protein and fibre are high, which will help you control your hunger and will promote a healthy gut environment. I've also included lots of good fats, and have kept the saturated fat low.

### AVERAGE PER DAY
Energy 7600kJ
(1800 cal)
Protein 99g
Carbohydrate 144g
Fat 84g
Saturated fat 19g
Fibre 40g

# 7-DAY MENU PLANNER

| DAY | BREAKFAST | SNACK | LUNCH | SNACK | DINNER |
|---|---|---|---|---|---|
| 1 | Creamy polenta porridge with roasted rhubarb & sweet dukkah (page 58) | 2 apple & pepita bliss balls (page 28) | Curried lentil soup with roast pumpkin seeds (page 85) | 50g mixed nuts + 1 apple | Sichuan beef noodles with creamy sesame dressing (page 166) |
| 2 | $1\frac{1}{2}$ serves Turkish-style scrambled eggs (page 67) | 1 apple | $1\frac{1}{2}$ serves Miso chicken noodle soup (page 90) | 50g almonds | Baked fish with cauliflower crumble (page 157) |
| 3 | Big mushrooms with fetta & spinach (page 34) + 1 extra slice soy and linseed toast | 1 cup red grapes + 30g cashews | Tuna pasta with pesto & tomatoes (page 131) | 2 macadamia & fig bliss balls (page 28) | $1\frac{1}{2}$ serves Fast lamb curry with sticky chickpea & cauliflower rice (page 149) |
| 4 | Cauliflower dhal with poached egg (page 49) + Half a wholemeal pitta bread | 2 macadamia & fig bliss balls (page 28) | Creamy broccoli soup with crispy quinoa (page 115) | 1 pear with 20g (1 slice) cheddar cheese | $1\frac{1}{2}$ serves Coq au vin with endive salad (page 192) |
| 5 | $1\frac{1}{2}$ serves Rose, cardamom & pistachio quinoa porridge (page 64) | 1 apple + 30g almonds | Curried lentil soup with roasted pumpkin seeds (page 85) (or, leftover broccoli soup from yesterday's lunch, if you prefer) | $\frac{1}{2}$ cup greek yoghurt + 1 orange | $1\frac{1}{2}$ serves Mustard-roasted lamb, roast cauliflower & minted greens (page 154) |
| 6 | $1\frac{1}{2}$ serves Polenta, corn & sausage pancakes (page 41) | 1 slice wholemeal toast topped with 1 tb natural peanut butter & $\frac{1}{2}$ banana sliced | Spanakopita quesadillas (page 112) | 50g mixed nuts & seeds + 1 mandarin | $1\frac{1}{2}$ serves Pasta with salmon & minty pea pesto (page 172) |
| 7 | Turkish-style scrambled eggs (page 67) | 1 apple | Creamy seafood soup (page 123) | 50g mixed nuts + 1 apple | Herb-roasted pork with sweet potato & turnip fries (page 141) + Ginger-poached rhubarb almond fillo tart (page 202) |

NOTE: While you need to pay attention to your blood sugar levels, especially if taking insulin, the snacks are optional. If you're not hungry, and your blood sugar levels are ok, you can skip the snacks.

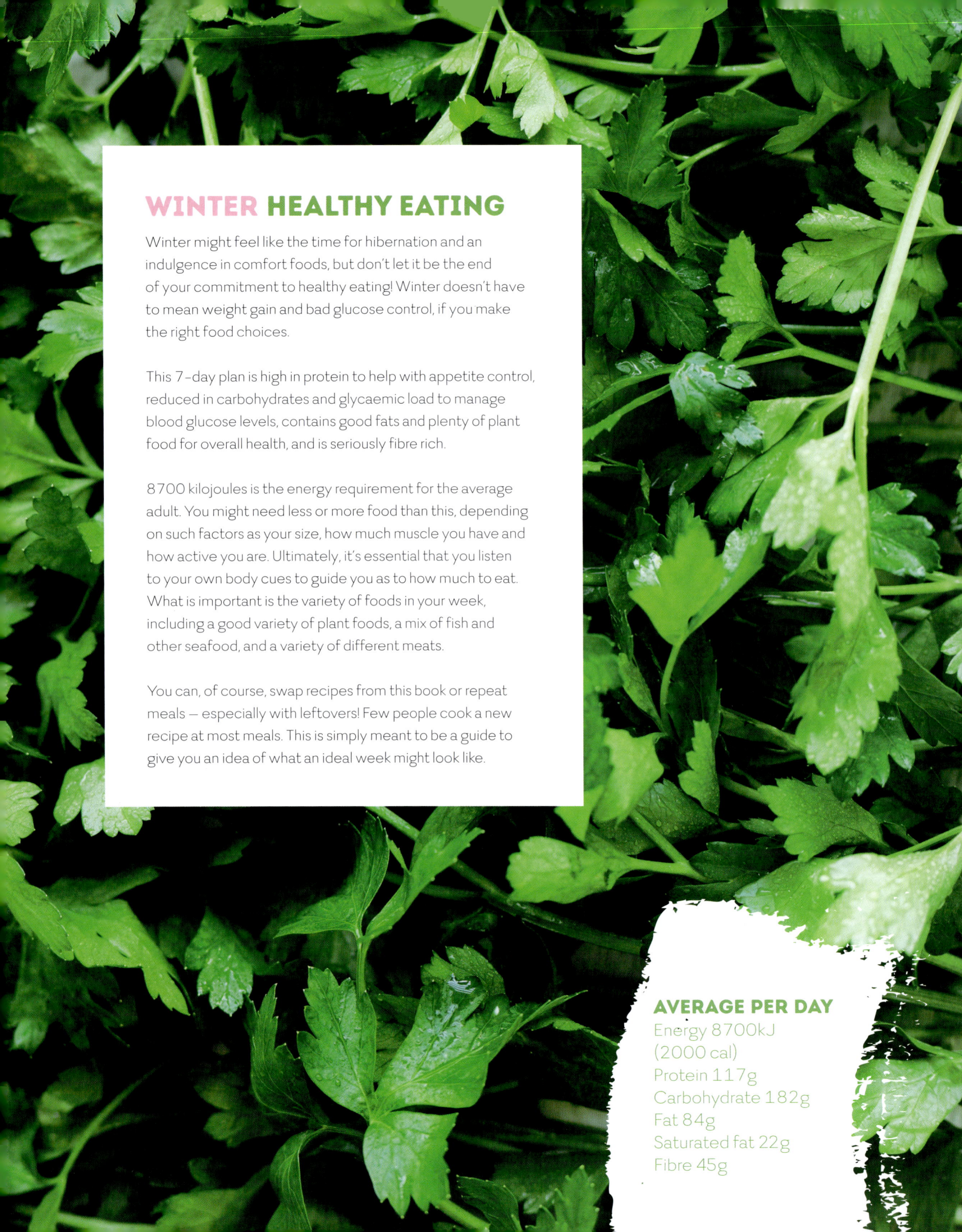

# WINTER HEALTHY EATING

Winter might feel like the time for hibernation and an indulgence in comfort foods, but don't let it be the end of your commitment to healthy eating! Winter doesn't have to mean weight gain and bad glucose control, if you make the right food choices.

This 7-day plan is high in protein to help with appetite control, reduced in carbohydrates and glycaemic load to manage blood glucose levels, contains good fats and plenty of plant food for overall health, and is seriously fibre rich.

8700 kilojoules is the energy requirement for the average adult. You might need less or more food than this, depending on such factors as your size, how much muscle you have and how active you are. Ultimately, it's essential that you listen to your own body cues to guide you as to how much to eat. What is important is the variety of foods in your week, including a good variety of plant foods, a mix of fish and other seafood, and a variety of different meats.

You can, of course, swap recipes from this book or repeat meals — especially with leftovers! Few people cook a new recipe at most meals. This is simply meant to be a guide to give you an idea of what an ideal week might look like.

**AVERAGE PER DAY**
Energy 8700kJ
(2000 cal)
Protein 117g
Carbohydrate 182g
Fat 84g
Saturated fat 22g
Fibre 45g

# 7-DAY MENU PLANNER

| DAY | BREAKFAST | SNACK | LUNCH | SNACK | DINNER |
|---|---|---|---|---|---|
| 1 | Turkish-style scrambled eggs (page 67) | 1 cup low-fat milk heated with 2 tsp pure cocoa powder<br>+<br>2 macadamia & fig bliss balls (page 28) | Pulled chicken tortillas (page 119)<br>+<br>1 apple | 200g greek yoghurt with 1 sliced banana<br>+<br>20g chopped almonds | Pasta with salmon & minty pea pesto (page 172)<br>+<br>2 cups mixed salad dressed with 2 tsp extra virgin olive oil & 1 tsp vinegar |
| 2 | 2 serves Open croque madame (page 46) | ½ cup frozen berries heated in microwave, served with 200g greek yoghurt | Spicy chicken, lettuce & avocado wrap (page 89) | 2 macadamia & fig bliss balls (page 28) | Sichuan beef & noodles with creamy sesame dressing (page 166) |
| 3 | Rose, cardamom & pistachio quinoa porridge (page 64) | 2 macadamia & fig bliss balls (page 28) | Spiced cauliflower soup with chickpea croûtons (page 128)<br>+<br>2 slices wholegrain sourdough with 1 tb light cream cheese | 2 slices wholemeal toast with 2 tb natural peanut butter<br>+<br>1 banana | Herb-roasted pork with sweet potato & turnip fries (page 141)<br>+<br>1½ serves Baked rice pudding with raspberries (page 217) |
| 4 | Creamy polenta porridge with roasted rhubarb & sweet dukkah (page 58) | 30g mixed nuts & seeds<br>+<br>1 apple | Spanakopita quesadillas (page 112) | 1 cup greek yoghurt<br>+<br>1 banana | 1½ serves Braised chicken with mushrooms & artichokes (page 187)<br>+<br>3 x 10g squares dark chocolate |
| 5 | Lentil omelette with braised capsicum & watercress (page 71) | 1 banana<br>+<br>30g almonds | Creamy broccoli soup with crispy quinoa (page 115) | 1 cup low-fat milk heated with 2 tsp pure cocoa powder<br>+<br>2 apple & pepita bliss balls (page 28) | Pot-roasted beef with mushrooms & thyme (page 175) |
| 6 | Baked pumpkin, tomato & egg skillet (page 38)<br>+<br>1 slice wholegrain sourdough toast spread with ¼ avocado | 1 apple<br>+<br>40g (2 slices) cheddar cheese | Chicken tacos with avocado salsa (page 98) | 1 cup low-fat milk heated with 2 tsp pure cocoa powder<br>+<br>2 apple & pepita bliss balls (page 28) | Teriyaki salmon with edamame & cucumber rice salad (page 169) |
| 7 | 1½ serves Cinnamon crumpets with autumn fruit (page 37) | 1 cup diced pineapple with 200g greek yoghurt | Prawns, roast pumpkin & warm black bean hummus (page 97) | 50g almonds<br>+<br>2 prunes | Rosemary lamb roast with yoghurt flatbread & tzatziki (page 184)<br>+<br>Berry & apple crumble with custard apple 'custard' (page 201) |

NOTE: While you need to pay attention to your blood sugar levels, especially if taking insulin, the snacks are optional. If you're not hungry, and your blood sugar levels are ok, you can skip the snacks.

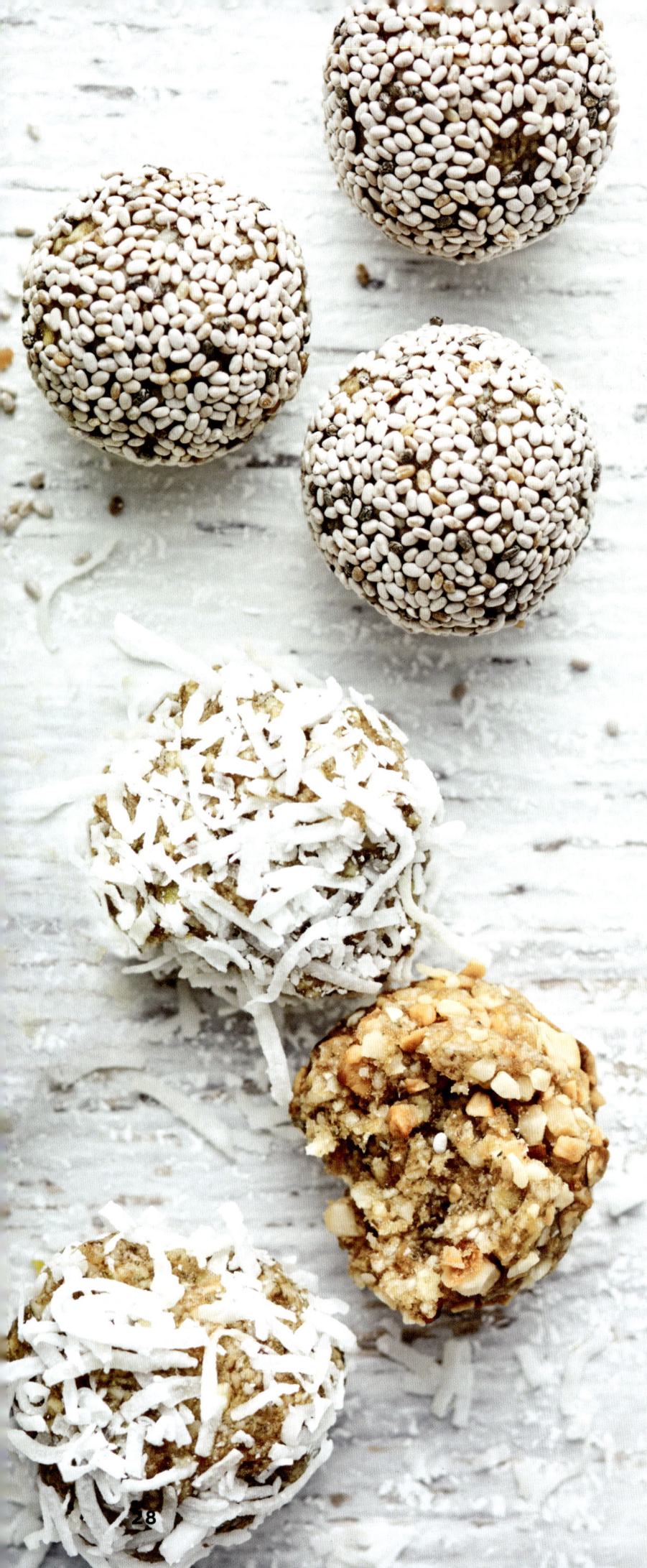

# SNACKS

Your snacking habits can make or break a healthy eating plan. Making the right choice as to when, or indeed if, to snack, as well as what to snack on, can make all the difference to your blood glucose control and your weight management.

## MACADAMIA & FIG BLISS BALLS

**PREP TIME** 20 MINUTES (+ REFRIGERATION) **MAKES** 30

Process 1 cup macadamia nuts until finely chopped. Add 200g (6½oz) chopped medjool dates, 75g (2½oz) soft and juicy dried figs, 2 tablespoons white chia seeds and ½ teaspoon ground cinnamon; process until well combined. Add about 2 teaspoons hot water; process until mixture comes together. With damp hands, roll 2 level teaspoons of mixture into balls. Roll balls in 1 cup white chia seeds to coat; place on a baking-paper-lined oven tray. Refrigerate for 1 hour.

**TIP** Bliss balls can be refrigerated in an airtight container for up to 2 weeks or frozen for up to one month.

**NUTRITIONAL COUNT PER BALL** 5.7g total fat (0.7g saturated fat); 374kJ (89 cal); 6.5g carbohydrate; 1.8g protein; 3.4g dietary fibre; 0mg sodium

## APPLE & PEPITA BLISS BALLS

**PREP TIME** 20 MINUTES (+ REFRIGERATION) **MAKES** 35

Process 1 cup natural sliced almonds until finely chopped. Add 200g (6½oz) chopped medjool dates, 50g (1½oz) coarsely chopped dried apple, ¼ cup shredded coconut and ½ cup pepitas (pumpkin seed kernels); process until well combined. Add about 2 teaspoons hot water; process until mixture comes together. With damp hands, roll 2 level teaspoons of mixture into balls. Rolls balls in 1 cup shredded coconut to coat; place on a baking-paper-lined oven tray. Refrigerate for 1 hour.

**TIP** Bliss balls can be refrigerated in an airtight container for up to 2 weeks or frozen for up to one month.

**NUTRITIONAL COUNT PER BALL** 5.7g total fat (2.1g saturated fat); 342kJ (81 cal); 5.5g carbohydrate; 1.7g protein; 1.6g fibre; 3mg sodium

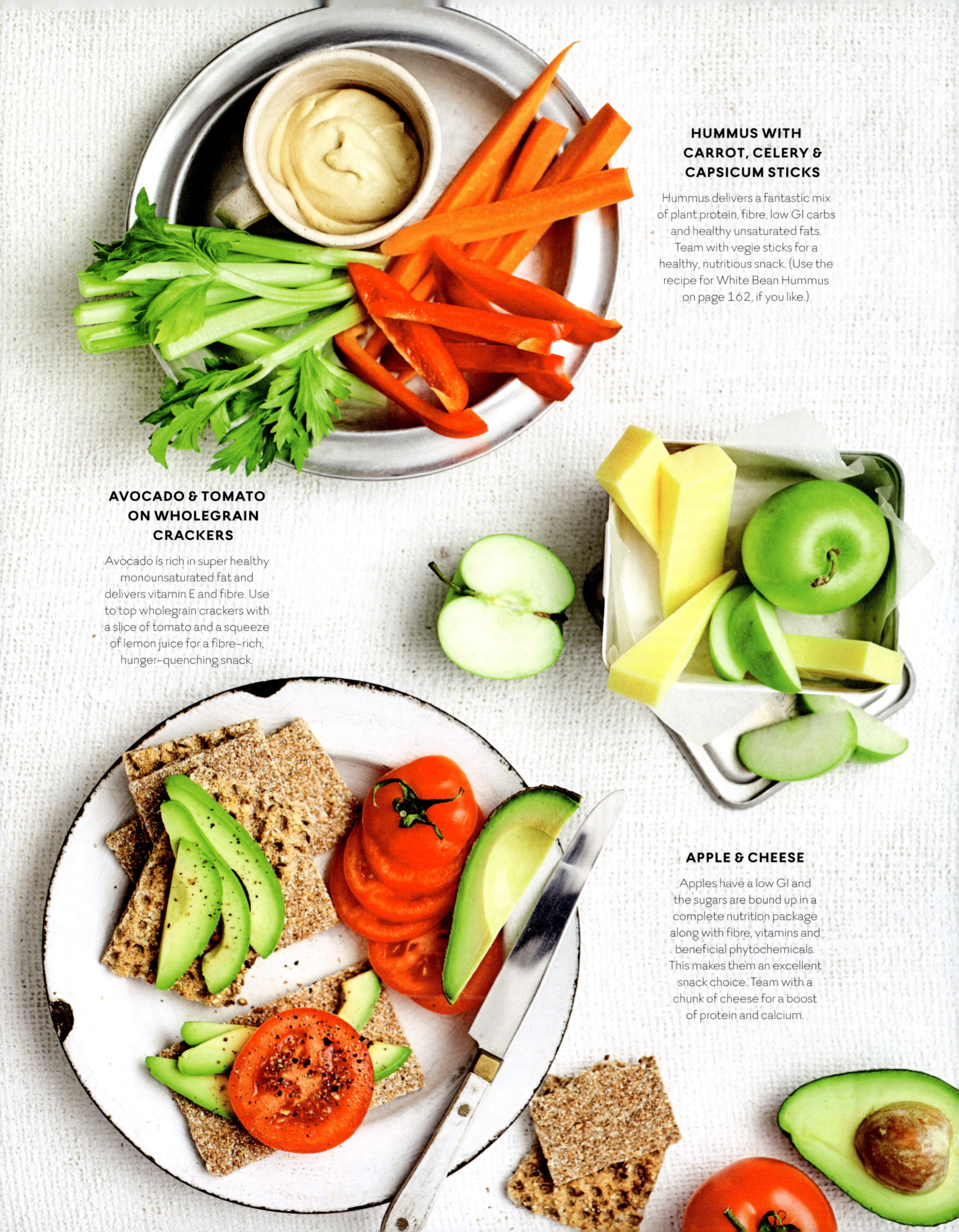

## HUMMUS WITH CARROT, CELERY & CAPSICUM STICKS

Hummus delivers a fantastic mix of plant protein, fibre, low GI carbs and healthy unsaturated fats. Team with vegie sticks for a healthy, nutritious snack. (Use the recipe for White Bean Hummus on page 162, if you like.)

## AVOCADO & TOMATO ON WHOLEGRAIN CRACKERS

Avocado is rich in super healthy monounsaturated fat and delivers vitamin E and fibre. Use to top wholegrain crackers with a slice of tomato and a squeeze of lemon juice for a fibre-rich, hunger-quenching snack.

## APPLE & CHEESE

Apples have a low GI and the sugars are bound up in a complete nutrition package along with fibre, vitamins and beneficial phytochemicals. This makes them an excellent snack choice. Team with a chunk of cheese for a boost of protein and calcium.

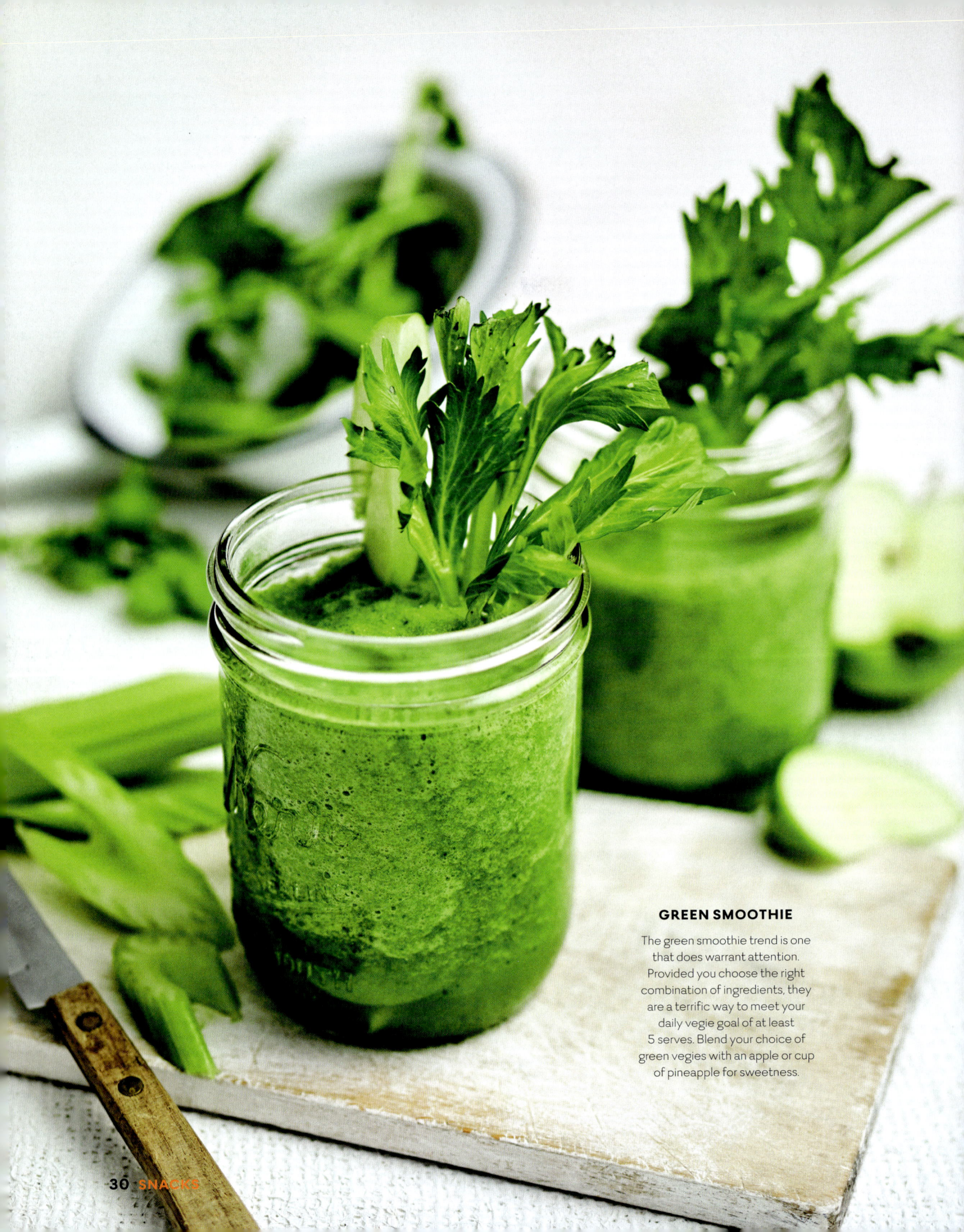

**GREEN SMOOTHIE**

The green smoothie trend is one that does warrant attention. Provided you choose the right combination of ingredients, they are a terrific way to meet your daily vegie goal of at least 5 serves. Blend your choice of green vegies with an apple or cup of pineapple for sweetness.

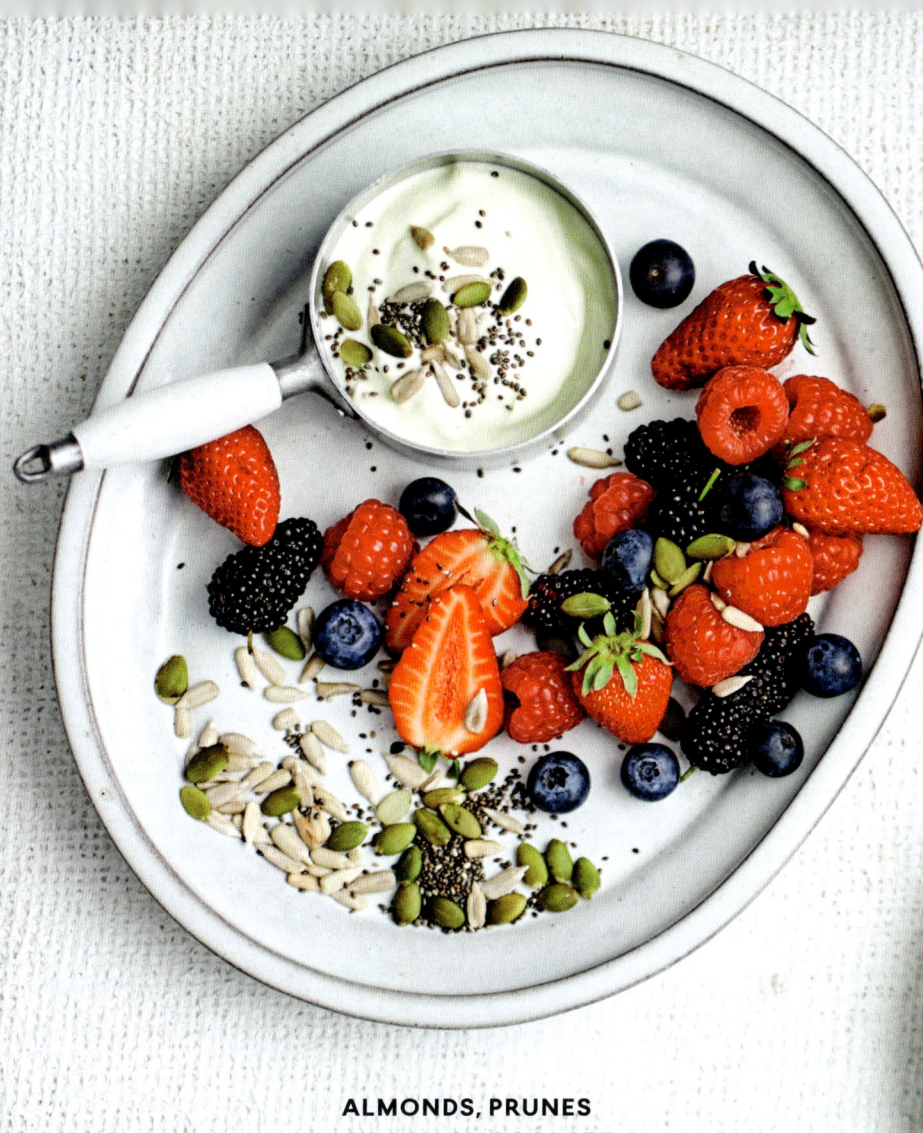

## GREEK YOGHURT, BERRIES & SEEDS

Greek-style yoghurt is high in protein and low GI, helping to keep hunger pangs at bay between meals. Team with antioxidant-rich berries and sprinkle with seeds such as pepitas, sunflower or chia seeds for extra fibre and healthy fats.

## ALMONDS, PRUNES & DARK CHOCOLATE

This combination is tasty, and feels decadent, yet is truly good for you! Dark chocolate has a higher cocoa content, and is, therefore, higher in protective polyphenols. Prunes are another antioxidant-rich food, and a handful of nuts a day reduces your risk of heart disease.

## BOILED EGGS

Boil a few eggs and keep in your fridge for fast, easy snacks. With no carbohydrate they won't affect your blood glucose levels, but the protein and fat content will help you to control your appetite. Sprinkle with chilli flakes, paprika or seaweed for extra flavour.

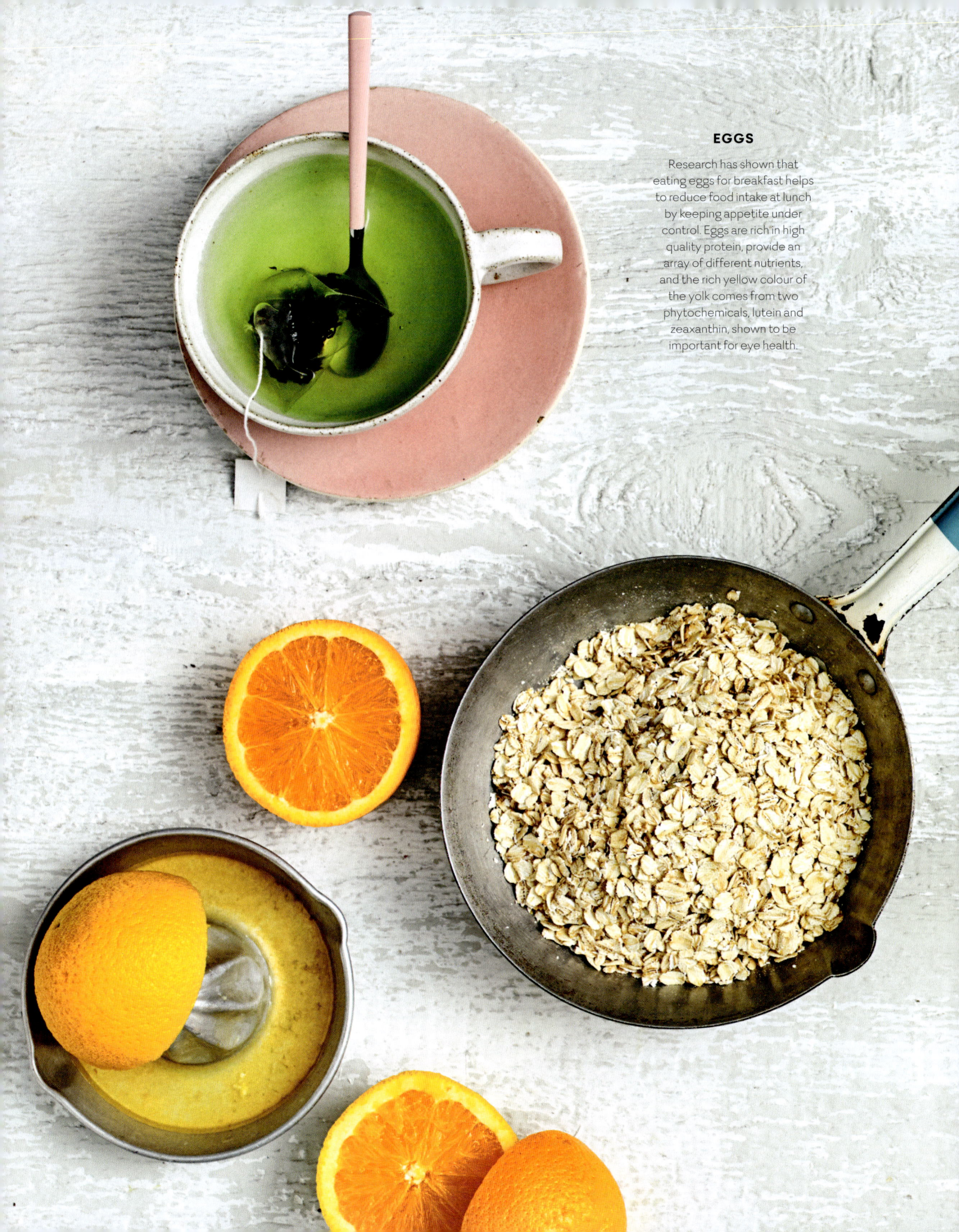

**EGGS**

Research has shown that eating eggs for breakfast helps to reduce food intake at lunch by keeping appetite under control. Eggs are rich in high quality protein, provide an array of different nutrients, and the rich yellow colour of the yolk comes from two phytochemicals, lutein and zeaxanthin, shown to be important for eye health.

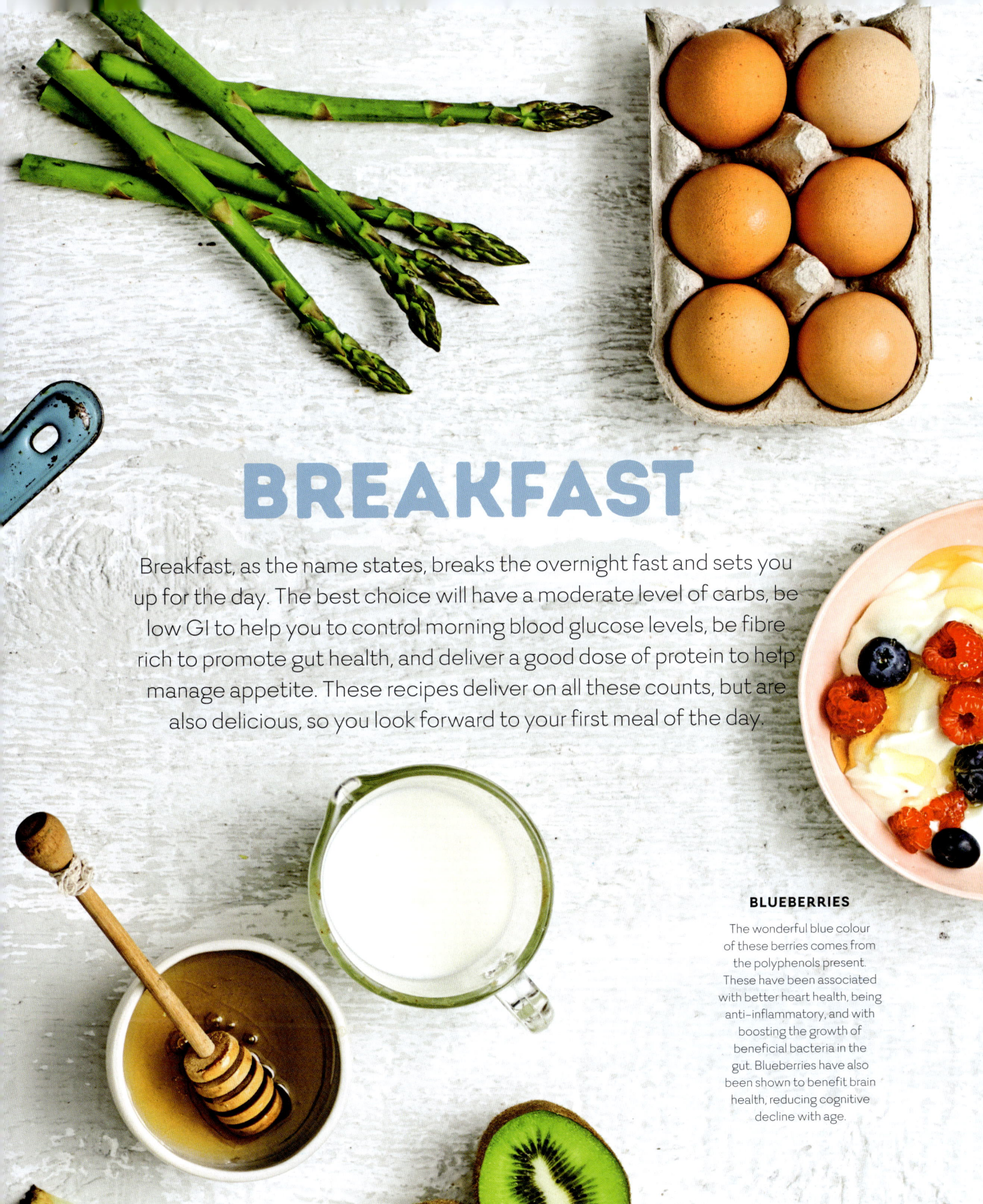

# BREAKFAST

Breakfast, as the name states, breaks the overnight fast and sets you up for the day. The best choice will have a moderate level of carbs, be low GI to help you to control morning blood glucose levels, be fibre rich to promote gut health, and deliver a good dose of protein to help manage appetite. These recipes deliver on all these counts, but are also delicious, so you look forward to your first meal of the day.

**BLUEBERRIES**

The wonderful blue colour of these berries comes from the polyphenols present. These have been associated with better heart health, being anti-inflammatory, and with boosting the growth of beneficial bacteria in the gut. Blueberries have also been shown to benefit brain health, reducing cognitive decline with age.

**NUTRITIONAL COUNT PER SERVING**

| 20.1g total fat (4.6g saturated fat) | 1522kJ (363 cal) | 24.2g carbohydrate | 17.1g protein | 7.7g fibre | 582 mg sodium |
|---|---|---|---|---|---|

# BIG MUSHROOMS
## with fetta & spinach

**PREP + COOK TIME** 30 MINUTES **SERVES** 4

4 portobello mushrooms (200g)
2 tablespoons extra virgin olive oil
1 shallot, chopped finely
½ teaspoon ground nutmeg
200g (6½oz) baby spinach leaves
1 tablespoon water
4 slices soy and linseed bread (280g)
1 clove garlic, peeled
100g (3oz) reduced-fat fetta, crumbled
2 tablespoons pepitas (pumpkin seed kernels), toasted

**1** Preheat oven to 200°C/400°F. Line an oven tray with baking paper.

**2** Place mushrooms on tray; bake for 15 minutes or until browned and softened slightly.

**3** Meanwhile, heat 1 tablespoon of the oil in a medium frying pan over medium heat. Cook shallot, stirring, for 4 minutes or until light golden. Add nutmeg; stir to combine. Add spinach and the water; cook, stirring, for 1 minute or until just wilted. Stir in any mushroom juices left on the tray.

**4** Heat a grill plate (or grill pan) over medium–high heat; grill bread for 2 minutes each side or until toasted and light grill marks appear. Rub garlic clove over one side of each piece of toast.

**5** Top each mushroom evenly with spinach mixture; sprinkle evenly with fetta and pepitas. Drizzle with remaining oil; serve with toast.

**DR JO SAYS**
Dark leafy greens, such as kale, silver beet and spinach, are rich in two antioxidants called lutein and zeaxanthin. These play an important role in protecting the eyes from oxidative damage and reducing the risk of age-related macular degeneration.

**TIP** Instead of the portobello mushrooms, use the same weight of button mushrooms and reduce the cooking time, checking after 5 minutes.

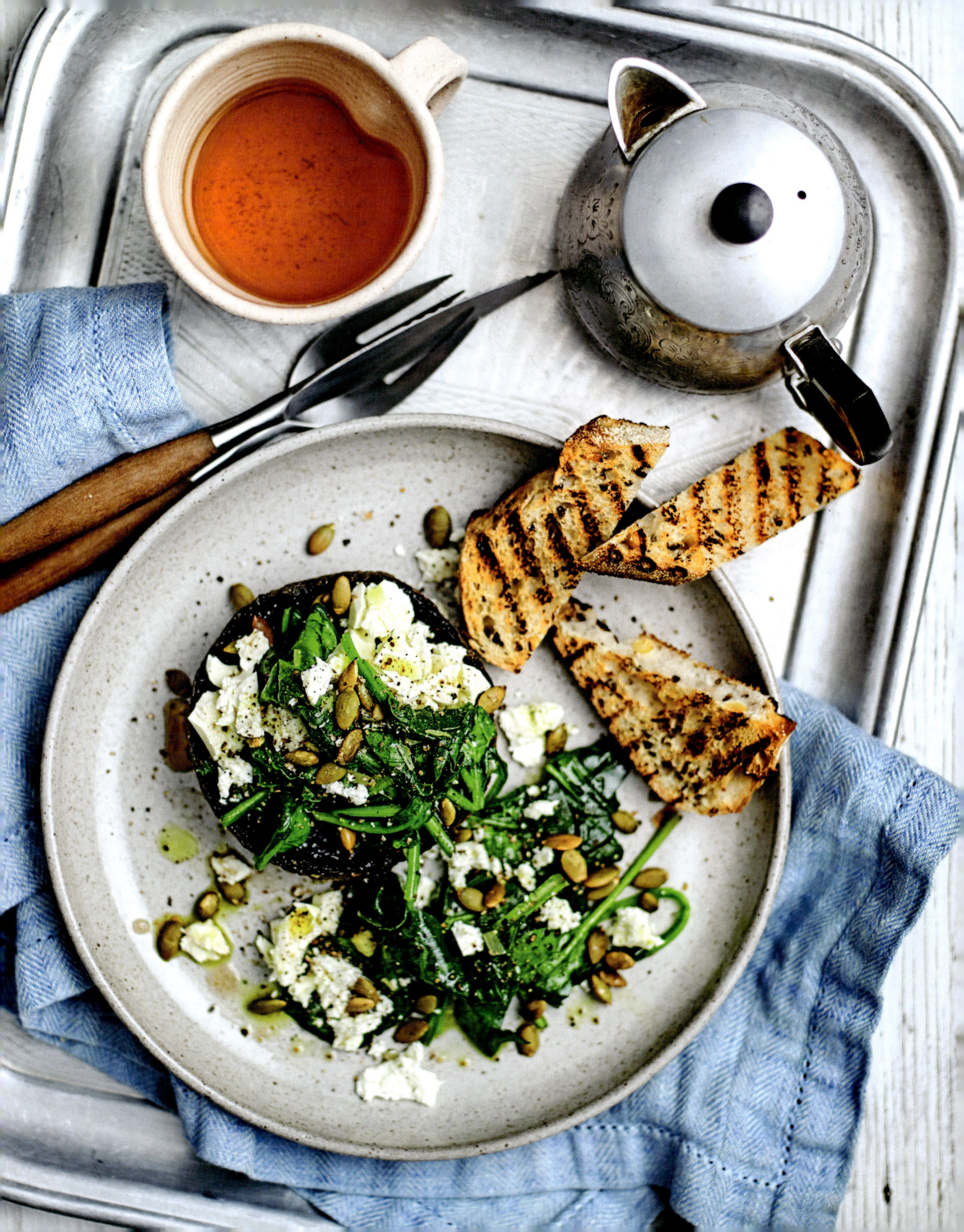

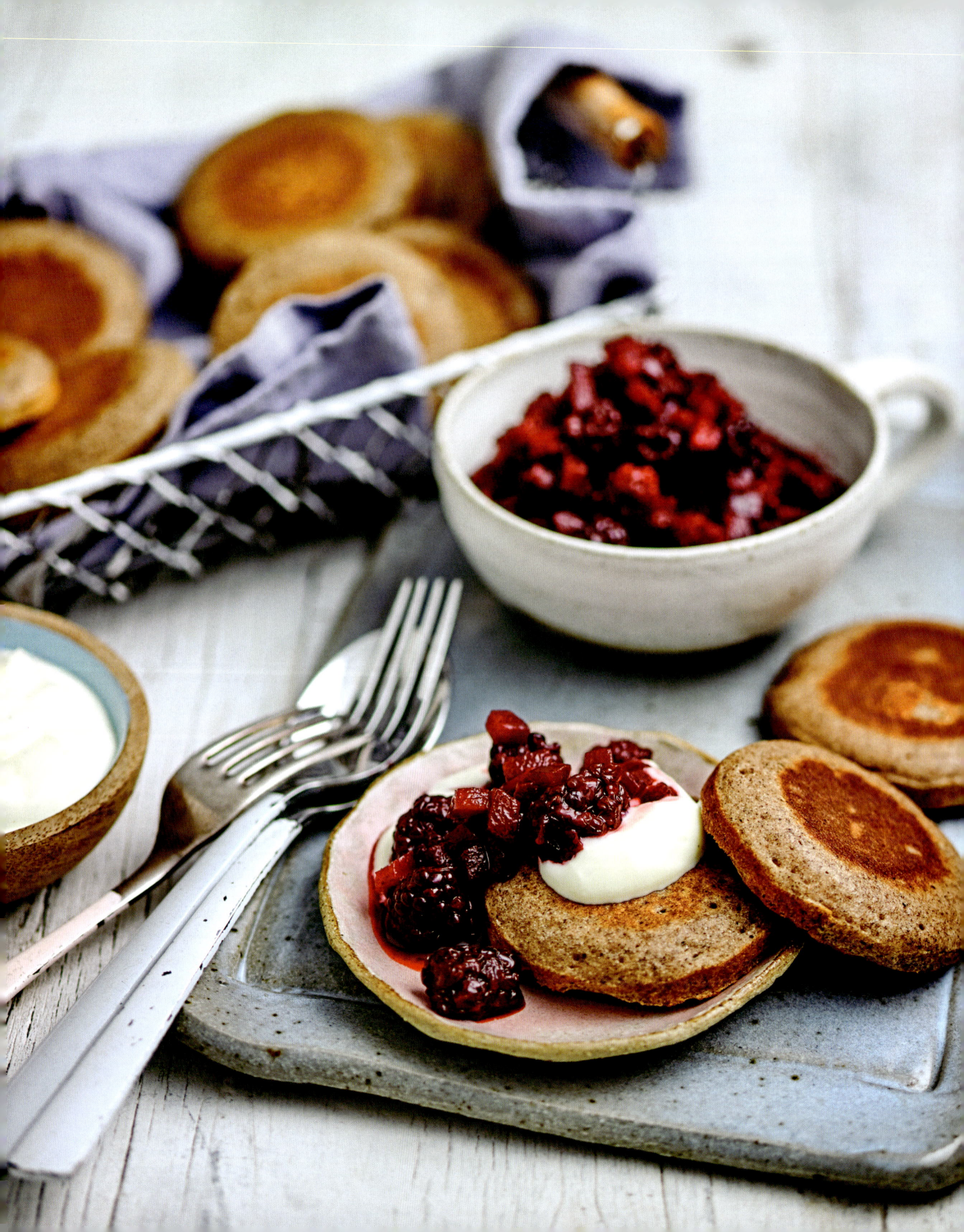

| ● 5.5g total fat (2.3g saturated fat) | ● 1342kJ (320 cal) | ● 48.2g carbohydrate | ● 13.9g protein | ● 7.6g fibre | ● 169mg sodium |
| --- | --- | --- | --- | --- | --- |

# CINNAMON CRUMPETS
## with autumn fruit

**PREP + COOK TIME** 40 MINUTES **SERVES** 4

1 cup (250ml) milk, lukewarm
2 teaspoons (7g) dried yeast
2 tablespoons brown sugar
1 cup (150g) buckwheat flour
1 teaspoon ground cinnamon
¼ teaspoon bicarbonate of soda (baking soda)
1 medium ripe pear (230g), diced finely
250g (8oz) blackberries
2 tablespoons water
olive-oil spray
¾ cup (210g) unsweetened vanilla-bean
   Greek-style yoghurt

**1** Combine milk, yeast and 1½ tablespoons of the sugar in a small jug; stand for 10 minutes or until frothy.

**2** Meanwhile, sift flour, cinnamon and soda into a large bowl; whisk in milk mixture until smooth. Stand at room temperature for at least 5 minutes but no longer than 10 minutes before cooking.

**3** Place pear, blackberries, the water and remaining sugar in a small heavy-based saucepan over high heat. Cook, covered, for 5 minutes or until fruit is just tender. Remove lid; cook for a further 4 minutes or until pear is soft but retains its shape and liquid reduces to a slightly syrupy consistency. Cool.

**4** Heat four 7cm (2¾in) egg rings in a large non-stick frying pan over low heat until hot; spray lightly with oil. Spoon 1½ tablespoons of batter into each ring; cover pan with a tight-fitting lid. Cook crumpets for 4 minutes or until bubbles appear on the surface; remove lid. Taking care, remove crumpets from pan; carefully remove from rings, using a sharp knife if necessary to release edges. Flip crumpets; cook for 30 seconds or until light golden. Repeat with remaining batter and oil spray to make a total of 12 crumpets.

**5** Divide crumpets among four plates; spoon over a quarter of the fruit and a little of the syrup. Serve with yoghurt.

| ● 16.1g total fat (3.4g saturated fat) | ● 1515kJ (361 cal) | ● 25.2g carbohydrate | ● 23.2g protein | ● 10.9g fibre | ● 414mg sodium |
|---|---|---|---|---|---|

# Baked pumpkin,
# TOMATO & EGG SKILLET

**PREP + COOK TIME** 1 HOUR **SERVES** 4

600g (1¼lb) butternut pumpkin, peeled,
   cut into 1.5cm (¾in) dice
1 tablespoon extra virgin olive oil
2 teaspoons coarsely chopped fresh sage
¼ teaspoon cracked black pepper
½ bunch silver beet (swiss chard) (375g) (see tips)
400g (12½oz) can cherry tomatoes (see tips)
400g (12½oz) can salt-reduced kidney beans,
   drained, rinsed
⅓ cup (80ml) water
8 eggs
1 tablespoon dukkah
1 tablespoon small fresh flat-leaf parsley leaves

**1** Preheat oven 200°C/400°F.

**2** Place pumpkin, oil, sage and pepper in a large ovenproof frying pan; stir to combine. Bake for 20 minutes or until pumpkin is just tender.

**3** Meanwhile, discard three-quarters of the silver beet stalks; finely chop remaining stalks and leaves. Add tomatoes, silver beet, kidney beans and the water to pan with pumpkin; press all ingredients down so as much of the silver beet is submerged as possible. Return to oven; bake, stirring halfway through cooking time, for a further 15 minutes or until bubbles appear.

**4** Using the back of a wooden spoon, make eight indents in the pumpkin mixture. Crack an egg into each one; return to the oven and bake for 12 minutes or until whites are set and yolks are runny. Sprinkle with dukkah and parsley to serve.

**TIPS** You will need 3½ cups of chopped silver beet for this recipe. Swap canned cherry tomatoes with a can of diced tomatoes, if you like.

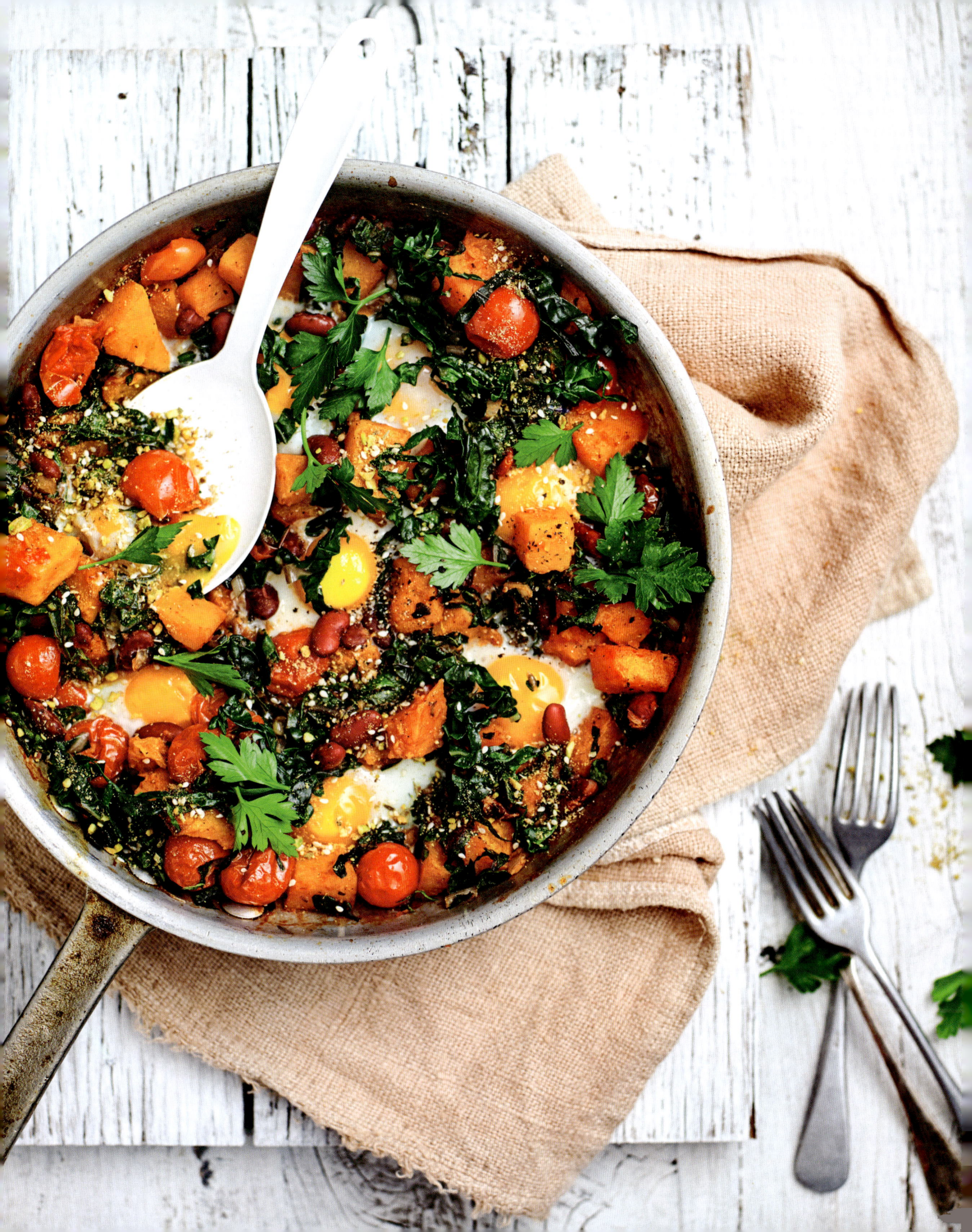

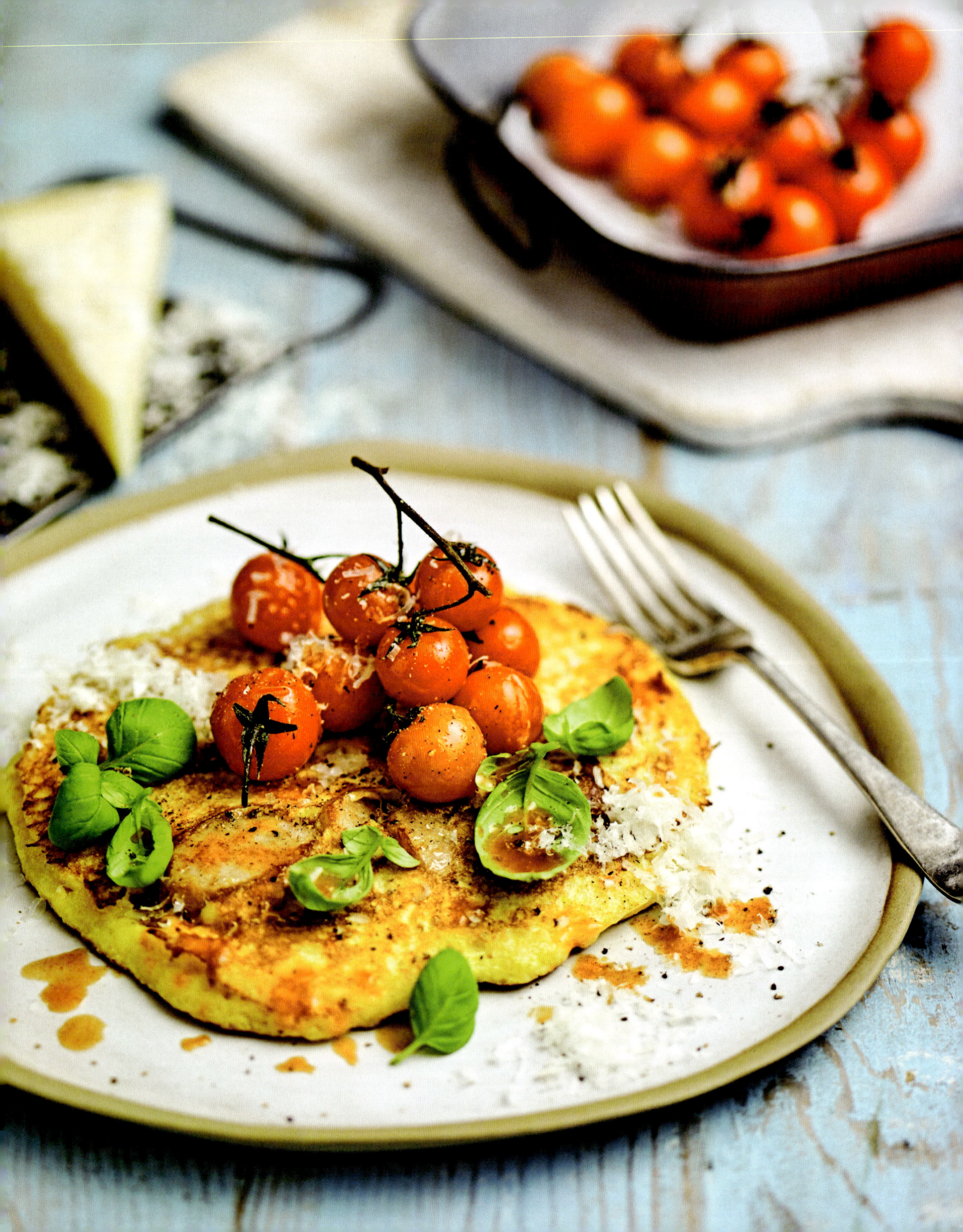

| 14.2g total fat (5g saturated fat) | 1420kJ (339 cal) | 30.1g carbohydrate | 20.6g protein | 4.1g fibre | 609mg sodium |

# Polenta, corn
# & SAUSAGE PANCAKES

**PREP + COOK TIME** 30 MINUTES **SERVES** 4

½ cup (85g) instant polenta (cornmeal)
¼ cup (40g) wholemeal self-raising flour
3 eggs
¼ cup (60ml) skim milk
125g (4oz) canned creamed corn
¾ cup (60g) finely grated low-fat parmesan
olive-oil spray
120g (4oz) low-fat chicken sausages
250g (8oz) cherry truss tomatoes (see tip)
¼ cup fresh baby basil leaves
1 teaspoon Tabasco sauce, to serve, optional

**1** Whisk polenta and flour in a large jug. Whisk eggs, milk, corn and ½ cup of the parmesan in a medium bowl. Add egg mixture to polenta mixture; whisk to combine. Season with pepper.

**2** Heat a large non-stick frying pan over medium heat; spray with oil. Cook sausages, turning, for 8 minutes or until browned. Remove from pan; slice thinly. Return to pan; cook for 2 minutes on each side or until cooked through and golden. Remove three-quarters of sausage from pan.

**3** Pour a quarter of the pancake batter (½ cup) over the remaining sausage in pan; cook for 2 minutes. Flip pancake over; cook for a further 1 minute or until golden and just cooked through. Remove from pan; cover to keep warm. Repeat three times with remaining sausage and pancake batter to make a total of four pancakes.

**4** Meanwhile, place tomatoes on a small oven tray. Cook under a preheated hot grill (broiler) for 3 minutes or until starting to soften and skins start to split.

**5** Sprinkle pancakes evenly with remaining parmesan and basil leaves. Serve pancakes with tomatoes and a dash of Tabasco sauce, if you like.

**DR JO SAYS**
Polenta is ground white or yellow corn. The yellow colour comes from the presence of carotenoids, including beta-carotene, lutein and zeaxanthin, all of which are important for eye health, which can be a concern for those with diabetes.

**TIP** Truss tomatoes are simply small vine-ripened tomatoes with the vine still attached. If cherry truss tomatoes are not available, use regular cherry tomatoes instead.

**NUTRITIONAL COUNT PER SERVING**

| ● 22.4g total fat (4.7g saturated fat) | ● 2005kJ (479 cal) | ● 50.7g carbohydrate | ● 15g protein | ● 7.7g fibre | ● 84mg sodium |
|---|---|---|---|---|---|

# Yoghurt, chia
# & APPLE OAT BIRCHER

**PREP + COOK TIME** 10 MINUTES (+ STANDING) **SERVES** 4

1⅓ cups (375g) natural Greek-style yoghurt
1 cup (250ml) milk
1 tablespoon chia seeds
1½ cups (135g) rolled oats
2 medium red apples (300g)
½ teaspoon ground cinnamon
¼ teaspoon ground cardamom
⅓ cup (45g) coarsely chopped roasted hazelnuts
¼ cup (40g) coarsely chopped roasted natural almonds
1 tablespoon honey

**1** Combine 1 cup of the yoghurt, milk, chia seeds and oats in a medium bowl. Stand for 15 minutes.

**2** Meanwhile, coarsely grate 1½ apples. Add grated apple and spices to oat mixture; stir to mix well. Cut remaining apple into eight thin wedges.

**3** Divide oat mixture evenly among four bowls; top with remaining yoghurt and apple. Sprinkle with nuts and drizzle with honey to serve.

**TIP** Swap nutmeg for cinnamon, if you like.

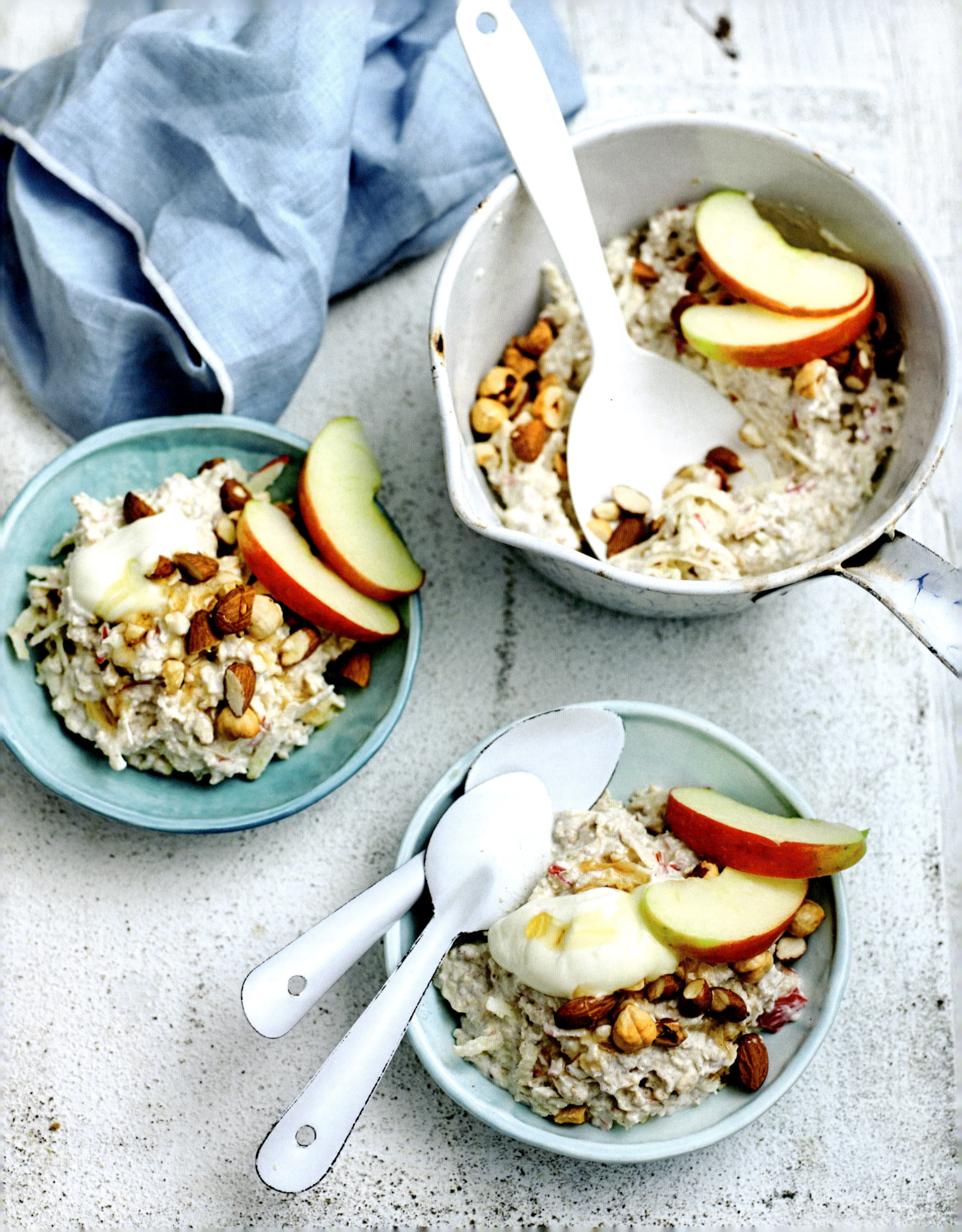

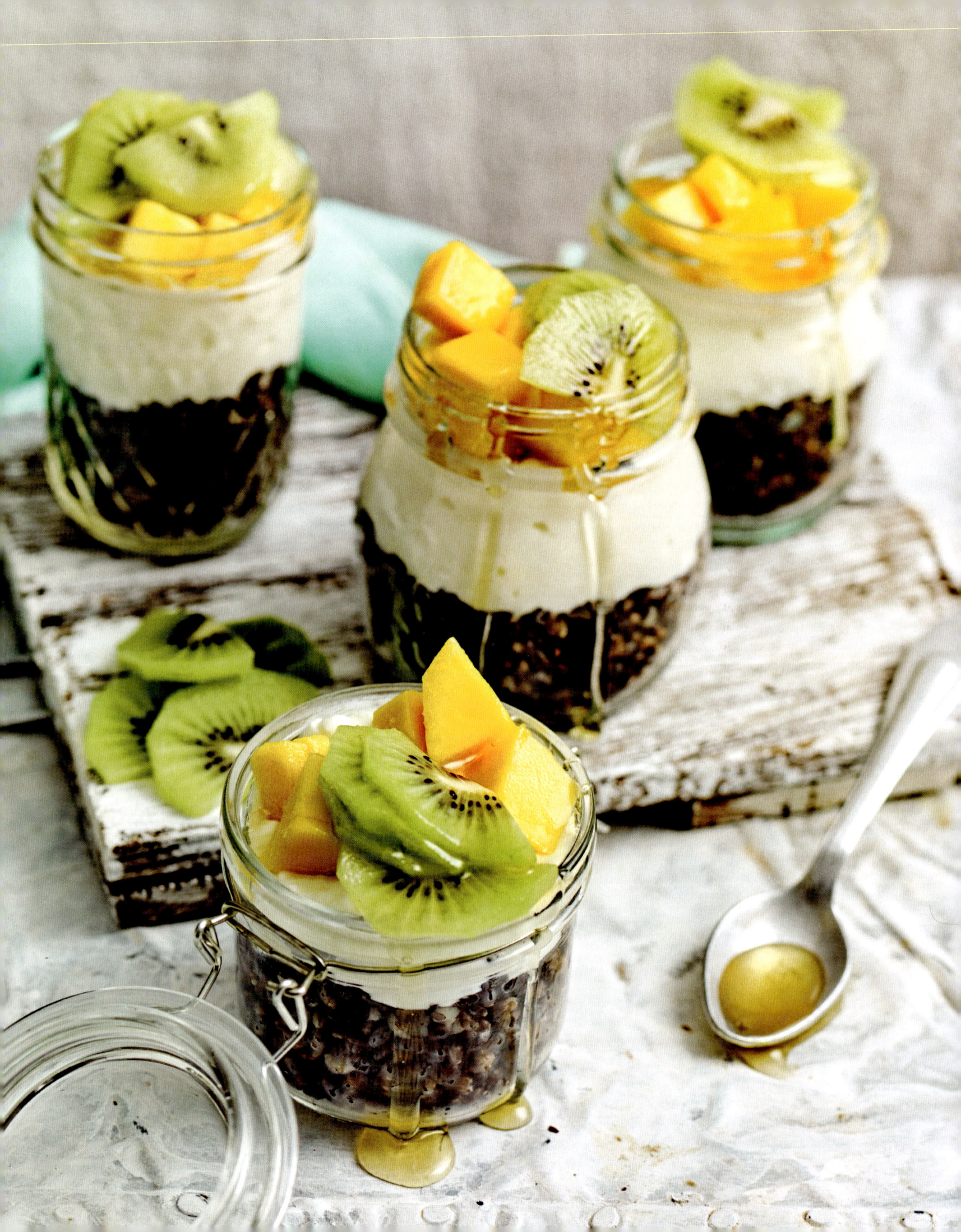

**NUTRITIONAL COUNT PER SERVING**

| ● 6.3g total fat (3.7g saturated fat) | ● 1360kJ (325 cal) | ● 44.7g carbohydrate | ● 20.3g protein | ● 6.7g fibre | ● 294mg sodium |
|---|---|---|---|---|---|

# Grab-n-go
# BREKKY JARS

**PREP + COOK TIME** 45 MINUTES (+ COOLING) **SERVES** 4

¾ **cup (150g) black barley**
**1.25 litres (5 cups) water**
**2 cups (400g) reduced-fat cottage cheese**
**1 small mango (300g), peeled, diced**
**200g (6½oz) kiwifruit, sliced**
**2 tablespoons manuka honey**

**1** Place barley and the water in a medium saucepan over medium-high heat; bring to the boil. Reduce heat to low; cook for 35 minutes or until barley is tender. Drain; stand until cool.

**2** Layer barley, cottage cheese and fruit evenly into four 1¼ cup (310ml) jars or airtight containers. Drizzle each with 2 teaspoons honey just before serving.

**TIP** The jars can be prepared the night before and refrigerated, covered, overnight for breakfast the next day; drizzle with honey just before serving.

**BLACK BARLEY** is an heirloom variety of barley. This high-fibre wholegrain has a dark mahogany colour, and a chewy, nutty taste. Add to soups, salads, pilafs, either on its own or in combination with other grains, and use instead of rice.

**DR JO SAYS**
Eating a snack with 20-30g of carbohydrate is a good idea an hour or so before you exercise. This will help to lift your energy levels, provide the fuel you need and prevent a hypo during your workout.

**NUTRITIONAL COUNT PER SERVING**

| ● 12.8g total fat (5g saturated fat) | ● 1234kJ (295 cal) | ● 21g carbohydrate | ● 21g protein | ● 4.3g fibre | ● 786mg sodium |
|---|---|---|---|---|---|

# OPEN CROQUE MADAME

**PREP + COOK TIME** 15 MINUTES **SERVES** 4

½ bunch asparagus (85g), sliced thinly lengthways
olive-oil spray
4 eggs
4 slices wholemeal sourdough bread (200g)
10g (½oz) butter, softened
1 tablespoon dijon mustard
100g (3oz) thinly sliced lean ham
⅓ cup (40g) grated gruyére cheese
25g (¾oz) baby rocket (arugula)

**1** Blanch asparagus in a saucepan of boiling water; drain.
**2** Heat a large non-stick frying pan over high heat; spray with oil. Fry eggs until cooked to your liking.
**3** Preheat a grill (broiler). Grill bread for 1 minute each side or until golden.
**4** Spread toast with butter and mustard. Top evenly with ham, asparagus and cheese.
**5** Place toasts under hot grill (broiler) for 1 minute or until cheese melts. Top with eggs and rocket leaves; season with pepper.

**TIP** You can poach or boil the eggs instead of frying, if you like.

**TO BLANCH** something, is to cook it in boiling water for a few minutes and then refresh it in cold water to stop the cooking process. This keeps the ingredients fresh, crisp and full of flavour.

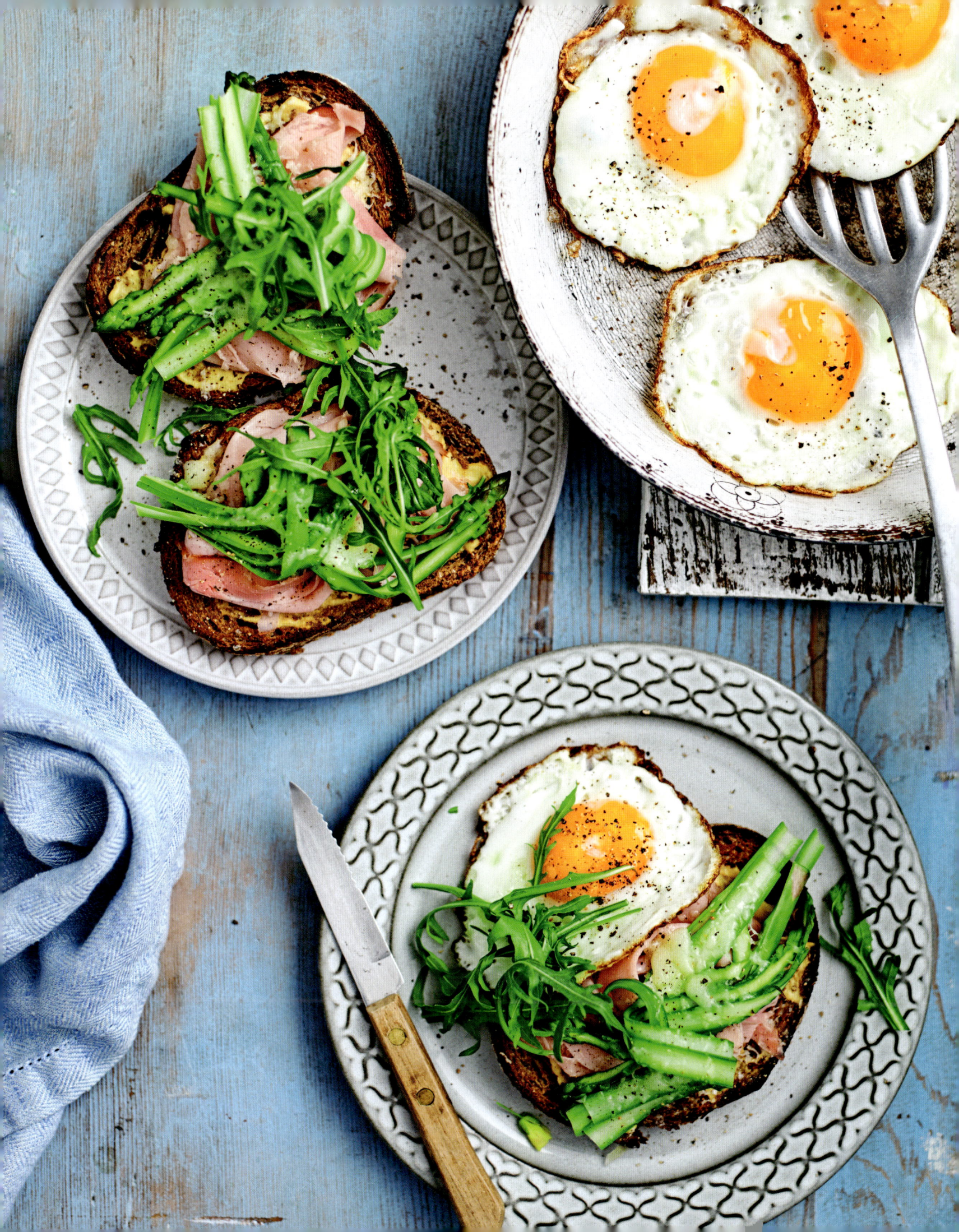

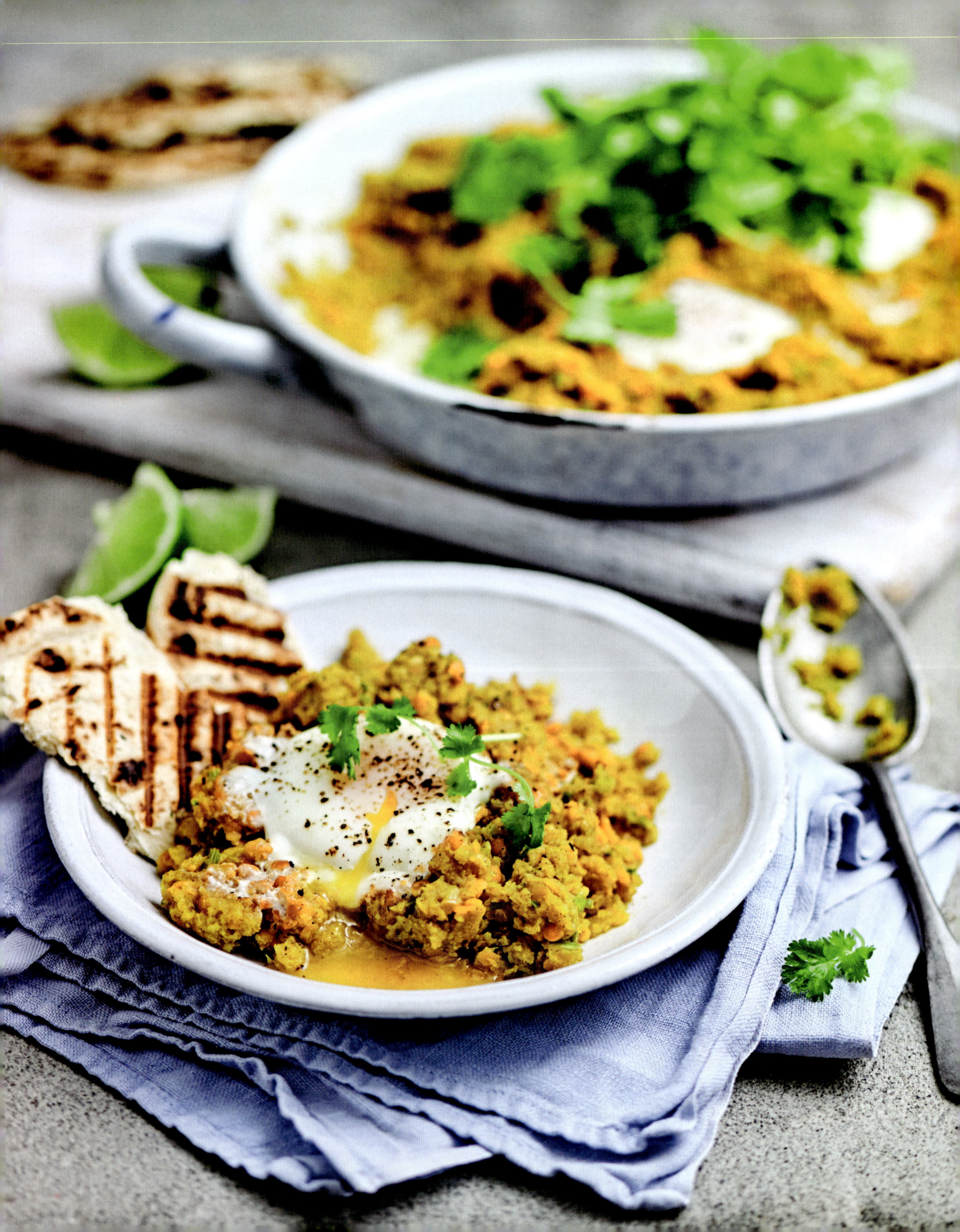

**NUTRITIONAL COUNT PER SERVING**

| 18.2g total fat (3.3g saturated fat) | 1755kJ (419 cal) | 36g carbohydrate | 21.7g protein | 10.5g fibre | 510mg sodium |
|---|---|---|---|---|---|

# CAULIFLOWER DHAL
## with poached eggs

**PREP + COOK TIME** 1 HOUR **SERVES** 4

½ medium cauliflower (750g), chopped coarsely
1½ cups (375ml) salt-reduced vegetable stock
1½ cups (375ml) water
2 teaspoons cumin seeds
1 teaspoon coriander seeds
1 teaspoon yellow mustard seeds
1 bunch fresh coriander (cilantro) (see tips)
2 tablespoons extra virgin olive oil
1 medium onion (150g), chopped coarsely
2 cloves garlic, crushed
4cm (1½in) piece fresh ginger, grated finely
2 teaspoons ground turmeric
¾ cup (115g) red lentils
1 stick cinnamon
4 large eggs
1 wholemeal pitta bread (125g), toasted, quartered
1 lime (65g), cut into wedges

**1** Place cauliflower, stock and the water in a medium saucepan; bring to the boil. Reduce heat to low; cook, covered, for 15 minutes or until cauliflower is tender. Cool slightly, then blend or process till smooth.

**2** Meanwhile, crush cumin seeds, coriander seeds and mustard seeds coarsely with a mortar and pestle. Separate coriander roots, stems and leaves. Finely chop roots and stems; reserve leaves.

**3** Heat oil in a large heavy-based frying pan over medium heat. Add crushed seeds; cook, stirring, for 1 minute or until fragrant. Add onion, garlic, ginger, turmeric and chopped coriander roots and stems. Cook, stirring occasionally, for a further 5 minutes or until onion softens.

**4** Add cauliflower, lentils and cinnamon stick to pan; stir to combine (take care as the mixture may spit). Cover; bring to the boil over high heat. Reduce heat to low; cook, covered, for 10 minutes or until mixture is thickened.

**5** Using the back of a wooden spoon, make four indents into the dhal mixture; crack an egg into each one. Cook, covered, for 12 minutes or until eggs are set. Discard cinnamon stick.

**6** Top dhal with coriander leaves; serve with pitta bread and lime wedges.

**DR JO SAYS**
Although studies have not been conclusive, there is some evidence that cinnamon may help blood glucose control for people with type 2 diabetes.

**TIPS** You need 4 coriander roots and 3 cups of leaves for this recipe. Wash coriander roots and stems well before using.

You can make this recipe up to the end of step 4 the day before serving; store, covered, in the fridge. Gently reheat the next day, then continue from step 5.

| 23.4g total fat (5g saturated fat) | 1567kJ (374 cal) | 17g carbohydrate | 20g protein | 11.2g fibre | 293mg sodium |

# ASPARAGUS, EGG
## & white bean smash

**PREP + COOK TIME** 20 MINUTES **SERVES** 4

2 bunches asparagus (340g)

2 tablespoons extra virgin olive oil

4 eggs

1 teaspoon ground sumac

1 tablespoon smoked almonds, chopped finely

1 tablespoon dukkah

**WHITE BEAN SMASH**

1 tablespoon extra virgin olive oil

3 cloves garlic, crushed

2 teaspoons finely grated lemon rind

2 x 400g (12½oz) cans salt-reduced cannellini beans, drained, rinsed

½ cup (125ml) water

¼ cup (20g) finely grated parmesan

1 tablespoon lemon juice

**1** Make white bean smash.

**2** Heat a grill plate (or grill pan or barbecue) on high. Wet the asparagus under cold running water. Grill asparagus, turning, for 5 minutes or until tender and grill marks appear.

**3** Heat oil in a large non-stick frying pan over high heat; fry eggs until cooked to your liking.

**4** To make the smoked almond dukkah, combine sumac, smoked almonds and dukkah in a small bowl.

**5** Serve asparagus and fried eggs on a bed of white bean smash, sprinkled with smoked almond dukkah.

**WHITE BEAN SMASH** Heat oil in a large heavy-based saucepan over medium heat. Cook garlic and lemon rind for 30 seconds or until fragrant. Add beans and the water to the pan; bring to the boil. Reduce heat to low-medium; cook for a further 3 minutes or until mixture thickens. Stir through parmesan and lemon juice; mash coarsely. Cover to keep warm. (Makes 3 cups)

**TIP** The white bean smash will thicken on standing, so add a little boiling water if a looser consistency is preferred.

**DR JO SAYS**
Eating garlic regularly can improve your cardiovascular health. Some evidence shows that garlic may lower blood pressure and slow the development of atherosclerosis.

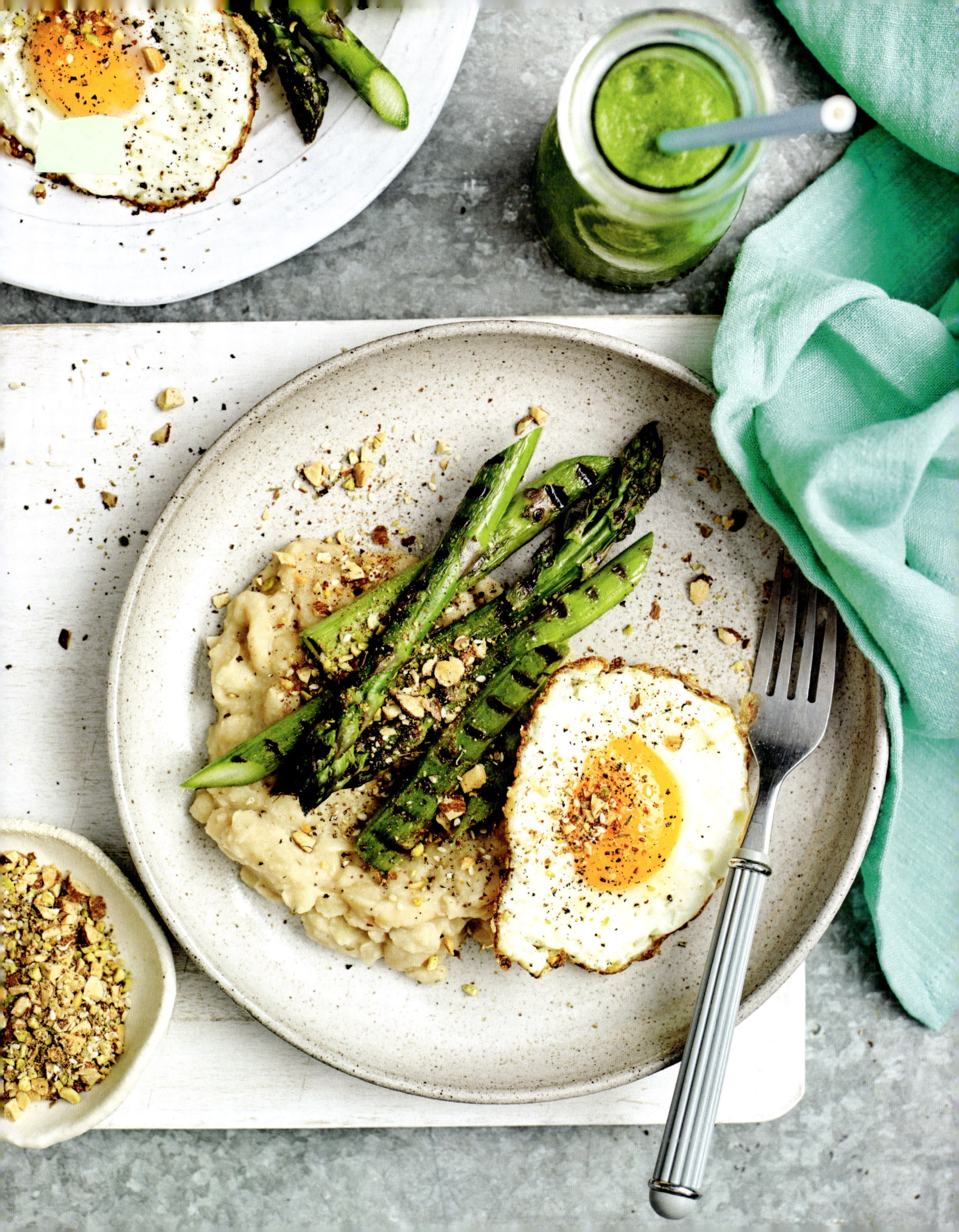

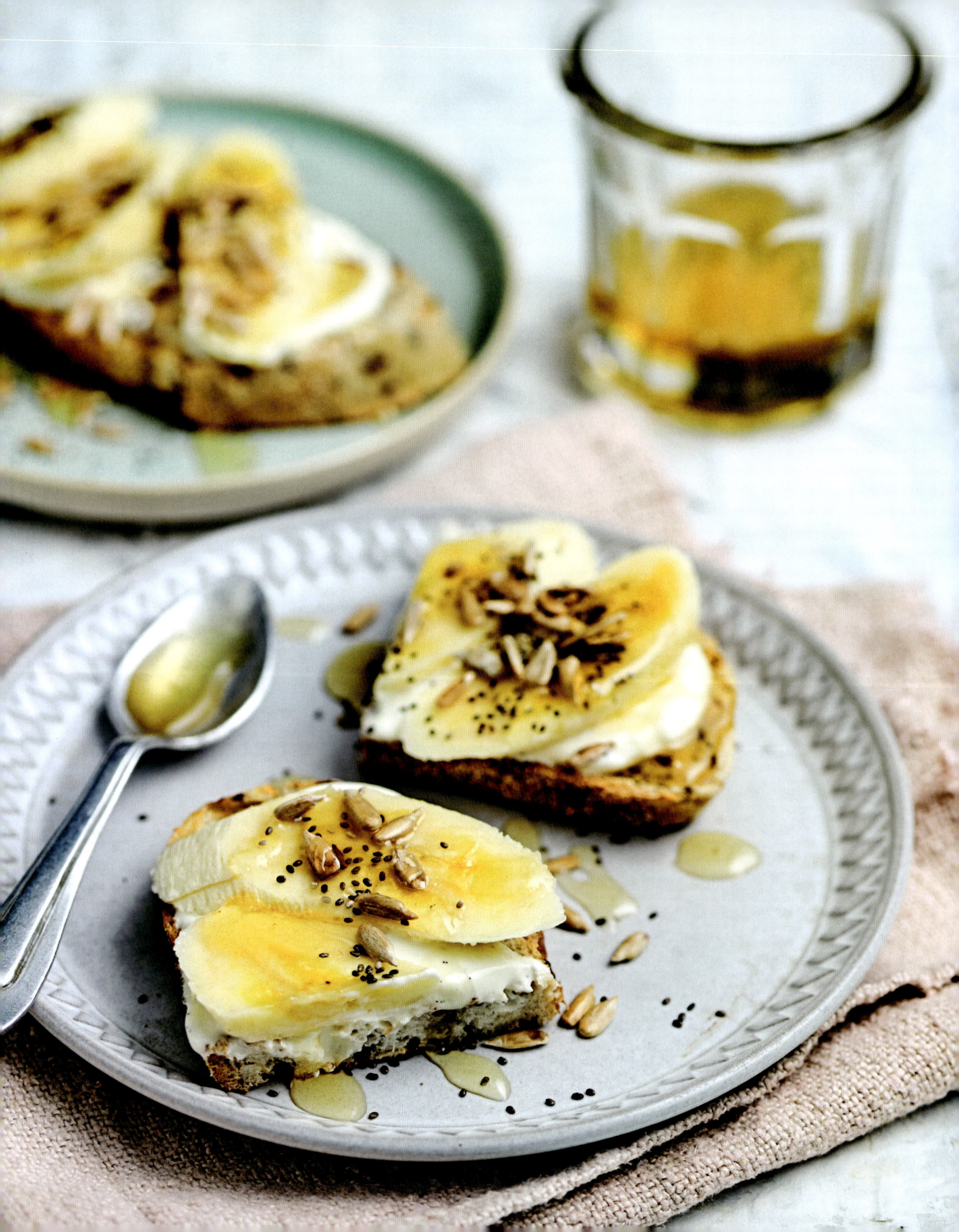

## NUTRITIONAL COUNT PER SERVING

| 5.7g total fat (1.5g saturated fat) | 1306kJ (312 cal) | 52.9g carbohydrate | 11.1g protein | 3.6g fibre | 332mg sodium |
|---|---|---|---|---|---|

# Crunchy banana &
# VANILLA TOASTS

**PREP + COOK TIME** 10 MINUTES **SERVES** 4

½ cup (140g) natural Greek-style yoghurt
1 teaspoon vanilla bean paste
4 slices soy and linseed sourdough bread (280g)
2 medium bananas (400g), sliced
1 teaspoon flaxseeds (linseeds), toasted
2 teaspoons sunflower seeds, toasted
1 teaspoon black chia seeds, toasted
1 tablespoon honey

**1** Combine yoghurt and vanilla in a small bowl.

**2** Toast bread; spread evenly with vanilla yoghurt. Top with banana slices and toasted seeds. Drizzle evenly with honey to serve.

**TIP** Choose a Greek-style yoghurt that doesn't contain added sugar.

**DR JO SAYS**
I don't recommend using seed oils, as these are highly processed and refined. Whole seeds, on the other hand, are wonderfully nutritious, adding good fats, fibre and several vitamins and minerals to your diet.

| ● 22.8g total fat (3.7g saturated fat) | ● 1796kJ (429 cal) | ● 32.1g carbohydrate | ● 18.5g protein | ● 9.5g fibre | ● 55mg sodium |
|---|---|---|---|---|---|

# MUESLI 'SOLDIERS'
## with yoghurt dipping sauce

**PREP + COOK TIME** 30 MINUTES (+ COOLING) **SERVES** 6

¾ cup (75g) lupin flakes (see tips)
⅔ cup (105g) natural almonds
½ cup (10g) puffed millet
⅓ cup (50g) sunflower seeds
⅓ cup (65g) pepitas (pumpkin seed kernels)
⅓ cup (45g) dried cranberries
2 rings dried pineapple (65g), chopped coarsely
1 teaspoon agar agar powder (see tips)
¼ cup (90g) honey

### YOGHURT DIPPING SAUCE

1 medium apple (150g)
1½ cups (420g) natural Greek-style yoghurt
¼ cup (60ml) water
1 teaspoon mixed spice

**1** Preheat oven to 180°C/350°F. Grease and line base and sides of a 20cm (8in) square cake pan.

**2** Mix lupin flakes, almonds, puffed millet, sunflower seeds, pepitas, cranberries and pineapple in a large bowl. Sprinkle with agar agar; drizzle with honey. Using clean hands, mix until well combined. Press mixture firmly into pan with wet hands or a spatula to flatten the surface. Bake, turning pan halfway through cooking time, for 20 minutes or until golden; the mixture will firm on cooling. Transfer to a wire rack to cool completely.

**3** Meanwhile, make yoghurt dipping sauce.

**4** Using a serrated knife, cut muesli slice in half, then cut each half into nine bars to yield 18 bars in total. Serve three 'soldiers' each, for dipping into yoghurt dipping sauce.

**YOGHURT DIPPING SAUCE** Dice apple finely. Combine ingredients in a medium bowl. Divide evenly among six bowls or glasses, cover; refrigerate until required.

**TIPS** Agar agar is a seaweed-based gelling agent available from major supermarkets, health food stores and Asian food stores. Leftovers make great muesli bars for a lunch-box snack. Store in an airtight container for up to 4 days; they may soften slightly on storing, resulting in a chewier muesli bar.

**LUPIN FLAKES** are made by processing whole dried lupin beans into flakes. They are a protein and fibre-rich legume (belonging to the same family as beans, peas, lentils and peanuts), and are gluten free. They are also low in carbohydrates and have a low GI. Lupin flakes are available from major supermarkets and health food stores.

### DR JO SAYS

Nuts are rich in magnesium, an essential mineral shown to reduce the risk of type 2 diabetes. In a review published in 2016, compared to those with the lowest magnesium intake, those with the highest had a 17% lower risk.

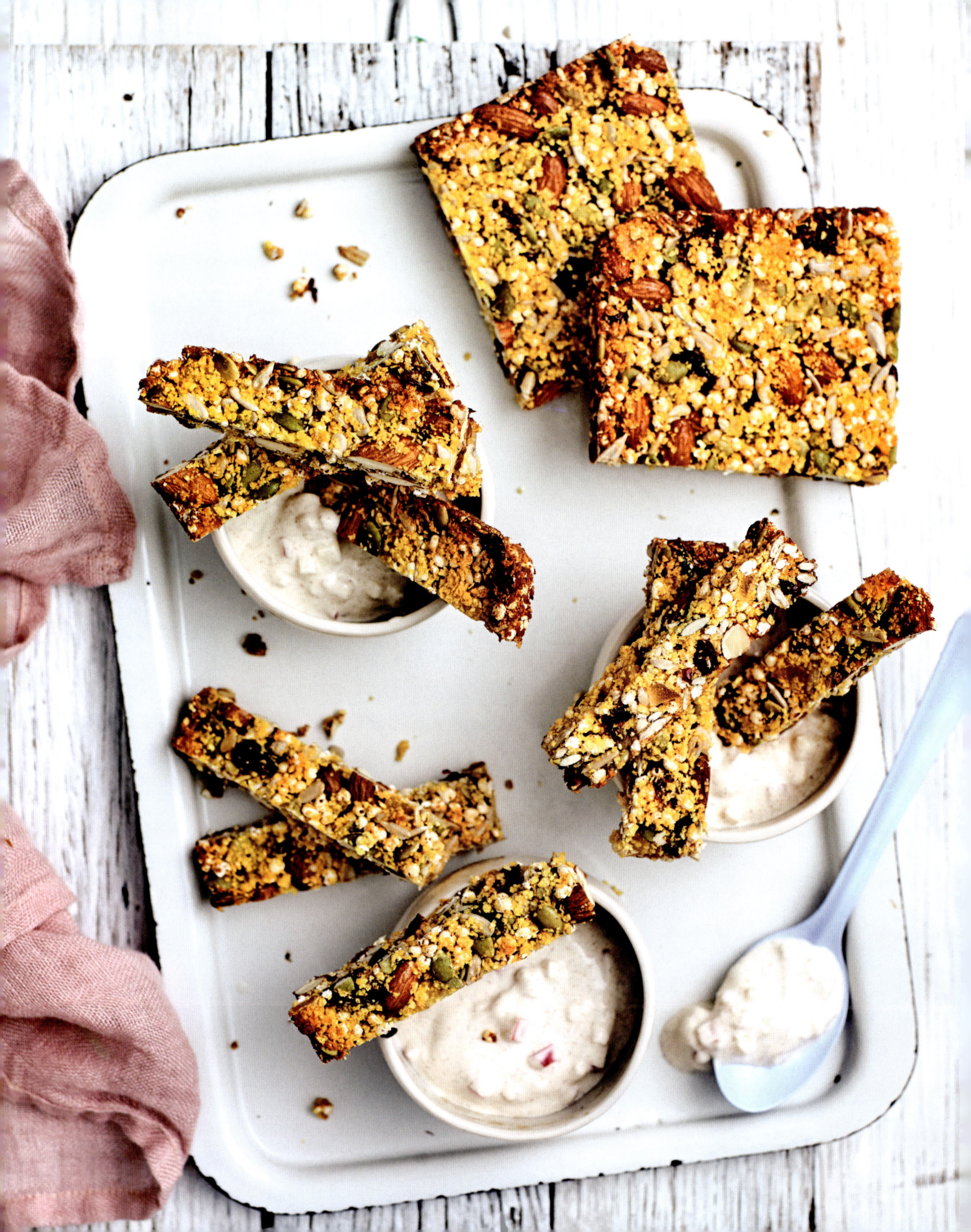

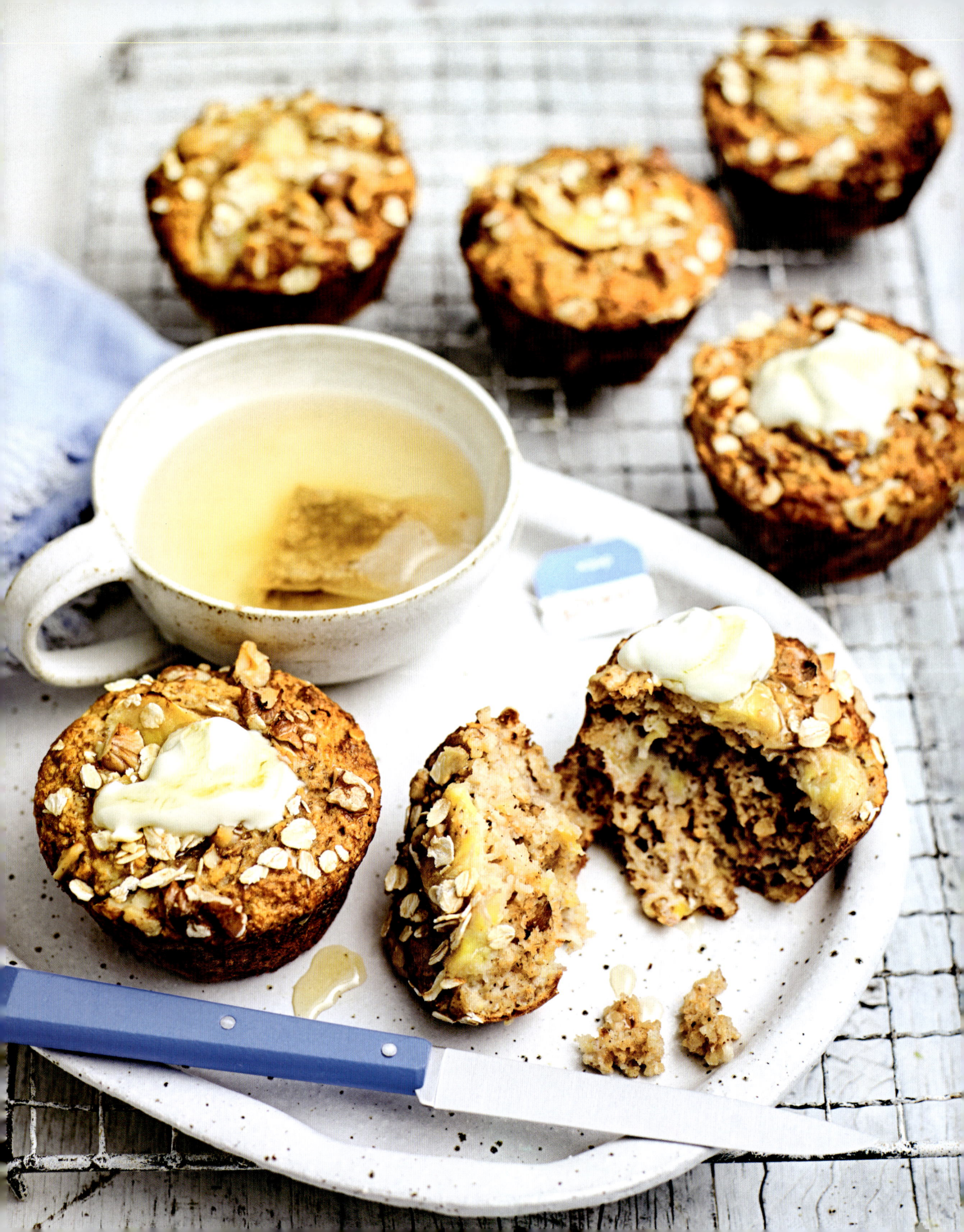

## NUTRITIONAL COUNT PER SERVING

| 16.3g total fat (5g saturated fat) | 1633kJ (390 cal) | 46.6g carbohydrate | 11.4g protein | 5.9g fibre | 228mg sodium |
|---|---|---|---|---|---|

# Banana oat MUFFINS

**PREP + COOK TIME** 40 MINUTES (+ COOLING) **SERVES** 6

$1\frac{1}{2}$ cups (135g) rolled oats
$\frac{1}{2}$ cup (80g) wholemeal plain (all-purpose) flour
1 teaspoon ground nutmeg
$\frac{1}{2}$ teaspoon bicarbonate of soda (baking soda)
1 teaspoon baking powder
$\frac{1}{2}$ cup (55g) coarsely chopped walnuts
120g (4oz) apple sauce
2 eggs, beaten lightly
$\frac{1}{4}$ cup (60ml) milk
$\frac{1}{2}$ cup (140g) natural Greek-style yoghurt
$\frac{3}{4}$ cup (210g) mashed ripe banana (see tip)
$1\frac{1}{2}$ tablespoons honey
1 medium banana (200g), extra, cut into 12 slices
2 teaspoons lemon juice
$\frac{2}{3}$ cup (185g) natural Greek-style yoghurt, extra

**1** Preheat oven to 200°C/400°F. Lightly spray a 6-hole ($\frac{3}{4}$ cup/180ml) texas muffin pan with oil spray; line base and side with 2 overlapping strips of baking paper.

**2** Reserve 1 tablespoon of the oats. Process remaining oats until chopped finely but still retaining some texture. Combine chopped oats, flour, nutmeg, soda, baking powder and half of the walnuts in a large bowl. Make a well in the centre; pour in combined apple sauce, egg, milk, yoghurt, mashed banana and 1 tablespoon of the honey. Stir until just combined, taking care not to over-mix. Spoon batter evenly into pan holes.

**3** Combine sliced banana and lemon juice in a small bowl. Place 2 banana slices on each muffin; sprinkle evenly with reserved oats and remaining walnuts.

**4** Bake for 25 minutes or until muffins are golden and cooked when a skewer inserted into the centre comes out clean. Cool muffins in pan for 5 minutes before turning, top-side up, onto a wire rack to cool completely.

**5** Drizzle remaining honey over top of muffins just before serving. Serve with extra yoghurt.

**TIP** You will need to mash about 2 medium bananas for this recipe.

| ● 11.6g total fat (5.3g saturated fat) | ● 1389kJ (332 cal) | ● 44.3g carbohydrate | ● 11.6g protein | ● 3.5g fibre | ● 18mg sodium |

# CREAMY POLENTA PORRIDGE
## with roasted rhubarb & sweet dukkah

PREP + COOK TIME 35 MINUTES SERVES 4

300g (9½oz) rhubarb (see tip)
2 tablespoons water
2½ cups (625ml) skim milk
½ cup (125ml) light coconut milk
¼ cup (90g) honey
1 cup water (250ml), extra
⅔ cup (110g) white polenta (cornmeal)

SWEET DUKKAH
1½ tablespoons unsalted hazelnuts
1½ tablespoons pistachios
1 tablespoon sesame seeds
3 teaspoons coriander seeds
2½ teaspoons brown sugar
¾ teaspoon ground cinnamon
¾ teaspoon ground cardamom

1 Preheat oven to 200°C/400°F.

2 Cut rhubarb into 8cm (3¼in) lengths. Place in a flameproof roasting pan, cover with foil; roast for 20 minutes or until rhubarb is soft but still holds its shape. Carefully transfer to a plate, leaving one piece of rhubarb in the pan.

3 Add the 2 tablespoons of water to rhubarb in pan; mash until mixture breaks up. Cook over low–medium heat, stirring, for 1 minute or until rhubarb breaks down into a sauce consistency. Remove from heat; cover to keep warm.

4 Make sweet dukkah before turning oven off.

5 Meanwhile, whisk milk, coconut milk, honey and the extra water in a medium saucepan; bring to the boil. Reduce heat to low, slowly add polenta; cook, whisking constantly, for 2 minutes or until thick.

6 Divide polenta evenly among four bowls; top evenly with rhubarb and rhubarb sauce; Sprinkle with dukkah to serve.

SWEET DUKKAH Place nuts and seeds on an oven tray lined with baking paper; roast for 5 minutes. Crush coarsely with a mortar and pestle; cool. Place sugar and spices in a small bowl, add nut mixture; mix well.

TIP Rhubarb cooking time may vary according to thickness and ripeness of the rhubarb, so check after 15 minutes, then continue to cook if necessary.

The rhubarb can be cooked the day before; store in an airtight container, large enough so the rhubarb holds its shape, in the fridge.

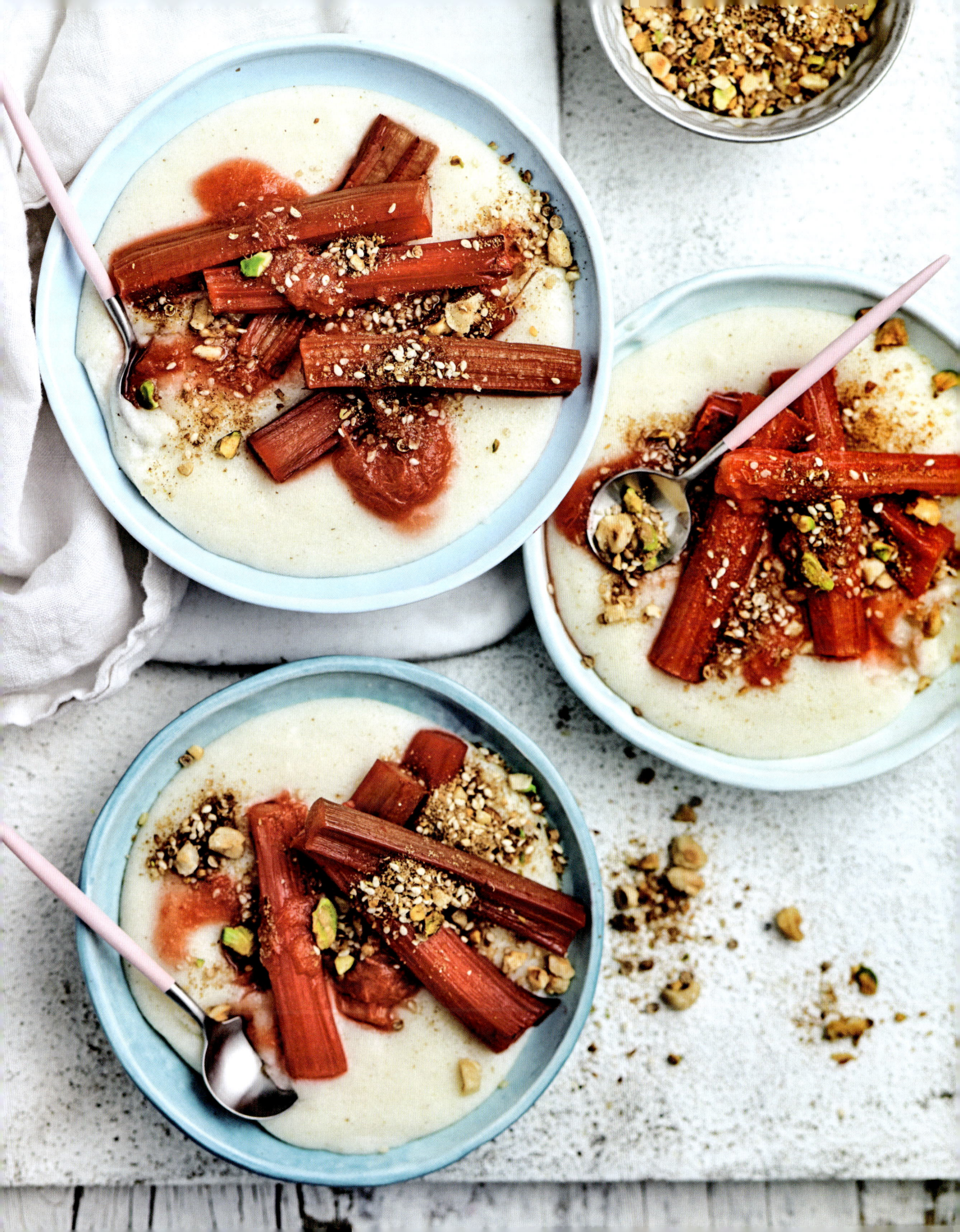

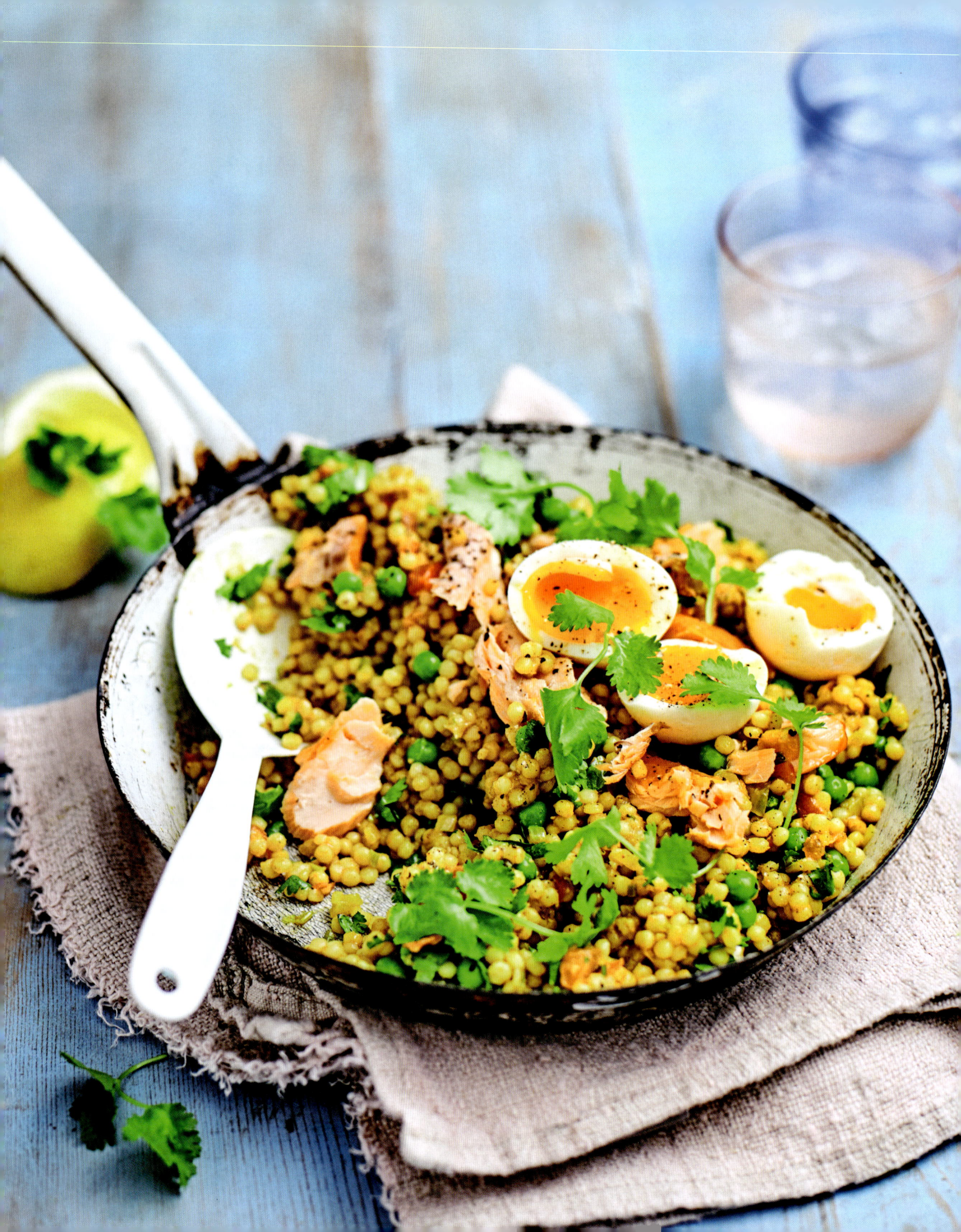

● 12.8g total fat (2.7g saturated fat) | ● 1771kJ (423 cal) | ● 49.8g carbohydrate | ● 23.4g protein | ● 5.2g fibre | ● 558mg sodium

# Pearl couscous
# & SALMON 'KEDGEREE'

**PREP + COOK TIME** 30 MINUTES **SERVES** 4

½ bunch fresh coriander (cilantro) (see tips)

2 eggs

1 tablespoon olive oil

½ small onion (40g), chopped finely

2 cloves garlic, crushed

4cm (1½in) piece fresh ginger, grated finely

1 fresh bay leaf

1 tablespoon curry powder

1 medium tomato (150g), diced finely

1¼ cups (250g) pearl couscous

1 cup (250ml) salt-reduced chicken stock (see tips)

1 cup (250ml) water

⅓ cup (40g) frozen peas, blanched

150g (4½oz) hot-smoked salmon, flaked

2 tablespoons lemon juice

1 tablespoon small fresh coriander (cilantro) leaves, extra, to serve

2 medium lemons (280g), cut into cheeks

**1** Separate coriander leaves from bunch; chop leaves coarsely and chop stems and roots finely; you need ½ cup firmly packed leaves and 2 tablespoons finely chopped stems and roots.

**2** Place eggs in a small saucepan; cover with cold water. Bring to the boil; cook for 3 minutes for soft-boiled. Remove, run under cold water; when cool enough to handle, peel, then cut in half.

**3** Heat oil in a large heavy-based non-stick frying pan over medium heat. Add coriander roots and stems, onion, garlic, ginger and bay leaf; cook for 4 minutes or until onion softens.

**4** Stir curry powder into pan; cook for 1 minute or until mixture is fragrant. Add tomato, couscous, stock and the water; bring to the boil. Reduce heat to low; cook, covered, for 7 minutes or until liquid is absorbed.

**5** Add peas, salmon, lemon juice and coriander leaves to pan; fluff through couscous with a fork.

**6** Divide couscous mixture among four bowls or plates; top each with half a boiled egg. Sprinkle with extra coriander; serve with lemon cheeks.

**DR JO SAYS**
The jury is still out on the impact of eggs on the health of those with diabetes. Eggs do provide terrific nutrition as part of a 'whole food' balanced diet, but currently the best advice is to be prudent and eat no more than six a week.

**TIPS** Wash coriander roots and stems well before using.
Omit the chicken stock and replace with an extra 1 cup (250ml) of water, if you like.

# *Beneficial* BERRIES

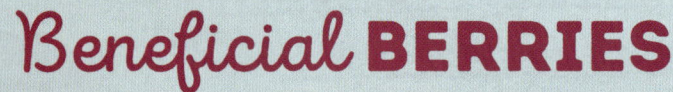

## BERRY RICOTTA TOAST

**PREP TIME** 10 MINUTES **SERVES** 2

Whisk 120g (4oz) low-fat ricotta, 1 tablespoon milk and 1 teaspoon finely grated lemon rind in a small bowl until smooth. Fold 30g (1oz) each fresh blueberries and raspberries through the ricotta mixture. Toast 2 x 40g (1½oz) slices dark rye bread. Spoon ricotta mixture onto toast. Top with 1 sliced small banana (130g) and another 30g (1oz) each fresh blueberries and raspberries. Serve sprinkled with 1 tablespoon white chia seeds.

**TIP** Recipe is best made just before serving.

**NUTRITIONAL COUNT PER SERVING** 5.3g total fat (1.7g saturated fat); 1076kJ (257 cal); 36.4g carbohydrate; 10.4g protein; 9.1g fibre; 286mg sodium

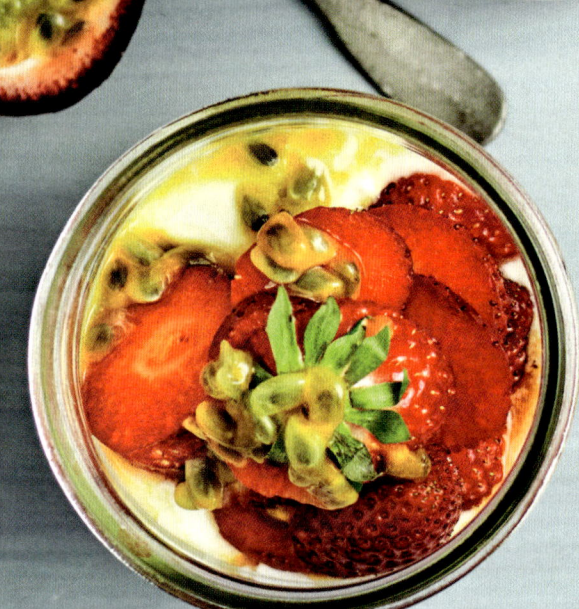

## PASSIONFRUIT & STRAWBERRY TRIFLE

**PREP TIME** 5 MINUTES **SERVES** 2

Divide 2 Weet-Bix (30g), broken into pieces and ¾ cup All-Bran cereal between two 1¼-cup serving glasses. Top evenly with 2 tablespoons fresh passionfruit pulp, 1 cup low-fat plain yoghurt and 140g (5oz) thinly sliced strawberries. Drizzle evenly with another 2 tablespoons fresh passionfruit pulp.

**TIPS** You will need about 4 passionfruit. You can make the trifle with any seasonal fruit combination or even with canned fruit in natural juices. Canned pears and frozen raspberries work well together, although this will alter the nutrition counts.

**NUTRITIONAL COUNT PER SERVING** 5.6g total fat (2.9g saturated fat); 1238kJ (295 cal); 45.2g carbohydrate; 11.4g protein; 11g fibre; 207mg sodium

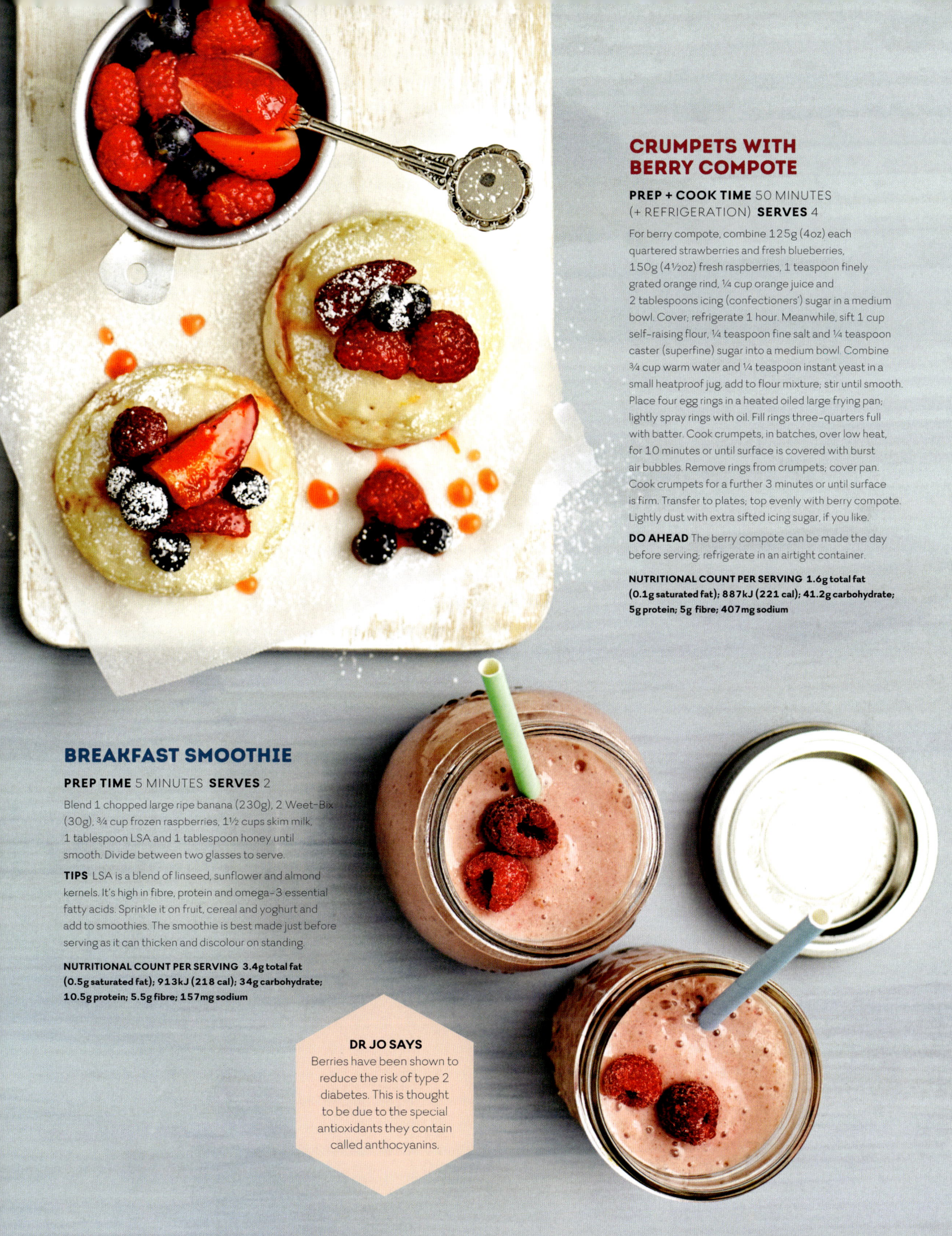

## CRUMPETS WITH BERRY COMPOTE

**PREP + COOK TIME** 50 MINUTES (+ REFRIGERATION) **SERVES** 4

For berry compote, combine 125g (4oz) each quartered strawberries and fresh blueberries, 150g (4½oz) fresh raspberries, 1 teaspoon finely grated orange rind, ¼ cup orange juice and 2 tablespoons icing (confectioners') sugar in a medium bowl. Cover; refrigerate 1 hour. Meanwhile, sift 1 cup self-raising flour, ¼ teaspoon fine salt and ¼ teaspoon caster (superfine) sugar into a medium bowl. Combine ¾ cup warm water and ¼ teaspoon instant yeast in a small heatproof jug, add to flour mixture; stir until smooth. Place four egg rings in a heated oiled large frying pan; lightly spray rings with oil. Fill rings three-quarters full with batter. Cook crumpets, in batches, over low heat, for 10 minutes or until surface is covered with burst air bubbles. Remove rings from crumpets; cover pan. Cook crumpets for a further 3 minutes or until surface is firm. Transfer to plates; top evenly with berry compote. Lightly dust with extra sifted icing sugar, if you like.

**DO AHEAD** The berry compote can be made the day before serving; refrigerate in an airtight container.

**NUTRITIONAL COUNT PER SERVING 1.6g total fat (0.1g saturated fat); 887kJ (221 cal); 41.2g carbohydrate; 5g protein; 5g fibre; 407mg sodium**

## BREAKFAST SMOOTHIE

**PREP TIME** 5 MINUTES **SERVES** 2

Blend 1 chopped large ripe banana (230g), 2 Weet-Bix (30g), ¾ cup frozen raspberries, 1½ cups skim milk, 1 tablespoon LSA and 1 tablespoon honey until smooth. Divide between two glasses to serve.

**TIPS** LSA is a blend of linseed, sunflower and almond kernels. It's high in fibre, protein and omega-3 essential fatty acids. Sprinkle it on fruit, cereal and yoghurt and add to smoothies. The smoothie is best made just before serving as it can thicken and discolour on standing.

**NUTRITIONAL COUNT PER SERVING 3.4g total fat (0.5g saturated fat); 913kJ (218 cal); 34g carbohydrate; 10.5g protein; 5.5g fibre; 157mg sodium**

### DR JO SAYS
Berries have been shown to reduce the risk of type 2 diabetes. This is thought to be due to the special antioxidants they contain called anthocyanins.

| 15.9g total fat (5g saturated fat) | 1430kJ (342 cal) | 31.6g carbohydrate | 15.9g protein | 4.5g fibre | 152mg sodium |

# Rose, cardamom & pistachio
# QUINOA PORRIDGE

PREP + COOK TIME 20 MINUTES **SERVES** 2

½ cup (100g) white quinoa, rinsed well
1 cup (250ml) milk
½ cup (125ml) water
1 teaspoon ground cardamom
½ teaspoon rosewater
⅔ cup (190g) low-fat natural Greek-style yoghurt
¼ cup (35g) coarsely chopped pistachios
2 teaspoons dried rose petals, optional (see tips)
3 teaspoons pure maple syrup

**1** Place quinoa, milk, the water, cardamom and rosewater in a medium heavy-based saucepan over medium heat; bring to the boil. Reduce heat to low; cook, stirring occasionally, for 15 minutes or until quinoa is softened and liquid absorbed.
**2** Divide porridge between two bowls; top evenly with yoghurt, pistachios and rose petals. Drizzle evenly with syrup to serve.

**TIPS** Ensure the dried rose petals are certified 'food grade', that is, fit to eat. Organic petals are grown without harmful chemicals or pesticides. You can find them at speciality food stores.

Serve immediately or, if making ahead of time, add a little extra water to loosen up the quinoa porridge when reheating, as it will thicken on standing.

**DR JO SAYS**
Eating about 60g nuts (a large handful) every day has been shown to improve blood glucose control in those with type 2 diabetes.

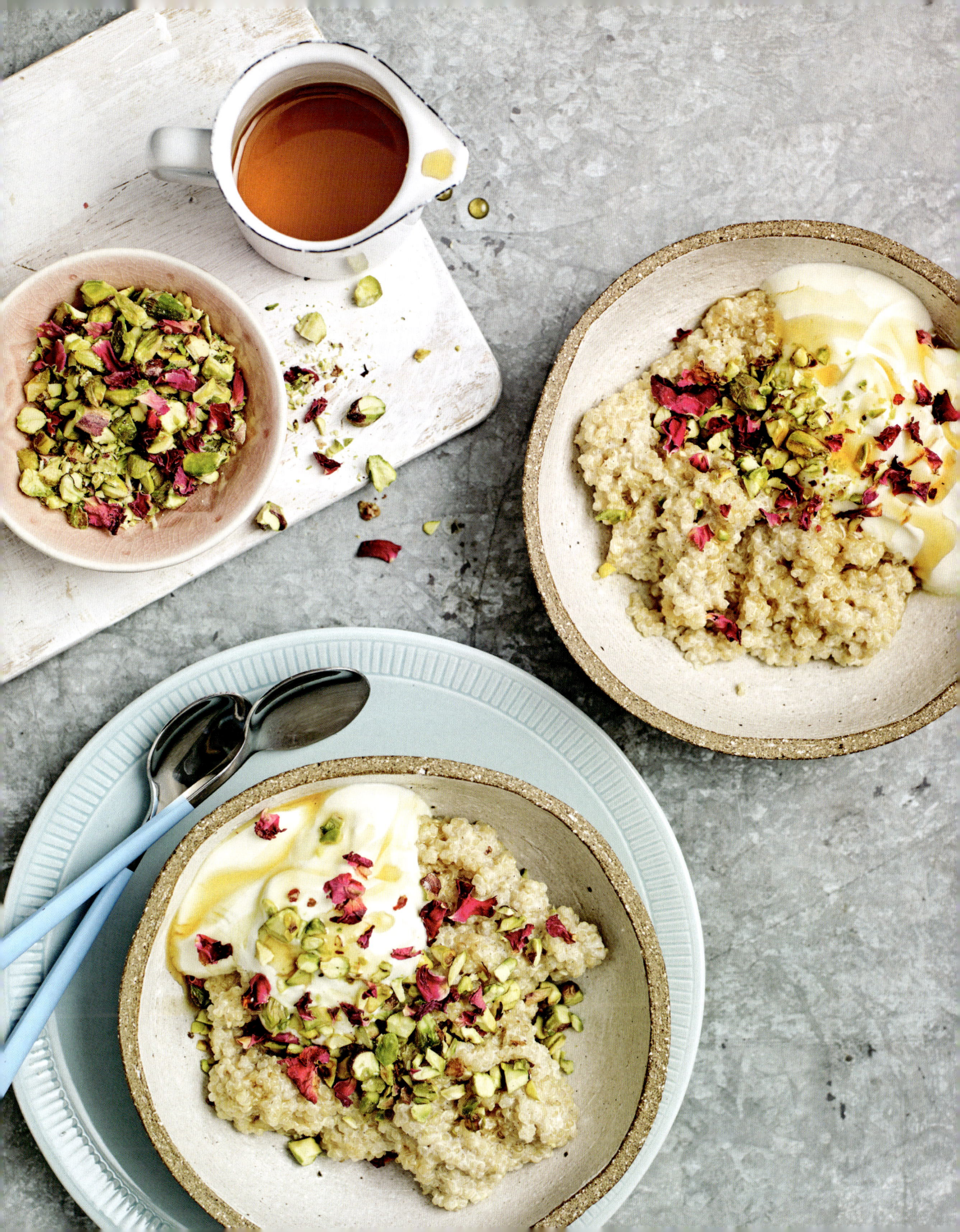

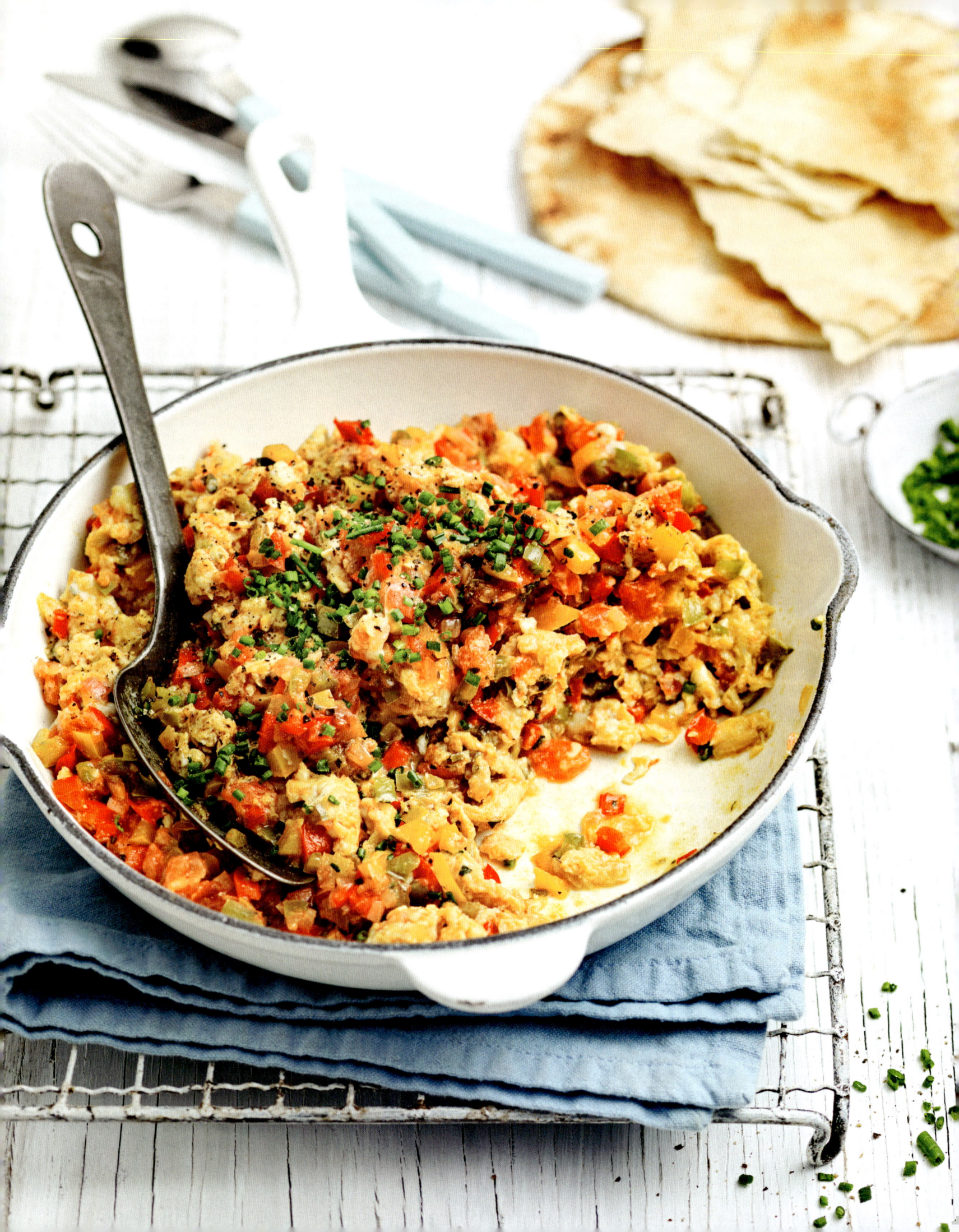

| ● 24.3g total fat (4.9g saturated fat) | ● 1767kJ (422 cal) | ● 29.1g carbohydrate | ● 20.6g protein | ● 5.3g fibre | ● 457mg sodium |
|---|---|---|---|---|---|

# Turkish-style
# SCRAMBLED EGGS

**PREP + COOK TIME** 25 MINUTES **SERVES** 4

¼ cup (60ml) olive oil
1 medium red onion (170g), chopped finely
1 medium red capsicum (bell pepper) (200g),
   chopped finely
1 medium green capsicum (bell pepper) (200g),
   chopped finely
1 medium yellow capsicum (bell pepper) (200g),
   chopped finely
1 teaspoon smoked paprika
¼ teaspoon cayenne pepper
2 tablespoons finely chopped fresh oregano leaves
3 medium ripe tomatoes (450g), peeled, seeded,
   chopped finely (see tips)
8 eggs, beaten lightly
2 tablespoons finely chopped fresh chives
2 small pitta breads (160g), toasted, halved
1 medium lemon (140g), cut into wedges

**1** Heat oil in a large heavy-based non-stick frying pan over low-medium heat. Cook onion, capsicum, paprika, cayenne and oregano, stirring frequently, for 8 minutes or until vegetables are very soft; add tomato. Increase heat to high; cook for a further 4 minutes or until tomato softens and mixture thickens. Transfer half the mixture to a medium bowl.

**2** Add egg to pan; cook, stirring frequently, for 40 seconds or until barely set. Remove from heat; gently fold in reserved vegetable mixture.

**3** Sprinkle egg mixture with chives; accompany with pitta bread and lemon wedges to serve.

---

**TIPS** To peel fresh tomatoes, cut a cross in the skins at the base, drop each one into simmering water for 30 seconds, then into a bowl of cold water. Peel tomatoes, starting from the cross; discard skins.

Use all red capsicums in this dish instead of the different colours, if preferred.

| ● 31.1g total fat (4.2g saturated fat) | ● 1891kJ (451 cal) | ● 25.6g carbohydrate | ● 15.1g protein | ● 7.1g fibre | ● 210mg sodium |
|---|---|---|---|---|---|

# Passionfruit, yoghurt & CANNELLINI BEAN LOAF

**PREP + COOK TIME** 55 MINUTES (+ COOLING) **SERVES** 8

400g (12½oz) can salt-reduced cannellini beans,
   drained, rinsed

⅓ cup (80ml) olive oil

4 eggs

2 tablespoons honey

2 teaspoons vanilla bean paste

1⅓ cups (375g) natural Greek-style yoghurt

2 cups (240g) almond meal

⅓ cup (55g) wholemeal plain (all-purpose) flour

1 teaspoon baking powder

1 tablespoon finely grated orange rind

½ cup passionfruit pulp (120g)

**1** Preheat oven to 180°C/350°F. Grease and line base and sides of a 21½cm x 11½cm (8½in x 4½in) loaf pan with baking paper.

**2** Process beans, oil, eggs, honey, vanilla and ⅓ cup of the yoghurt until smooth.

**3** Place almond meal, flour, baking powder and orange rind in a large bowl. Add bean mixture and ¼ cup of the passionfruit; fold until just combined.

**4** Spoon mixture into pan; bake for 45 minutes or until a skewer inserted into the centre comes out clean (cover with foil if over-browning). Leave in pan to cool completely.

**5** Turn loaf out; cut into 8 thick slices. Top evenly with remaining yoghurt and passionfruit to serve.

**TIPS** You will need approximately 6 passionfruit and 1 orange for this recipe.
Grill the sliced loaf under a heated grill (broiler) for 2 minutes on each side or until golden, if you like.

**DO AHEAD** You can make this loaf a day ahead; cool the loaf completely, then store in an airtight container. Individual slices can be wrapped in plastic wrap and frozen for up to three months, then thawed and grilled to serve.

**DR JO SAYS**
Using nut meals to replace some flour in a baking recipe is a great way to reduce the carbohydrate content, and therefore the glycaemic load, while adding fibre, protein and healthy fats.

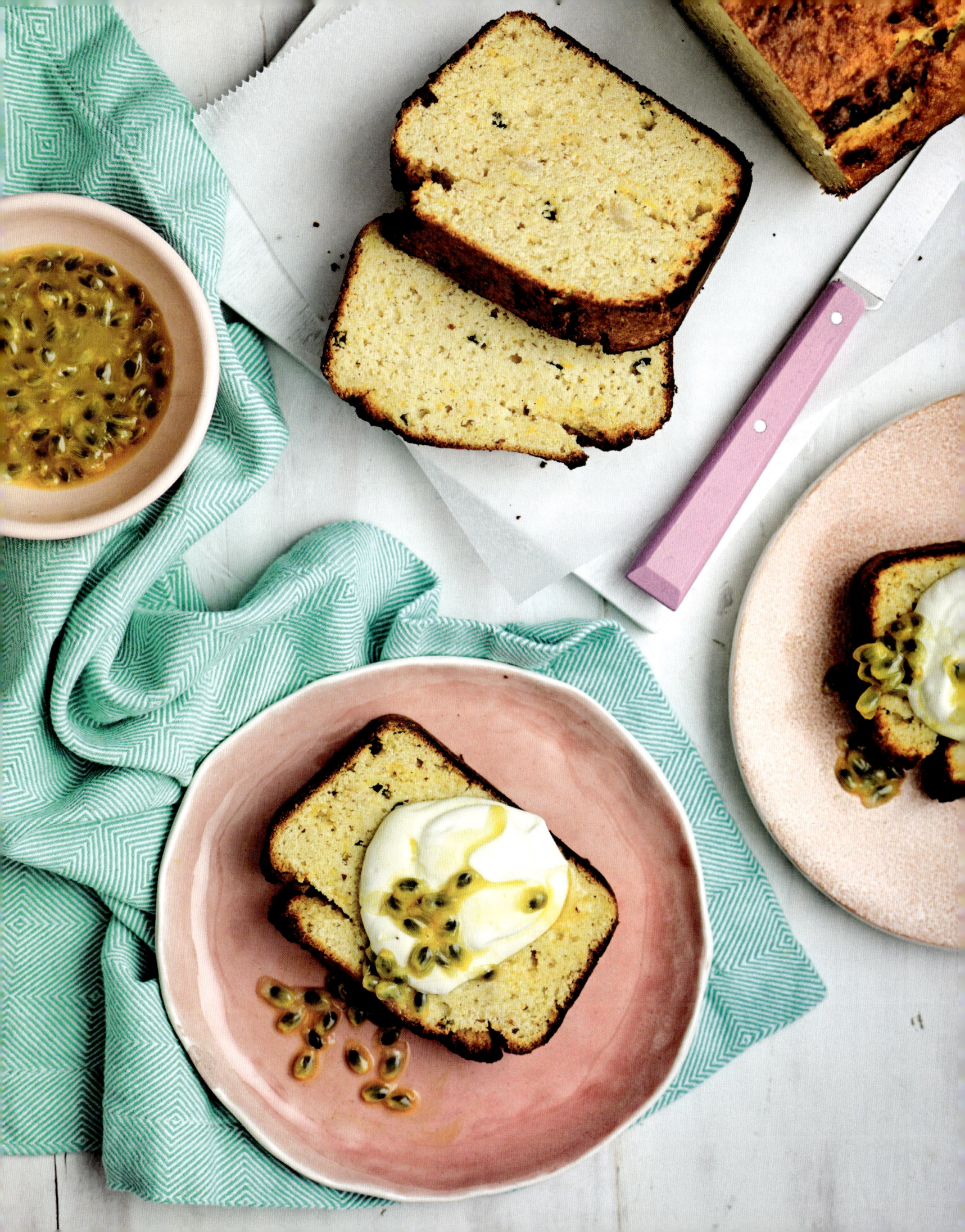

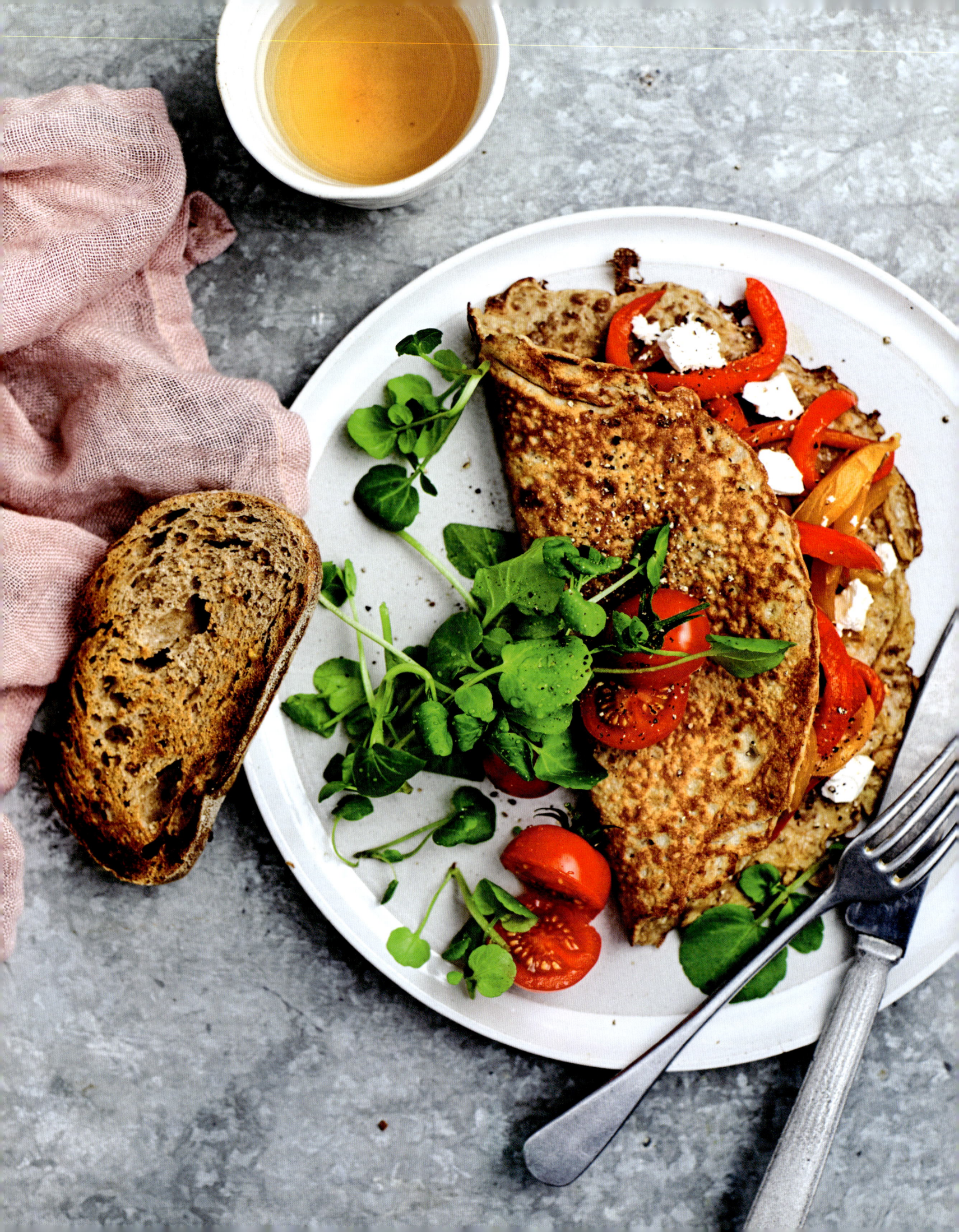

| ● 15.6g total fat (4.7g saturated fat) | ● 1376kJ (328 cal) | ● 21.9g carbohydrate | ● 21.5g protein | ● 6.5g fibre | ● 337mg sodium |
|---|---|---|---|---|---|

# LENTIL OMELETTES WITH
## braised capsicum & watercress

**PREP + COOK TIME** 40 MINUTES **SERVES** 4

1½ teaspoons coriander seeds (see tips)

1½ teaspoons cumin seeds

1 tablespoon extra virgin olive oil

1 medium red capsicum (bell pepper) (200g), seeded, sliced thinly

2 medium yellow capsicums (bell peppers) (400g), seeded, sliced thinly

1 fresh long green chilli, sliced thinly

1½ tablespoons red wine vinegar

6 eggs

400g (12½oz) can salt-reduced lentils, drained, rinsed

⅓ cup (80ml) milk

¼ teaspoon cracked black pepper

2 tablespoons soft fetta

200g (6½oz) cherry truss tomatoes, halved

60g (2oz) trimmed watercress

4 slices wholemeal sourdough bread (45g), toasted

**1** Heat a small heavy-based non-stick frying pan over medium heat, add seeds; cook, stirring, for 2 minutes or until fragrant. Crush seeds with a mortar and pestle; set aside. Wipe pan clean.

**2** Heat oil in a large heavy-based saucepan over low-medium heat. Cook capsicum, covered, stirring occasionally, for 15 minutes or until very soft and golden brown. Stir in chilli and vinegar; remove from heat.

**3** Meanwhile, place eggs, lentils, crushed seeds, milk and pepper in a large bowl. Pulse with a stick blender until almost smooth, with some coarsely crushed lentils still visible.

**4** Heat a small frying pan over medium heat. Add a quarter of the egg mixture; cook for 2 minutes, using a spatula to pull egg inwards from edge of the pan towards the centre to create folds, letting raw egg mixture fill any gaps. Sprinkle a quarter of the capsicum mixture and 2 teaspoons fetta over one half of the omelette. Cook for 1 minute; flip uncovered half over top to cover capsicum mixture. Slide carefully onto a plate. Repeat three times with remaining egg mixture, capsicum mixture and fetta to make three more omelettes.

**5** Top omelettes with tomatoes and watercress. Serve with toast.

**TIPS** Swap ground cumin and coriander for the seeds and omit step 1, if you like.
If you don't have a stick blender, use a blender or small food processor.

### DR JO SAYS
Tomatoes are rich in lycopene – a powerful antioxidant associated with a reduced risk of certain cancers and heart disease. You can absorb more lycopene by cooking your tomatoes in extra virgin olive oil, as is traditional in the Mediterranean.

| ● 14g total fat (5g saturated fat) | ● 1403kJ (335 cal) | ● 32g carbohydrate | ● 19g protein | ● 6g fibre | ● 191mg sodium |
|---|---|---|---|---|---|

# Baked berry
# GERMAN PANCAKE

**PREP + COOK TIME** 25 MINUTES **SERVES** 4

**6 eggs**
**1 cup (250ml) milk**
**1 teaspoon ground cinnamon**
**½ cup (80g) wholemeal plain (all-purpose) flour**
**1 tablespoon black chia seeds**
**¼ cup (60ml) pure maple syrup**
**125g (4oz) frozen mixed berries, thawed, patted dry**
**olive-oil spray**
**125g (4oz) strawberries, halved or quartered if large**
**½ cup (125ml) unsweetened vanilla-bean**
**Greek-style yoghurt**

**1** Preheat oven to 220°C/425°F.

**2** Blend eggs, milk, cinnamon, flour, chia seeds and
1 tablespoon of the maple syrup until smooth. Fold
through thawed berries.

**3** Lightly spray a large 25cm (10in) ovenproof frying pan
with oil. Pour batter into pan; bake, in oven, for 20 minutes
or until puffed and golden.

**4** Top pancake with strawberries and yoghurt; serve hot,
drizzled with remaining maple syrup.

**DO AHEAD** The pancake batter,
without the chia seeds and berries,
can be made the night before and
refrigerated; stir in chia seeds and
berries just before cooking.

**TIPS** For individual serves, divide
the batter evenly among four 1 cup
(250ml) ovenproof dishes, then
bake for 10 minutes or until puffed
and golden.
This recipe needs to be eaten hot
for best results.

**DR JO SAYS**
Snacks are not compulsory
and should not be used to
prevent low blood glucose.
This can result in weight gain
from overeating. If you
regularly experience hypos,
talk with your doctor or
diabetes educator.

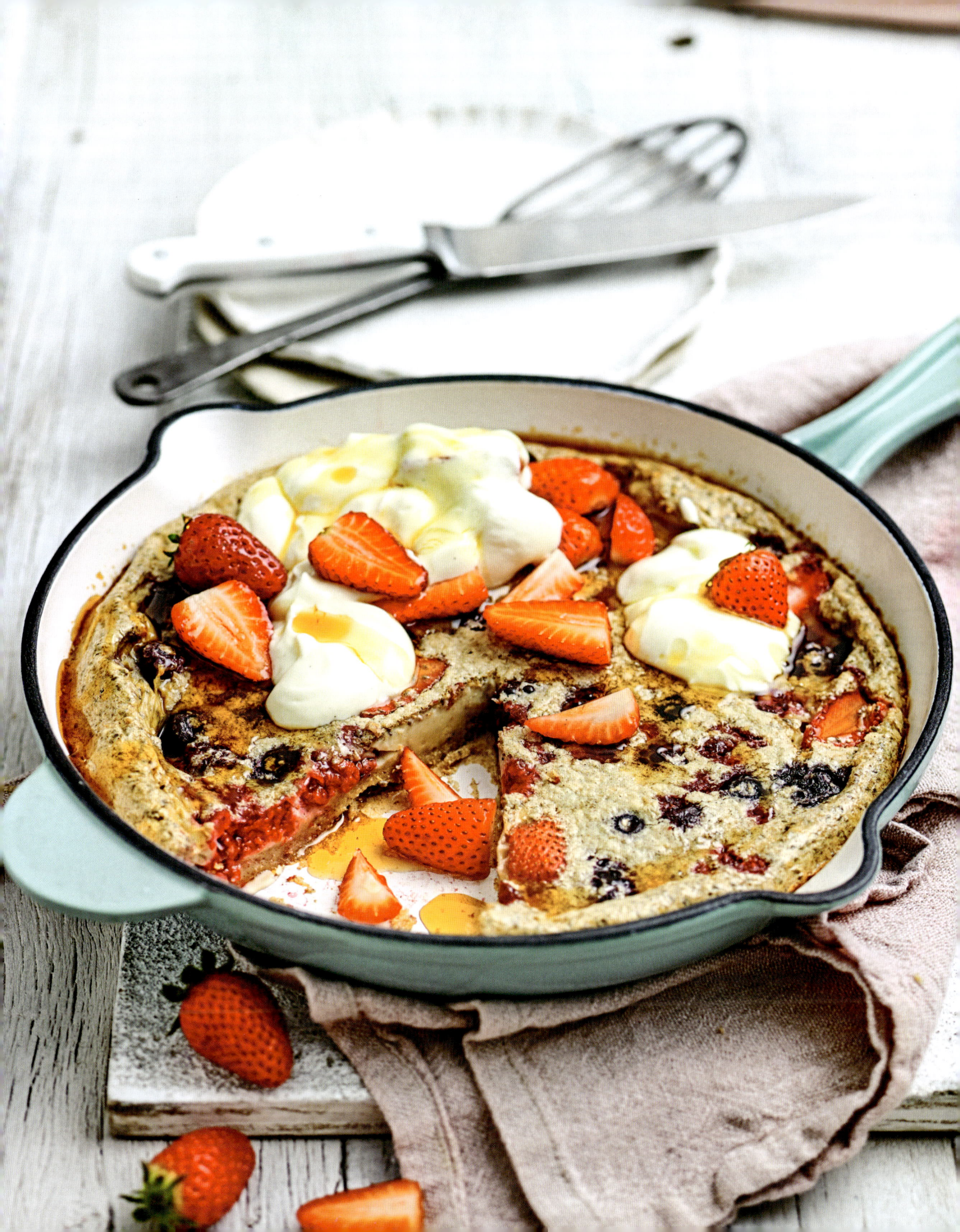

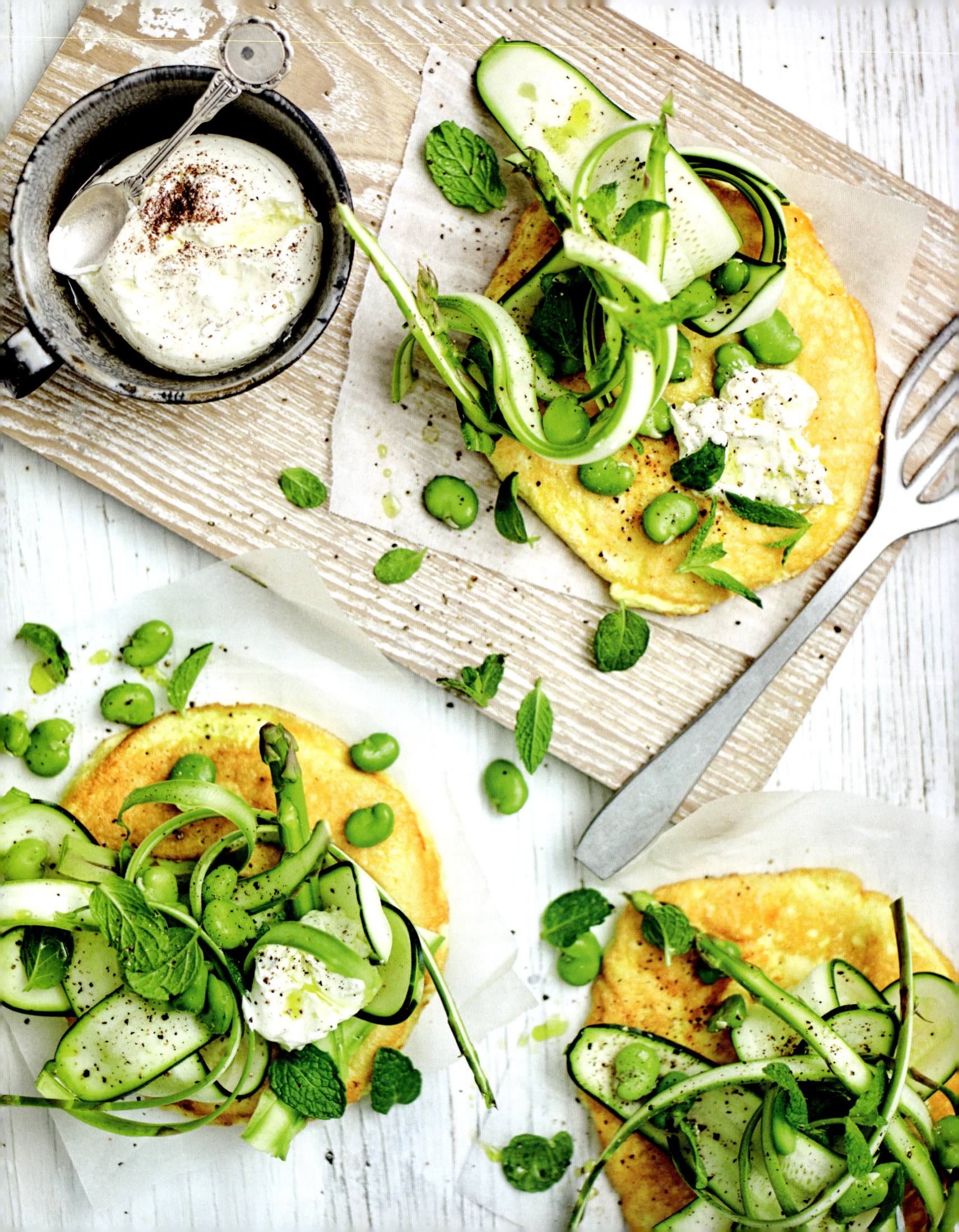

**NUTRITIONAL COUNT PER SERVING**

| | | | | | |
|---|---|---|---|---|---|
| ● 19.7g total fat (4.1g saturated fat) | ● 1123kJ (268 cal) | ● 3.1g carbohydrate | ● 18.6g protein | ● 4g fibre | ● 221mg sodium |

# Spring vegetable & mint
# SOUFFLÉ OMELETTES

**PREP + COOK TIME** 25 MINUTES **SERVES** 4

**8 eggs, separated (see tips)**
**olive-oil spray**
**2 small zucchini (180g), peeled into thin ribbons**
**1 bunch asparagus (170g), sliced thinly**
**1 cup (150g) frozen broad (fava) beans, blanched, peeled (see tips)**
**$\frac{1}{3}$ cup small fresh mint leaves**
**2 tablespoons extra virgin olive oil**
**1 tablespoon lemon juice**
**$\frac{1}{3}$ cup (95g) labne**

**1** Whisk egg whites in a large clean dry bowl with an electric mixer until stiff peaks form. Lightly whisk egg yolks in a medium bowl. Using a large metal spoon, gently fold egg yolk into egg white, taking care not to knock out too much air from the egg white.

**2** Lightly spray a 24cm (9½in) non-stick frying pan with oil; heat over medium heat. Add a quarter of the egg mixture, increase heat to medium-high; cook for 1 minute or until egg starts to set and come away from the edge of the pan. Turn carefully; cook for a further 1 minute. Transfer to a plate. Repeat with the remaining egg mixture to make three more omelettes.

**3** Place zucchini, asparagus, broad beans and mint in a medium bowl. Whisk oil and lemon juice together in a small bowl. Add to vegetables; toss gently to combine. Season to taste with pepper.

**4** Arrange vegetable mixture evenly on top of omelettes; top each with 1 tablespoon labne and serve immediately.

**DR JO SAYS**
Broad beans deliver plant protein, several nutrients, including folate, iron and magnesium, and are also a fantastic source of fibre, making them a terrific choice for those with diabetes.

**TIPS** Whisking the egg whites, then combining them with the egg yolks, aerates the mixture, creating a soufflé-like effect.
The recipe can be made even faster by simply beating the whole eggs together and cooking a quarter of the mixture at a time. While not giving the same soufflé effect, the resulting omelettes are just as tasty.

To blanch the beans, place them in boiling water for a couple of minutes, then refresh in cold water to stop the cooking process. This will loosen the tough beige-green inner shell, making it easier peel.

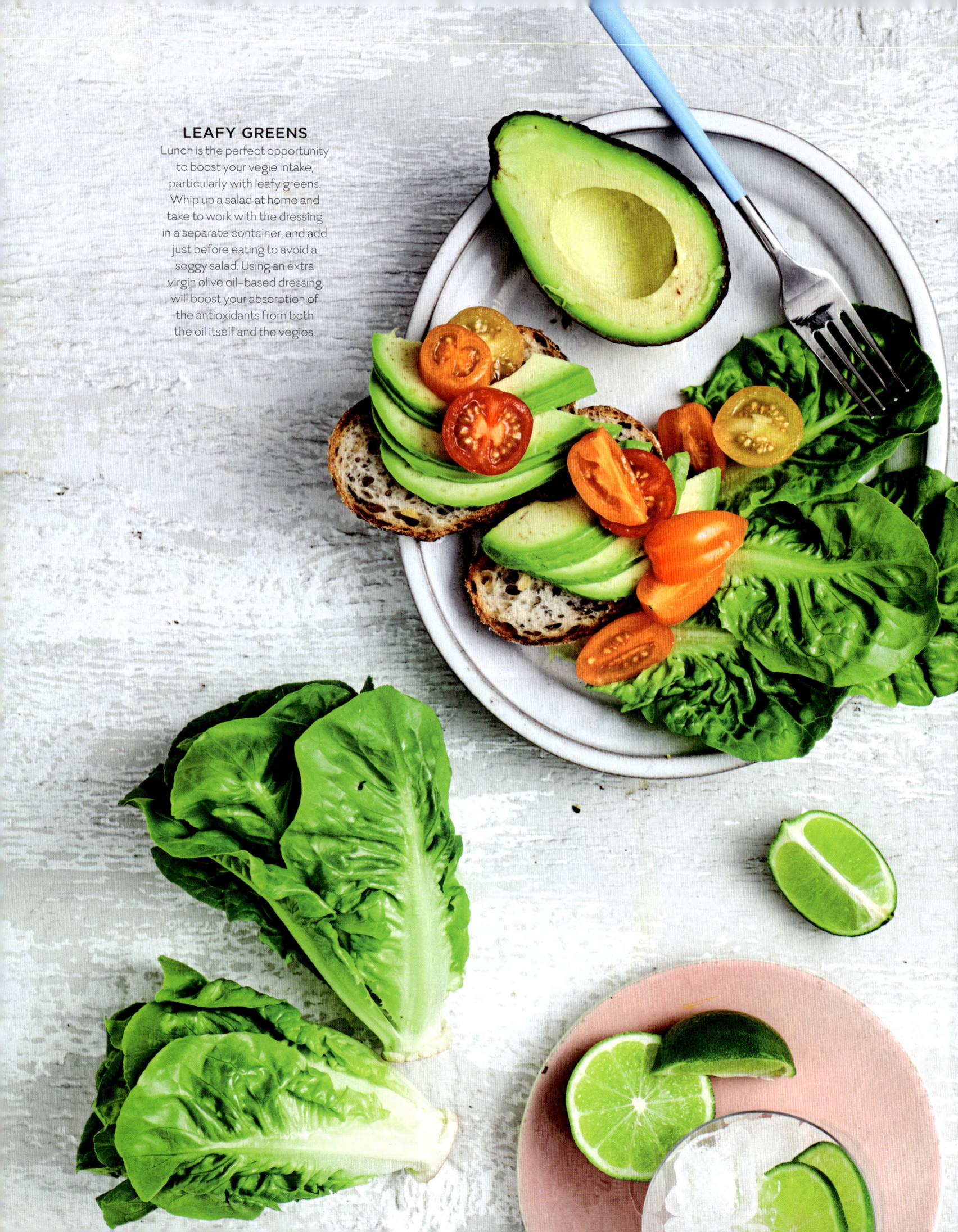

**LEAFY GREENS**
Lunch is the perfect opportunity to boost your vegie intake, particularly with leafy greens. Whip up a salad at home and take to work with the dressing in a separate container, and add just before eating to avoid a soggy salad. Using an extra virgin olive oil–based dressing will boost your absorption of the antioxidants from both the oil itself and the vegies.

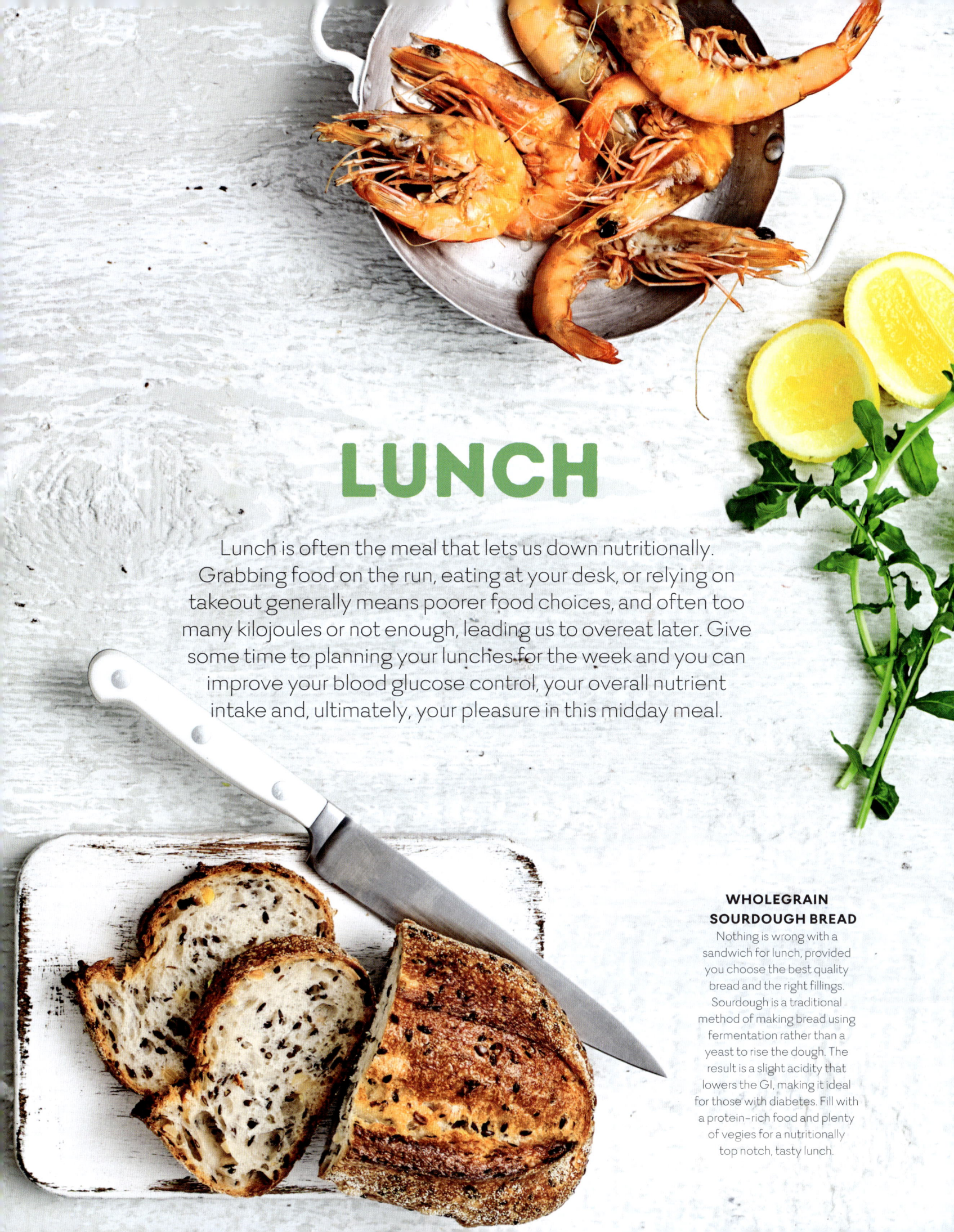

# LUNCH

Lunch is often the meal that lets us down nutritionally. Grabbing food on the run, eating at your desk, or relying on takeout generally means poorer food choices, and often too many kilojoules or not enough, leading us to overeat later. Give some time to planning your lunches for the week and you can improve your blood glucose control, your overall nutrient intake and, ultimately, your pleasure in this midday meal.

## WHOLEGRAIN SOURDOUGH BREAD

Nothing is wrong with a sandwich for lunch, provided you choose the best quality bread and the right fillings. Sourdough is a traditional method of making bread using fermentation rather than a yeast to rise the dough. The result is a slight acidity that lowers the GI, making it ideal for those with diabetes. Fill with a protein-rich food and plenty of vegies for a nutritionally top notch, tasty lunch.

| 13.6g total fat (3.2g saturated fat) | 1268kJ (303 cal) | 21.7g carbohydrate | 18.3g protein | 8.8g fibre | 655mg sodium |

# Mediterranean
# BEEF SALAD

**PREP + COOK TIME** 25 MINUTES **SERVES** 4

2 tablespoons extra virgin olive oil

1 clove garlic, crushed

1 large red onion (300g), cut into 8 wedges

1 medium eggplant (300g), cut into wedges

1 medium zucchini (120g), halved lengthways

1 medium red capsicum (bell pepper) (200g),
   quartered, seeds removed

400g (12½oz) can salt-reduced chickpeas
   (garbanzo beans), drained, rinsed

200g (6½oz) rare roast beef, torn coarsely (see tip)

100g (3oz) mixed salad leaves

3 medium roma (egg) tomatoes (225g),
   cut into 8 wedges

## OREGANO YOGHURT DRESSING

½ cup (140g) natural Greek-style yoghurt

¼ cup fresh oregano leaves, chopped finely

2 tablespoons lemon juice

1 teaspoon finely grated lemon rind

**1** Combine oil and garlic in a small bowl; brush onion, eggplant, zucchini and capsicum with garlic oil. Heat a grill plate (or grill pan or barbecue) over high heat; cook onion for 2 minutes each side and eggplant for 4 minutes each side or until grill marks appear; transfer to a tray. Cook zucchini and capsicum for 2 minutes each side or until grill marks appear; transfer to tray. Cut vegetables into chunks.

**2** Make oregano yoghurt dressing.

**3** Combine chickpeas, roast beef, salad leaves, tomato and chargrilled vegetables in a large bowl or platter; drizzle with oregano yoghurt dressing. Season with pepper.

**OREGANO YOGHURT DRESSING** Combine ingredients in a small bowl; season with pepper.

---

**TIP** Rare roast beef can be bought from a delicatessen or the deli counter at major supermarkets. You can also use leftover roast beef from the pot roast on page 175, if you have some.

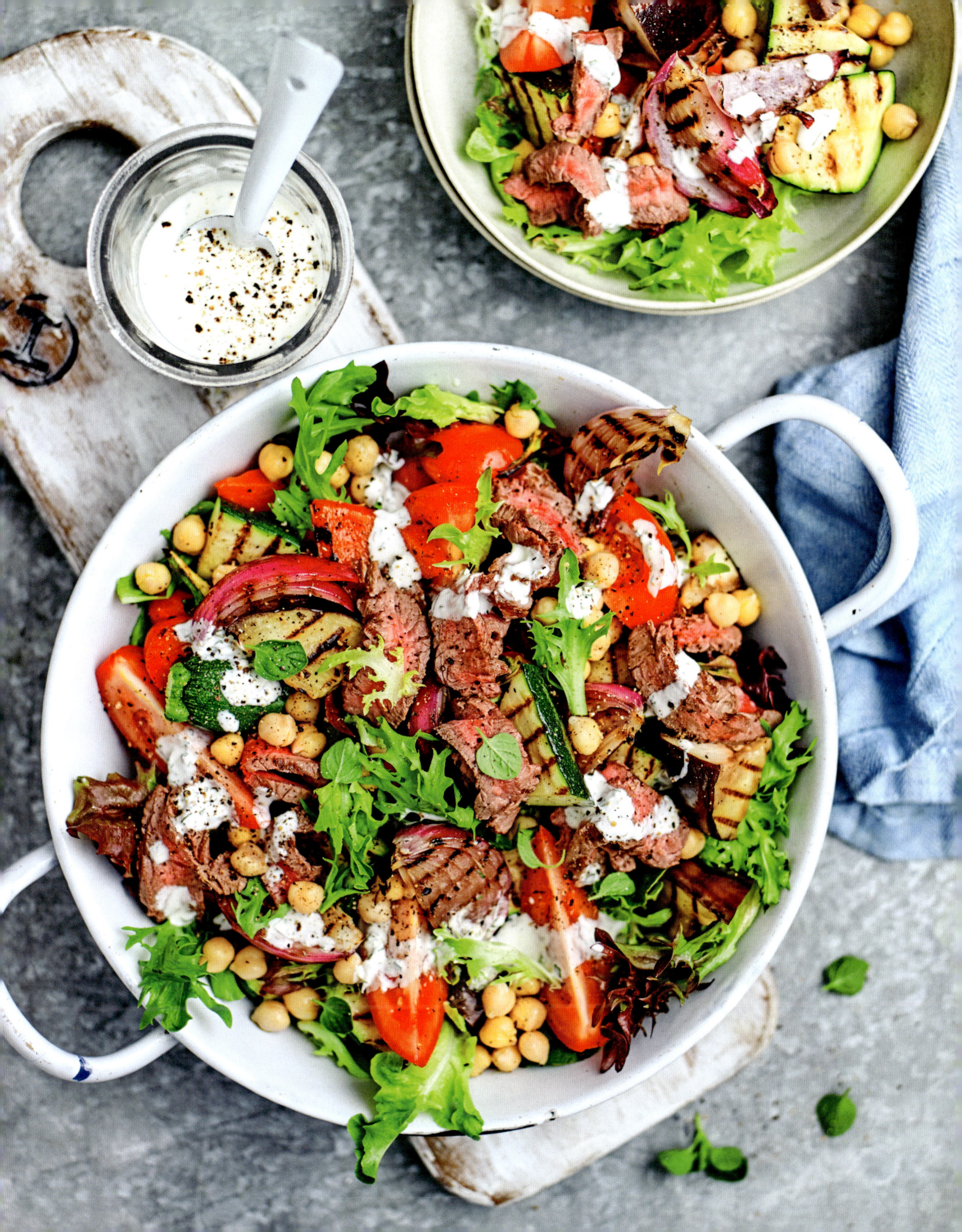

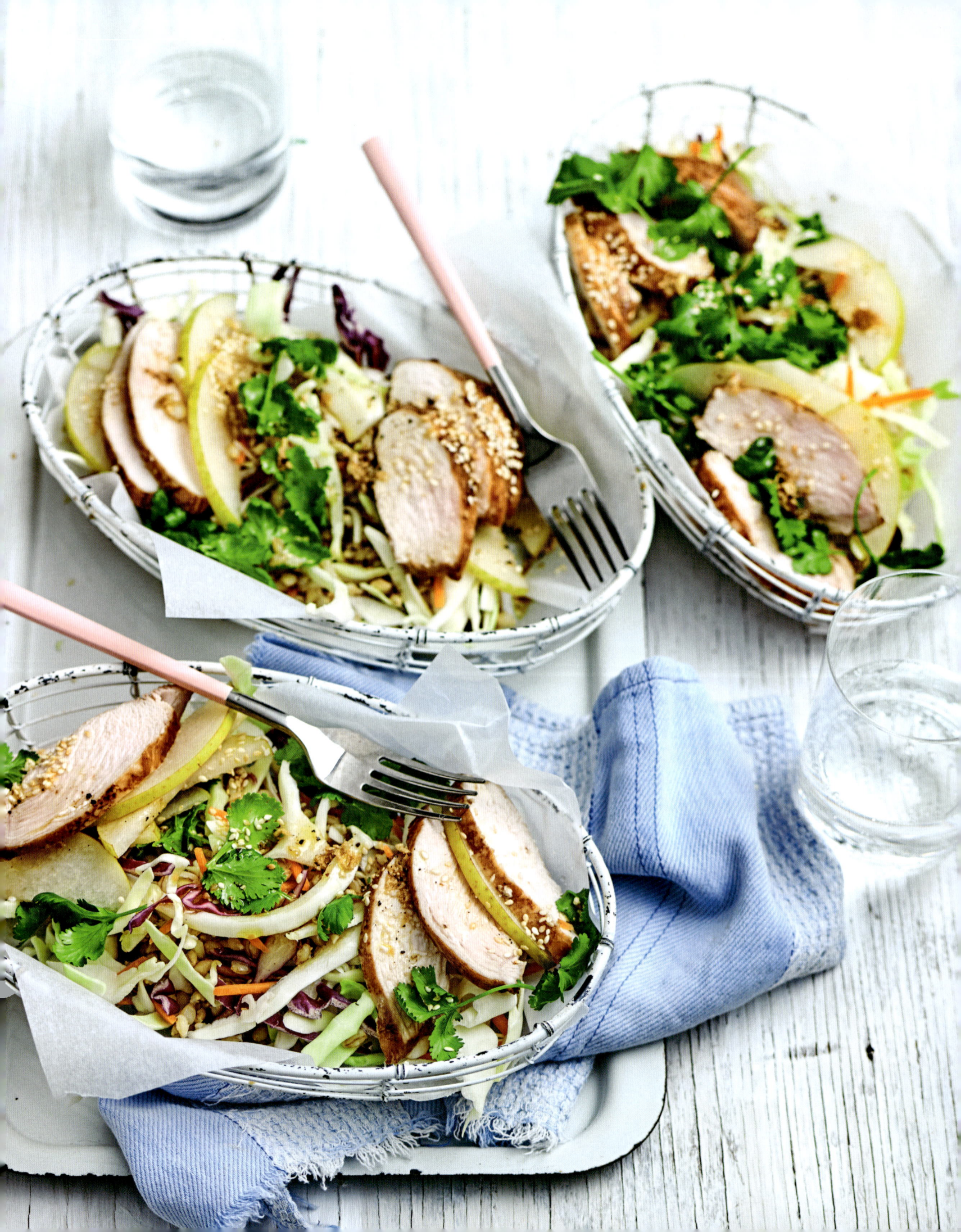

| | | | | | |
|---|---|---|---|---|---|
| ● 17.6g total fat (3.1g saturated fat) | ● 1812kJ (433 cal) | ● 31.1g carbohydrate | ● 33.8g protein | ● 6.8g fibre | ● 587mg sodium |

# Sesame chicken &
# BARLEY SALAD

**PREP + COOK TIME** 50 MINUTES **SERVES** 4

¾ cup (150g) pearl barley
2¼ cups (560ml) water
2 chicken breast fillets (400g)
2 teaspoons olive oil
2 teaspoons reduced-salt soy sauce
½ teaspoon sesame oil
1 medium (200g) nashi pear
250g (8oz) coleslaw salad mix
1 cup fresh coriander (cilantro) leaves
2 teaspoons sesame seeds, toasted

**SESAME DRESSING**
¼ cup (60ml) rice wine vinegar
2 tablespoons extra virgin olive oil
2 teaspoons reduced-salt soy sauce
½ teaspoon sesame oil
2 teaspoons finely grated fresh ginger
1 clove garlic, crushed

**1** Place barley and the water in a medium saucepan; bring to the boil. Reduce heat to low; cook, covered, for 35 minutes or until tender. Drain; transfer to a large bowl.

**2** Meanwhile, preheat oven to 240°C/475°F. Line an oven tray with baking paper.

**3** Place chicken, olive oil, soy sauce and sesame oil in a large bowl, season with pepper; toss to coat. Place chicken and marinade on the lined oven tray. Roast for 15 minutes or until cooked through. Cover loosely with foil; rest for 5 minutes, then slice thinly.

**4** Meanwhile, make sesame dressing.

**5** Thinly slice nashi pear. Add coleslaw mix, nashi pear, coriander, sesame dressing and any tray juices to barley; stir to mix. Top barley salad with chicken; sprinkle with sesame seeds to serve.

**SESAME DRESSING** Combine ingredients in a small bowl; season with pepper.

**DO AHEAD** This salad can be made a few hours ahead and refrigerated. Slice and add the nashi pear just before serving.

| ● 11g total fat (2.4g saturated fat) | ● 1197kJ (286 cal) | ● 8.7g carbohydrate | ● 34.1g protein | ● 7.1g fibre | ● 451mg sodium |
|---|---|---|---|---|---|

# Turkey
# SAN CHOY BAU

**PREP + COOK TIME** 25 MINUTES (+ STANDING) **SERVES** 4

1 cup (30g) dried shiitake mushrooms
½ cup (125ml) boiling water
2 tablespoons olive oil
1 medium onion (150g), sliced thinly
4cm (1½in) piece fresh ginger, peeled, grated finely
3 cloves garlic, crushed
500g (1lb) minced (ground) turkey
2 green onions (scallions), sliced thinly
2 tablespoons salt-reduced soy sauce
1 tablespoon lime juice
250g (8oz) bean sprouts
1 cup fresh coriander (cilantro) leaves
1 cup fresh dill tips
1 cup fresh mint leaves
1 cup fresh thai basil leaves
8 small iceberg lettuce leaves
2 medium carrots (240g), cut into matchsticks
   (see tips)
1 fresh long red chilli, sliced thinly
1 lime (65g), cut into wedges

**1** Place mushrooms and the boiling water in a medium bowl; stand for 15 minutes. Drain, discard stems; slice mushrooms thinly.

**2** Heat a large wok over medium heat. Add oil and onion; stir-fry for 2 minutes or until onion is softened but not coloured. Add mushroom, ginger and garlic; stir-fry for 1 minute. Remove onion mixture from wok.

**3** Add turkey mince to wok; stir-fry for 5 minutes, using a wooden spoon to break up any clumps, or until turkey is cooked through. Return onion mixture to wok with green onion, soy sauce and lime juice; stir-fry for 2 minutes or until well combined. Remove from heat; stir in bean sprouts.

**4** Combine herbs in a medium bowl.

**5** Divide turkey mixture among lettuce cups; top with carrot, herbs and chilli. Serve with lime wedges.

**TIPS** You can grate the carrot using a box grater, if preferred. If you don't have a wok, use a large frying pan instead.

This healthier take on the Chinese restaurant classic 'san choy bau' uses lean turkey mince as well as salt-reduced soy sauce.

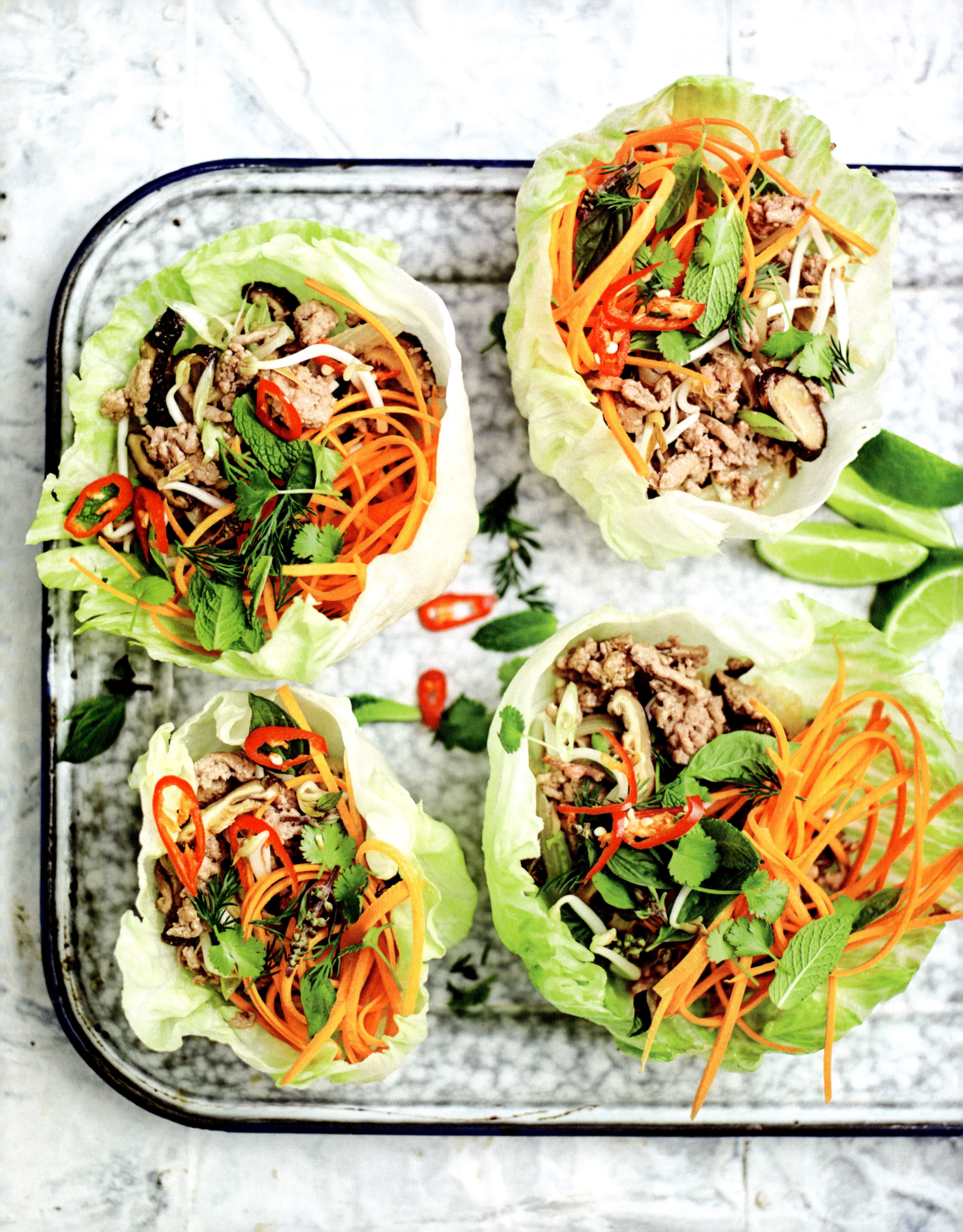

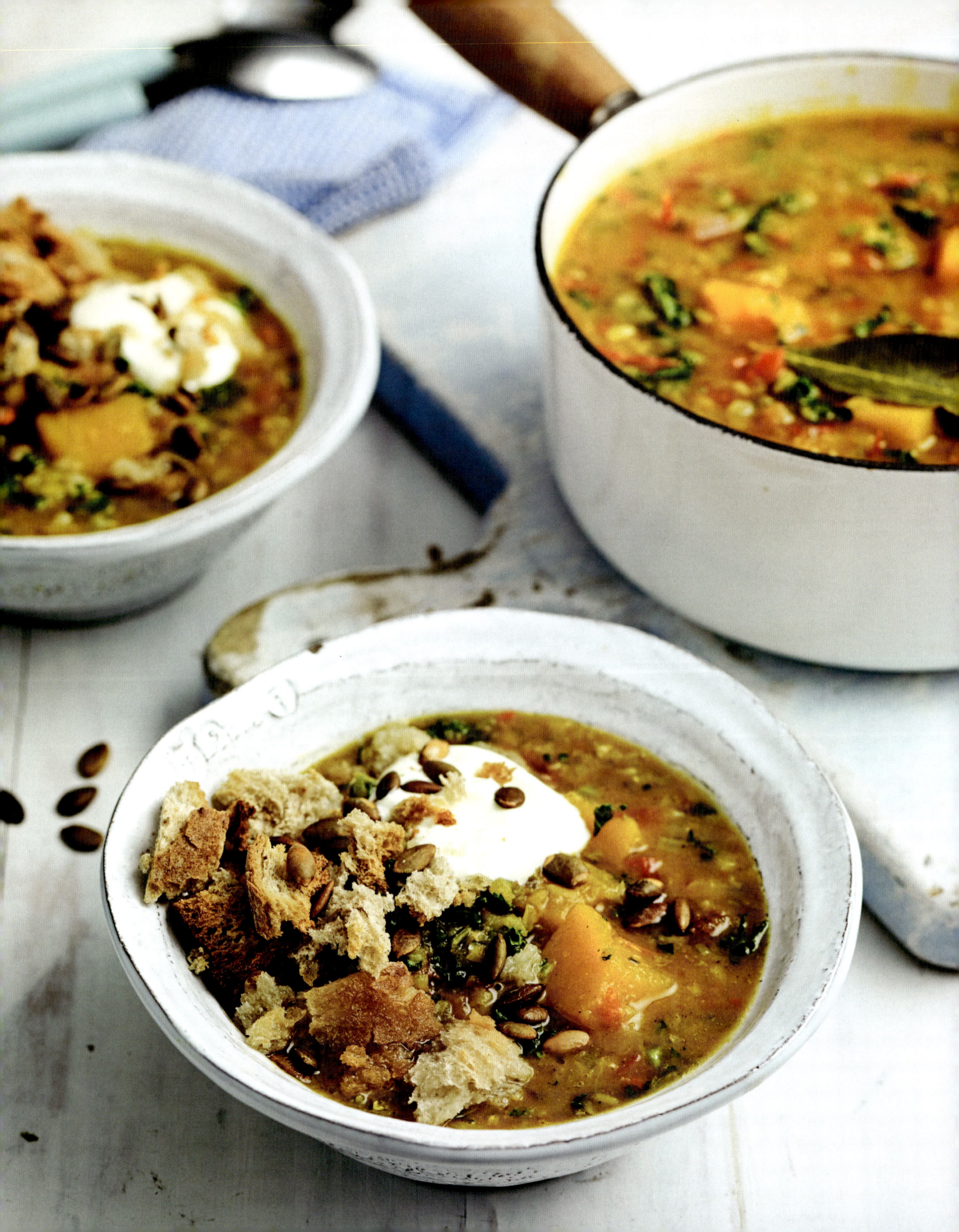

| | | | | | |
|---|---|---|---|---|---|
| ● 10.3g total fat (2.1g saturated fat) | ● 1484kJ (354 cal) | ● 42.3g carbohydrate | ● 18g protein | ● 8.6g fibre | ● 767mg sodium |

# CURRIED LENTIL SOUP
## with roast pumpkin seeds

**PREP + COOK TIME** 1 HOUR **SERVES** 4

½ bunch fresh coriander (cilantro)
1 tablespoon olive oil
1 medium onion (150g), chopped finely
2 cloves garlic, crushed
1 fresh long red chilli, seeded, chopped finely
4cm (1½in) piece fresh ginger, grated finely
2 teaspoons grated fresh turmeric (see tip)
1 teaspoon ground cumin
1 teaspoon garam masala
2 fresh bay leaves
1 cup (150g) red lentils
300g (9½oz) jap pumpkin, cut into 2cm (¾in) cubes
4 medium tomatoes (600g), seeded, diced finely
1 litre (4 cups) salt-reduced vegetable stock
2 cups (500ml) water
1½ cups shredded curly kale
80g (2½oz) light rye bread, torn
2 tablespoons pepitas (pumpkin seed kernels)
½ cup (140g) reduced-fat plain yoghurt

1  Separate coriander roots, stems and leaves. Wash and finely chop roots and stems (reserve leaves for another use).
2  Heat oil in a large heavy-based saucepan over medium heat. Add chopped coriander, onion, garlic, chilli and ginger; cook, stirring, for 4 minutes or until softened. Add turmeric, cumin, garam masala and bay leaves; cook, stirring, for 1 minute or until fragrant.
3  Add lentils, pumpkin, tomato, stock and the water to pan; bring to the boil over high heat. Reduce heat to low; cook, covered, for 25 minutes or until lentils and pumpkin are very tender. Remove lid; cook for a further 10 minutes or until thickened, adding kale for the last 2 minutes of cooking time to wilt.
4  Meanwhile; preheat oven to 180°C/350°F. Grease and line two large oven trays.
5  Tear bread coarsely into small pieces. Spread over one tray; spread pepitas over second tray. Bake, stirring once halfway through cooking time, for 10 minutes or until bread and pepitas are dry and crisp.
6  Divide soup into four bowls; top each with 1 tablespoon yoghurt. Sprinkle with roasted pepitas and rye croûtons to serve.

**DR JO SAYS**
Lentils are among the lowest GI foods measured, and they deliver a serious dose of mixed fibres that boost the growth of good gut bacteria, which assists with blood glucose control.

**TIP**  If fresh turmeric is not available, use 1 teaspoon ground turmeric instead. Fresh turmeric should be peeled before use, but needs to be handled with care, as it can stain anything – your skin, clothes, bench top and plastic cooking equipment and utensils.

| ● 3.7g total fat (1.3g saturated fat) | ● 1213kJ (289 cal) | ● 36.4g carbohydrate | ● 21.9g protein | ● 7.7g fibre | ● 794mg sodium |
|---|---|---|---|---|---|

# Pumpernickel with
# SMOKY TOMATO LIPTAUER

**PREP + COOK TIME** 30 MINUTES **SERVES** 4

300g (9½oz) pumpernickel bread
¾ cup (180g) reduced-fat soft ricotta
2 tablespoons semi-dried tomatoes (see tips),
    chopped coarsely
1 tablespoon chopped fresh chives
2 teaspoons lemon juice
¼ teaspoon smoked paprika
1 large tomato (220g), halved, sliced thinly
200g (6½oz) cooked peeled medium prawns (shrimp),
    sliced thinly lengthways (see tips)
6 small red radishes (90g), sliced thinly
40g (1½oz) baby rocket (arugula)
1 medium lemon (140g), cut into wedges

**1** Preheat oven to 200°C/400°F. Line an oven tray with baking paper.

**2** Place pumpernickel on the tray; bake, turning halfway through baking time, for 20 minutes or until crisp.

**3** Meanwhile, to make liptauer, blend or process ricotta, semi-dried tomato, chives, lemon juice and paprika until well combined. Season to taste with pepper.

**4** Spread liptauer on pumpernickel slices. Top with tomato, prawns, radish and rocket. Serve with lemon wedges.

**TIPS** We used the semi-dried tomatoes not packed in oil.
You will need to buy 440g (14oz) cooked unpeeled whole prawns to get the amount of peeled prawns needed for this recipe.

**DID YOU KNOW?** Liptauer is a spicy cheese spread made from soft cheeses, most often, but not always, using sheep-milk cheeses; it is popular in Hungary and other parts of Europe.
You can make the liptauer a day ahead. Cover and refrigerate until required. To save time, simply spread the liptauer on untoasted pumpernickel.

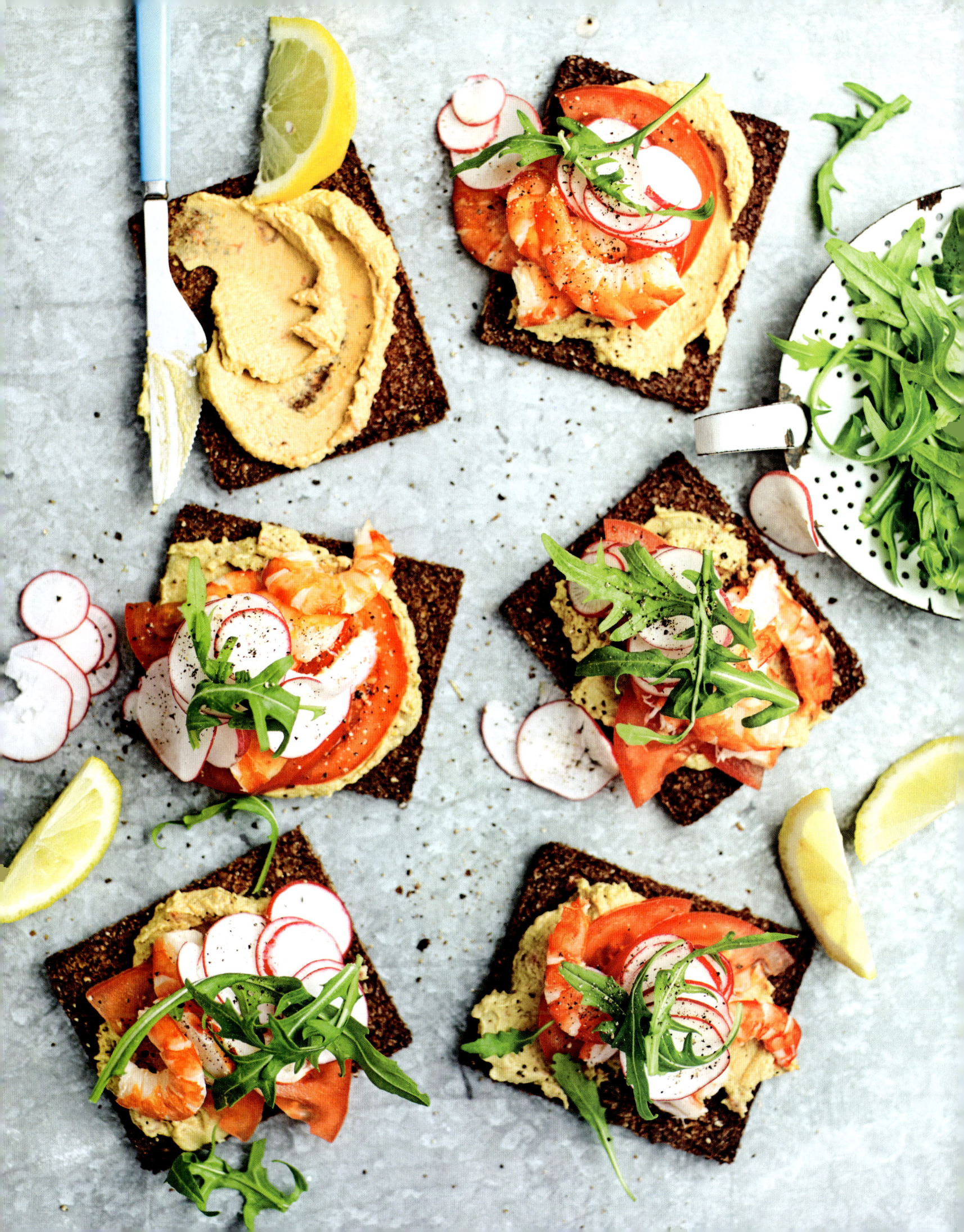

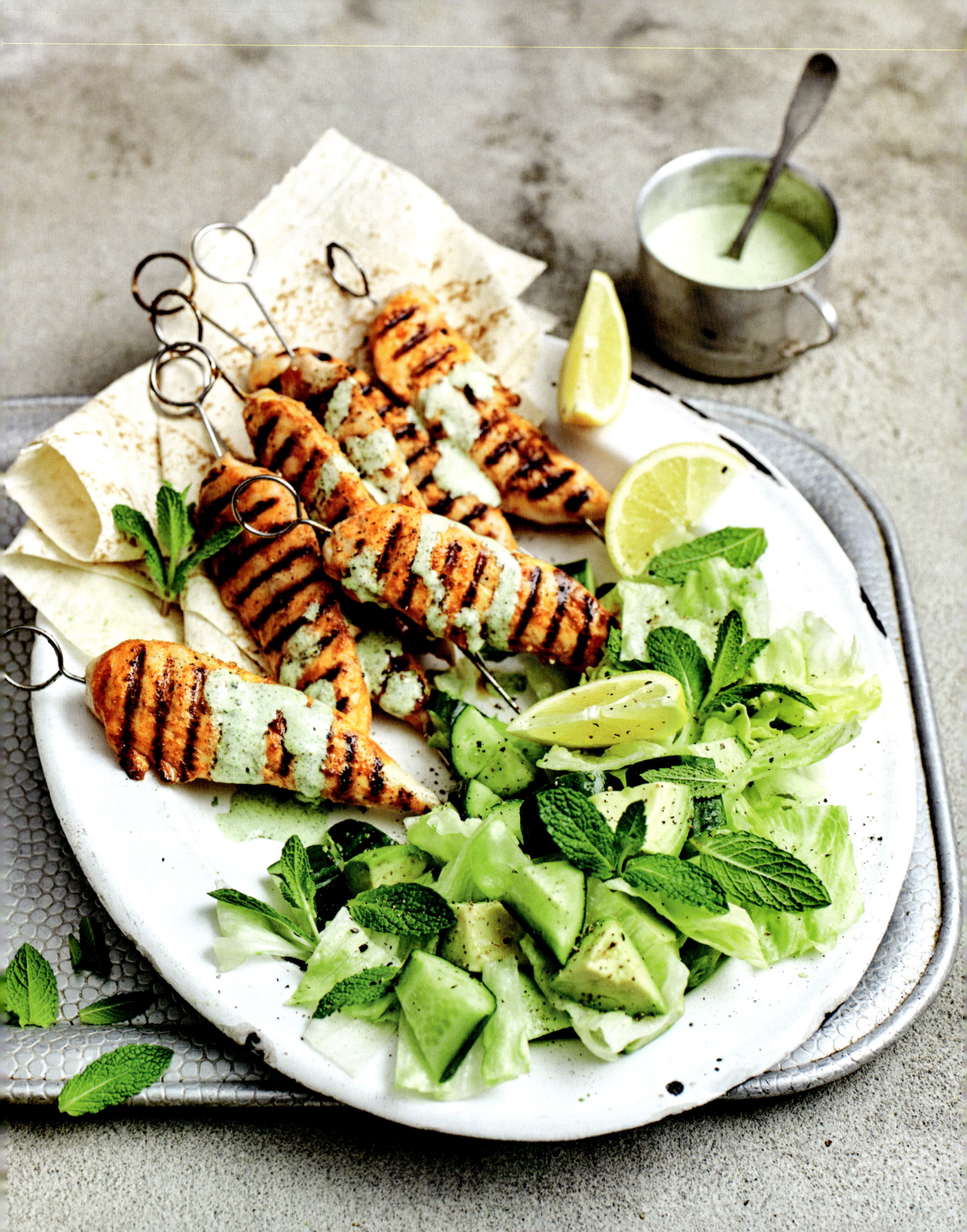

| ● 11.9g total fat (3.4g saturated fat) | ● 1552kJ (370 cal) | ● 27.3g carbohydrate | ● 34.6g protein | ● 5.4g fibre | ● 525mg sodium |
|---|---|---|---|---|---|

# Spicy chicken, lettuce
# & AVOCADO WRAPS

**PREP + COOK TIME** 20 MINUTES  **SERVES** 4

**500g (1lb) chicken tenderloins**
**¼ cup (60ml) sambal chilli sauce (see tips)**
**²/₃ cup (190g) natural Greek-style yoghurt**
**2 cups fresh mint leaves**
**½ large iceberg lettuce (350g), sliced roughly**
**2 lebanese cucumbers (260g), chopped coarsely**
**1 small avocado (200g), chopped coarsely**
**2 tablespoons lemon juice**
**4 slices mountain bread (100g)**
**1 medium lemon (140g), cut into wedges**

**1** Place chicken and sauce in a medium bowl; mix to coat chicken well. Thread skewers into chicken; place on a tray lined with plastic wrap.

**2** To make the yoghurt sauce, process yoghurt and 1 cup of the mint until smooth. Transfer to a bowl, cover; refrigerate until required.

**3** Heat a grill plate (or grill pan) over medium heat; line with baking paper. Cook chicken for 3 minutes each side or until cooked through. Transfer to a plate; cover loosely with foil to keep warm.

**4** Meanwhile, place lettuce, cucumber, avocado and remaining mint in a large bowl; toss gently with lemon juice.

**5** Divide chicken, salad and yoghurt sauce among bread wraps; serve with lemon wedges.

---

**TIPS** You need 8 skewers for this recipe. You can use either metal or bamboo skewers. We used sambal asli, a Malaysian-style chilli sauce, but your favourite chilli sauce would work just as well. The chicken can be marinated 1 day ahead; store, covered, in the fridge.

**DR JO SAYS**
Don't be scared of including good fats, such as avocado, nuts, seeds and extra virgin olive oil, in your daily diet. These foods are beneficial for blood glucose and insulin control, while helping you to control your appetite.

| • 7.9g total fat (1.5g saturated fat) | • 1517kJ (362 cal) | • 25.3g carbohydrate | • 36.2g protein | • 9.9g fibre | • 674mg sodium |
|---|---|---|---|---|---|

# *Miso chicken* NOODLE SOUP

**PREP + COOK TIME** 40 MINUTES (+ COOLING) **SERVES** 4

2 trimmed corn cobs (500g)

400g (12½oz) chicken breast fillets

½ cup (100g) frozen shelled edamame (soya beans), thawed

2 teaspoons sesame oil

450g (14½oz) kelp noodles

1 bunch baby buk choy (500g), shredded

½ cup fresh coriander (cilantro) leaves, chopped coarsely

4 green onions (scallions), sliced thinly

2 fresh long red chillies, sliced thinly

2 tablespoons reduced-salt soy sauce

⅓ cup (15g) dried seaweed (see tips)

4 dried shiitake mushrooms (15g), grated finely

⅓ cup (3g) dried bonito flakes

2 tablespoons finely grated fresh ginger

1 tablespoon dashi miso paste

2 teaspoons shichimi togarashi (see tips)

2 litres (8 cups) boiling water

**1** Bring a large saucepan of water to the boil; cook corn for 6 minutes or until tender. Transfer to a plate; cool.

**2** Meanwhile, return water to the boil; add chicken. Reduce heat to low; cook, covered, for 12 minutes or until chicken is cooked through. Using tongs, transfer chicken to a plate; leave to cool completely, then shred into bite-sized pieces.

**3** Blanch edamame in same pan of boiling water for 1 minute, drain; cool.

**4** Cut kernels from corn cobs; place in a bowl. Add oil, mix until kernels are separated.

**5** Rinse noodles in cold water to separate; divide among four large bowls. Top noodles with chicken, corn, edamame, buk choy, coriander, green onion and chilli.

**6** Add a quarter each of the soy sauce, seaweed, shiitake, bonito, ginger, miso and togarashi to each bowl.

**7** Just before serving, add 2 cups boiling water to each bowl, cover; set aside for 1 minute to heat through. Stir before serving.

**TIPS** Togarashi, also known as Japanese seven spice or simply seven-spice mix, is a Japanese blend of seven spices commonly used to flavour soups and noodles. If unavailable, substitute dried chilli flakes instead.
Dried seaweed is often sold as kelp, nori or yaki nori (toasted seaweed). These are the dark green wrappings around sushi rolls. Available in Asian food stores and larger supermarkets.

**FOR A PORTABLE OPTION**, this recipe can be prepared up to the end of step 6 the night before and refrigerated in four 1 litre (4 cup) glass jars with an airtight lid to take as a portable soup for lunch the next day. When ready to eat, add the boiling water to each jar, reseal and set aside for 1 minute to heat through. Stir before eating.

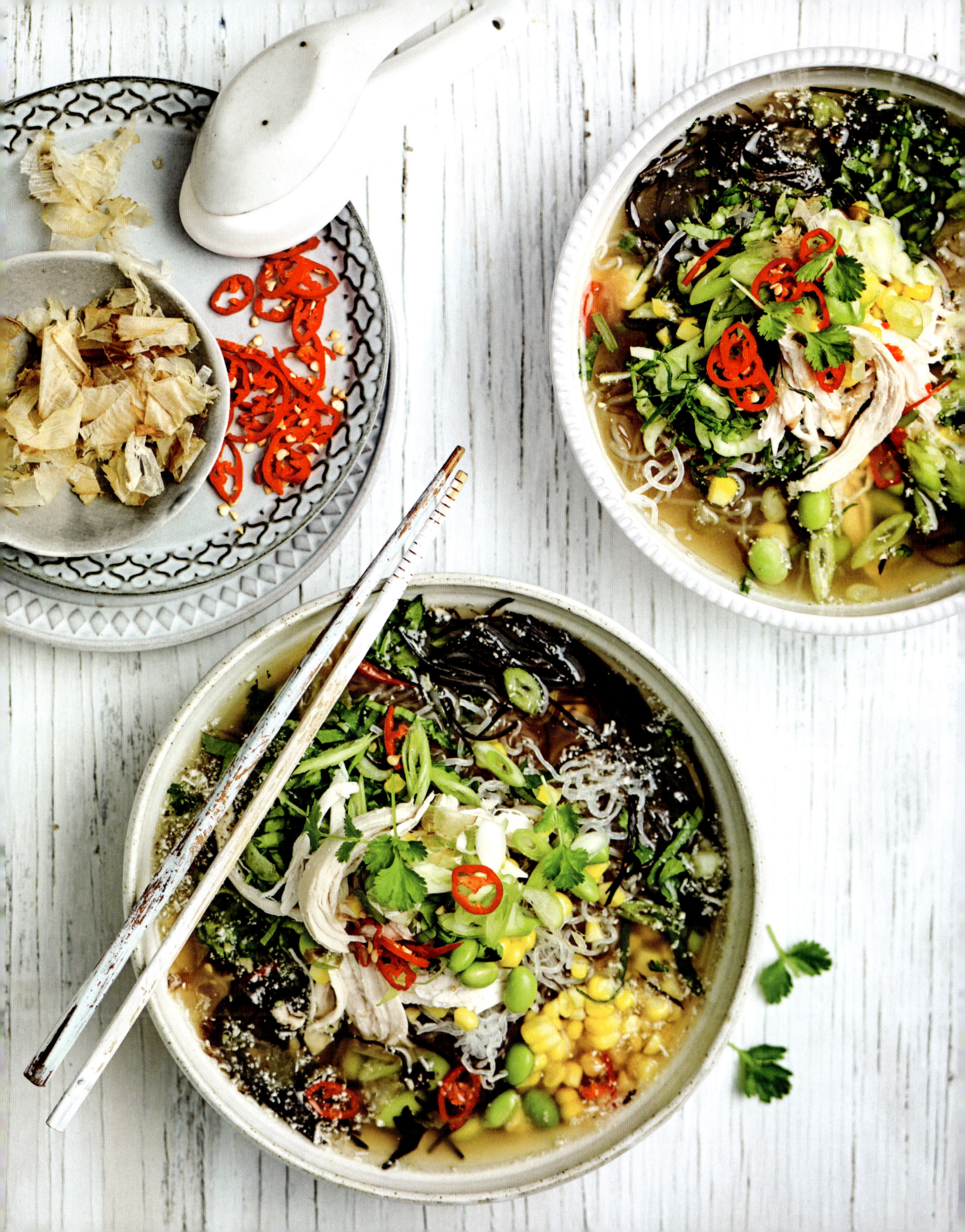

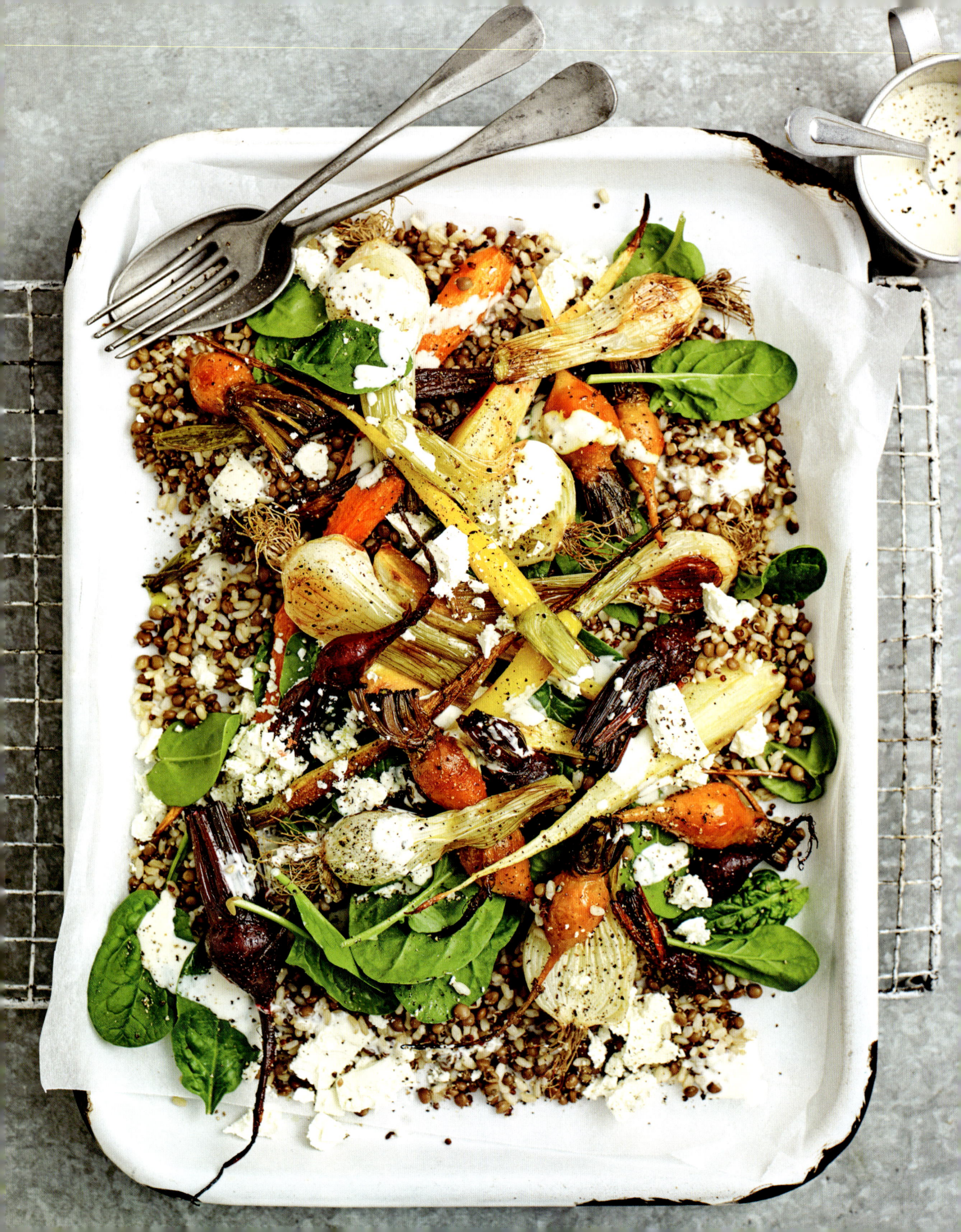

**NUTRITIONAL COUNT PER SERVING**

| 14.6g total fat (4.1g saturated fat) | 1708kJ (408 cal) | 44.3g carbohydrate | 17.2g protein | 9.6g fibre | 397mg sodium |
|---|---|---|---|---|---|

# ROASTED ROOT VEGETABLES
## & rice salad with spiced yoghurt

**PREP + COOK TIME** 1 HOUR **SERVES** 4

200g (6½oz) multi-coloured baby carrots, trimmed, peeled (see tip)
½ bunch baby golden beetroot (beets) (150g), trimmed (see tip)
½ bunch baby beetroot (beets) (250g), trimmed
1 small parsnip (120g), quartered lengthways
1 bunch spring onions (400g)
2 tablespoons extra virgin olive oil
250g (8oz) microwave brown rice and quinoa
400g (12½oz) can no-added-salt lentils, drained, rinsed
60g (2oz) baby spinach leaves
80g (2½oz) reduced-fat fetta, crumbled

**SPICED YOGHURT**
⅔ cup (190g) reduced-fat plain yoghurt
1 teaspoon finely grated lemon rind
2 tablespoons lemon juice
1 teaspoon moroccan seasoning

**1** Preheat oven to 200°C/400°F.

**2** Place vegetables and oil in a large roasting pan; toss to coat vegetables in oil. Roast, turning halfway through cooking time, for 45 minutes or until golden. When beetroot are cool enough to handle, peel, discarding skins.

**3** Meanwhile, cook rice and quinoa according to packet directions; when cool enough to open fully, tip rice into a medium bowl. Add lentils to rice; stir gently to combine.

**4** Make spiced yoghurt.

**5** Place rice mixture on a platter or divide among four plates or bowls; top with spinach, roasted vegetables and fetta. Spoon over spiced yoghurt to serve.

**SPICED YOGHURT** Combine ingredients in a small bowl.

**TIP** If multi-coloured (rainbow) baby carrots and golden beetroot are not available, use regular baby carrots and beetroot instead.

**DR JO SAYS**
Microwavable wholegrain rice sachets are terrific to keep in your panty for quick easy meals. In fact, the pre-cooking and reheating increases the level of resistant starch — a type of fibre that boosts the growth of good gut bacteria.

| ● 9.8g total fat (2.2g saturated fat) | ● 1905kJ (455 cal) | ● 45.7g carbohydrate | ● 36.1g protein | ● 7.6g fibre | ● 258mg sodium |

# TURKEY & RICE KOFTA
## with beetroot hummus

**PREP + COOK TIME** 30 MINUTES **SERVES** 4

250g (8oz) microwave brown rice

1 tablespoon ground cumin

2 teaspoons ground coriander

400g (12½oz) minced (ground) turkey

2 tablespoons finely chopped fresh coriander (cilantro)

2 teaspoons finely grated lemon rind

1 clove garlic, crushed

1 egg

2 wholegrain tortillas (80g), quartered

olive-oil spray

60g (2oz) baby rocket (arugula)

½ cup fresh coriander (cilantro) leaves

**BEETROOT HUMMUS**

400g (12½oz) can no-added-salt chickpeas
   (garbanzo beans), drained, rinsed

1 tablespoon tahini

50g (1½oz) cooked beetroot (beets)

½ cup (125ml) water

1 tablespoon lemon juice

1 small clove garlic, crushed

1 teaspoon ground cumin

**1** Make beetroot hummus.

**2** Cook rice according to packet directions. Place half in a large bowl; cool slightly. Refrigerate remaining rice in an airtight container for another use (see tips).

**3** Heat a small frying pan over medium heat; dry-fry cumin and coriander for 1 minute or until fragrant.

**4** Add turkey, spices, chopped coriander, lemon rind, garlic and egg to rice; stir until well combined. Divide turkey mixture into eight portions; mould each portion around a metal skewer into a log shape. Place on an oven tray lined with baking paper.

**5** Heat a grill plate (or grill pan or barbecue) over high heat. Lightly spray tortillas with oil; cook for 30 seconds each side or until grill marks appear. Transfer to a plate; cover with a clean tea towel to keep warm.

**6** Reduce heat to medium. Lightly spray koftas with oil; cook, turning occasionally, for 10 minutes or until golden and cooked through.

**7** Divide koftas, tortillas, rocket and coriander leaves among four plates. Serve with ¼ cup hummus per person.

**BEETROOT HUMMUS** Process ingredients until smooth. Season with black pepper. Transfer to a bowl, cover; refrigerate until required. (Makes 2 cups; see tips.)

**DR JO SAYS**

Cooking more of your own meals at home makes it much easier to eat healthily. You are in control of the quality and amounts of ingredients, plus you usually save money, too.

**TIPS** You only need 1 cup of the beetroot hummus for this recipe. If you serve with extra hummus, this will alter the nutrition counts. Store remaining hummus in an airtight container in the fridge for 3 days.

Leftover rice can be used to make the zucchini, spinach & sweet potato frittata slice on page 120, or the kale & brown rice nasi goreng on page 170.

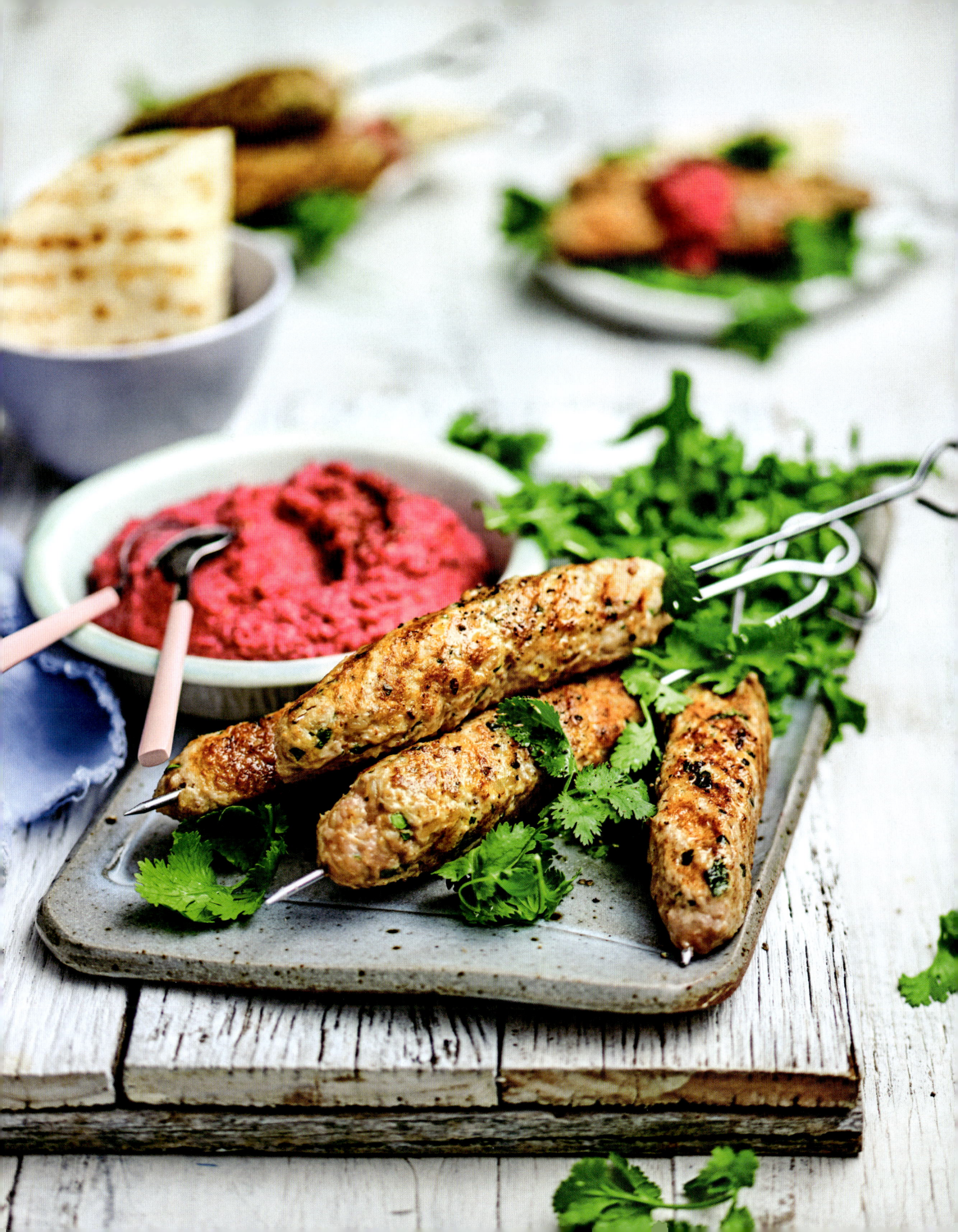

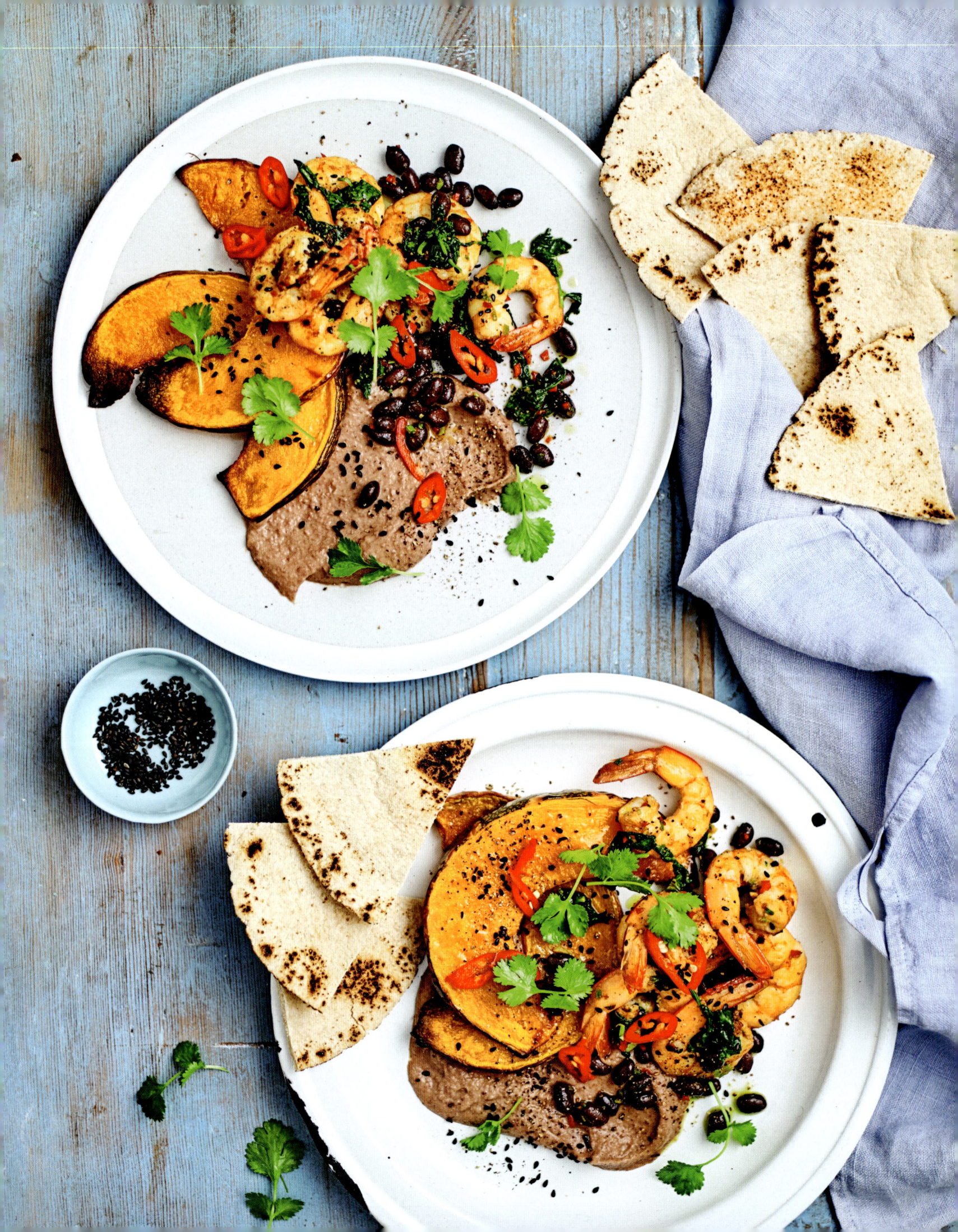

| ● 9.1g total fat (1.4g saturated fat) | ● 1644kJ (392 cal) | ● 36.3g carbohydrate | ● 32.6g protein | ● 13.6g fibre | ● 540mg sodium |

# PRAWNS, ROAST PUMPKIN
## & warm black bean hummus

**PREP + COOK TIME** 50 MINUTES **SERVES** 4

500g (1lb) jap pumpkin, unpeeled, seeded,
  cut into thin wedges
400g (12½oz) can black beans, drained, rinsed
2 cloves garlic, crushed
1½ tablespoons lemon juice
1 teaspoon tahini
2 tablespoons water
2 fresh long red chillies
800g (1½lb) uncooked king prawns (shrimp), shelled,
  deveined, with tails intact
1 bunch fresh coriander (cilantro), leaves picked,
  roots and stems washed, chopped finely
2 teaspoons finely grated lemon rind
1 tablespoon extra virgin olive oil
1 tablespoon black sesame seeds, toasted
150g (4½oz) wholemeal pitta bread, warmed,
  cut into wedges

**1** Preheat oven to 180°C/350°F. Line a large oven tray with baking paper.

**2** Place pumpkin on oven tray, season with pepper; roast for 35 minutes or until golden and tender.

**3** Meanwhile, to make the black bean hummus, process half the beans, 1 clove garlic, 1 tablespoon lemon juice and all the tahini and the water until smooth. Transfer mixture to a small saucepan.

**4** Seed and finely chop one chilli; thinly slice remaining chilli. Place prawns, chopped coriander roots and stems and a third of the leaves, lemon rind, chopped chilli and remaining garlic in a large bowl; stand for 5 minutes.

**5** Heat oil in a large non-stick frying pan over high heat. Add prawns; cook for 2 minutes or until golden and cooked through. Remove pan from heat, immediately add remaining beans, another third of the coriander leaves, sliced chilli and remaining lemon juice; stir to combine.

**6** Heat hummus over medium heat for 2 minutes or until warmed through. Spread hummus on a platter; top with pumpkin and prawn mixture. Sprinkle with sesame seeds and remaining coriander leaves; serve with warmed pitta.

**TIP** Swap lime juice and rind for lemon, if you like.

**DR JO SAYS**
Black beans are low GI, high in protein and fibre, and one of the best plant sources of iron. The wonderful colour comes from the presence of flavonoids, known to be important for good health.

| 18.4g total fat (2.6g saturated fat) | 1912kJ (456 cal) | 34.4g carbohydrate | 30.6g protein | 11.8g fibre | 664mg sodium |
|---|---|---|---|---|---|

# CHICKEN TACOS
## with avocado salsa

**PREP + COOK TIME** 35 MINUTES **SERVES** 4

2 trimmed corn cobs (500g)

olive-oil spray

4 wholegrain tortillas (160g)

500g (1lb) chicken tenderloins

3 teaspoons mexican chilli powder

1 medium red capsicum (bell pepper) (200g),
chopped finely

½ medium avocado (125g), diced

4 green onions (scallions), chopped finely

2 tablespoons lime juice

¼ cup coarsely chopped fresh coriander
(cilantro) leaves

1 tablespoon sweet chilli sauce

¼ cup (60g) light sour cream

1 lime (65g), cut into wedges

**1** Spray corn with oil; cook on a heated grill plate (or barbecue) over high heat, turning occasionally, for 10 minutes or until charred and tender. Cool.

**2** Place tortillas on heated oiled grill plate (or barbecue) for 30 seconds each side or until golden and grill marks appear. Transfer to a plate; cover with a clean tea towel to prevent drying out.

**3** Coat chicken evenly with chilli powder; grill for 4 minutes each side or until cooked through. Cover loosely with foil; rest for 10 minutes, then slice diagonally in half.

**4** When corn is cool enough to handle, cut kernels from cobs, in sections if possible.

**5** To make salsa, place capsicum, avocado, onion, lime juice, 2 tablespoons of the coriander and half the sweet chilli sauce in a bowl; stir gently to combine. Combine remaining chilli sauce and sour cream in a small bowl.

**6** Fill tacos evenly with salsa and chicken; top with corn, sour cream mixture and remaining coriander. Serve with lime wedges.

**DR JO SAYS**

Watch your portion size, particularly when eating out, to help you control your weight and blood glucose levels. Eating slowly and putting your cutlery down between mouthfuls can help you identify when you are satisfied and prevent overeating.

**TIPS** The chicken, avocado salsa and the sour cream mixture can be prepared up to a day ahead and stored, separately, in the fridge. Warm tortillas just before serving.

If you're not a fan of spicy food, simply reduce the amount of mexican chilli powder.

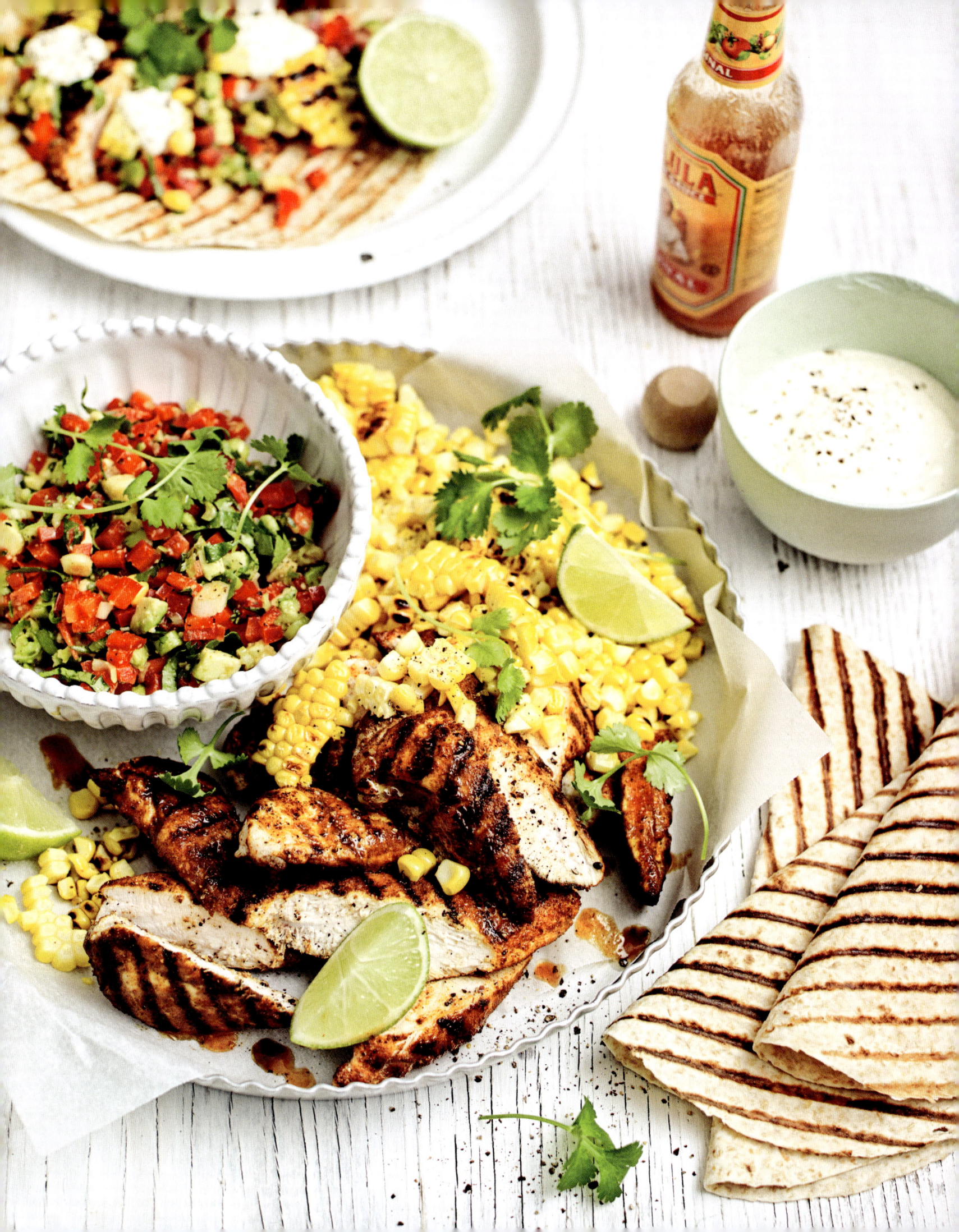

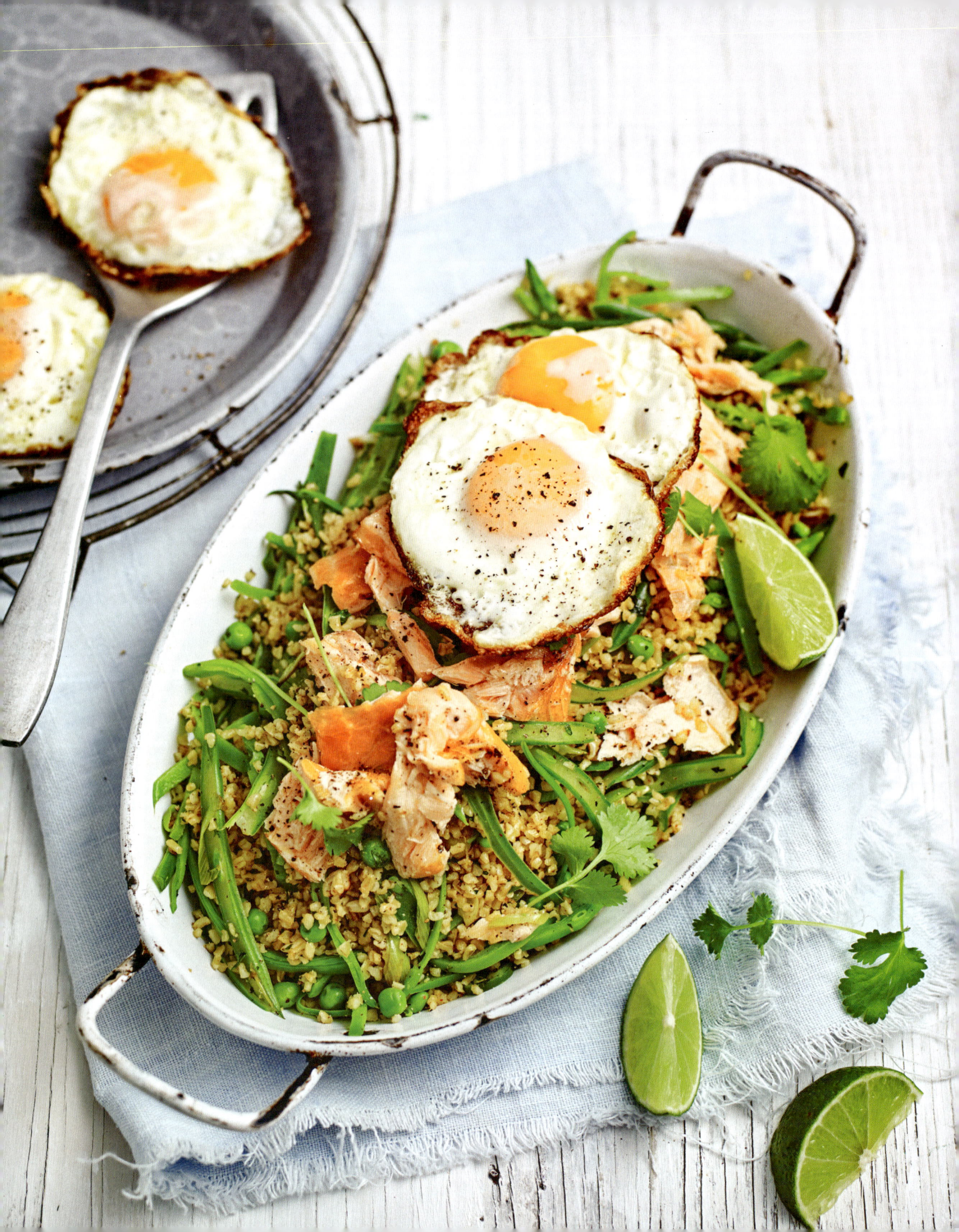

● 14g total fat (3.4g saturated fat) | ● 1935kJ (462 cal) | ● 47.1g carbohydrate | ● 34.2g protein | ● 5g fibre | ● 588mg sodium

# Salmon freekeh
# 'NASI GORENG'

**PREP + COOK TIME** 40 MINUTES **SERVES** 4

1¼ cups (250g) freekeh
3 cups (750ml) water
4 spring onions (100g), sliced thinly, green ends and
   roots reserved
olive-oil spray
200g (6½oz) green beans, sliced thinly lengthways
100g (3oz) snow peas, sliced thinly
¾ cup (90g) frozen peas
½ teaspoon smoked paprika
¼ teaspoon cracked black pepper
1 fresh long green chilli, sliced thinly
1 teaspoon reduced-salt soy sauce
⅓ cup fresh coriander (cilantro) leaves,
   chopped finely, plus extra leaves to serve
150g (4½oz) hot-smoked salmon, flaked
2 tablespoons water, extra
4 eggs
1 lime (65g), cut into wedges

**1** Place freekeh, the water and reserved green ends and roots of the spring onions in a medium saucepan; bring to a simmer. Cook freekeh following packet directions. Drain; set aside until needed. Discard spring onion roots and ends.
**2** Heat a large non-stick frying pan over medium heat; spray lightly with oil. Add spring onion, beans, snow peas and peas; cook for 2 minutes or until vegetables start to soften. Add freekeh, paprika, pepper, chilli, soy, chopped coriander and half of the salmon; stir gently to combine. Increase heat to high; cook for 2 minutes or until heated through. Stir in the extra water. Divide among four bowls.
**3** Wipe frying pan clean and return to medium heat; spray lightly with oil. Fry eggs until cooked to your liking.
**4** Top freekeh mixture evenly with remaining salmon; sprinkle with extra coriander, and top each bowl with an egg. Serve with lime wedges.

This is our twist on the traditional Indonesian fried rice recipe, in which we replace rice with freekeh.

**FREEKEH** is young (green) wheat that has been dried and roasted. It has a low GI, and is high in fibre and protein. It's available from Middle-Eastern food stores, and some major supermarkets, health food stores and greengrocers.

| ● 11.4g total fat (2.2g saturated fat) | ● 1098kJ (262 cal) | ● 20.3g carbohydrate | ● 15.7g protein | ● 7.6g fibre | ● 569mg sodium |

# Japanese-style vegie
# FRITTERS

**PREP + COOK TIME** 50 MINUTES **SERVES** 4

200g (6½oz) green cabbage, sliced thinly (see tips)
150g (4½oz) snow peas, sliced thinly
1 medium red capsicum (bell pepper) (200g),
   seeds removed, sliced thinly
4 green onions (scallions), sliced thinly
1½ cups fresh coriander (cilantro) leaves, plus
   2 tablespoons finely chopped stems
½ cup (75g) wholemeal spelt flour
4 eggs, whisked lightly
olive-oil spray
125g (4oz) snow pea sprouts, trimmed
2 teaspoons pickled pink ginger
1 tablespoon sesame seeds, toasted

**MISO DRESSING**
1 small carrot (70g), chopped coarsely
¼ cup (60ml) water
2 tablespoons white (shiro) miso
¼ cup (60ml) lime juice
2 teaspoons pickled pink ginger
1 teaspoon sesame oil

**1** Make miso dressing.

**2** Combine cabbage, snow peas, capsicum, half the green onion and the chopped coriander stems in a large bowl. Finely chop ¼ cup coriander leaves; add to bowl.

**3** Sprinkle flour over vegetables; toss to mix well. Stir in egg to coat the vegetables evenly.

**4** Spray a small heavy-based frying pan with oil; heat over medium heat. Add a quarter of the vegetable batter; cook for 4 minutes or until golden. Turn, cook for a further 5 minutes or until golden. Repeat with remaining mixture, lightly spraying pan with oil as needed, to make a total of four fritters.

**5** Top each fritter with a quarter each of the sprouts, pickled ginger and remaining coriander and green onion; drizzle with miso dressing. Sprinkle with sesame seeds to serve.

**MISO DRESSING** Blend or process ingredients until smooth.

**TIPS** You need 4 cups shredded cabbage for this recipe.
To make one large fritter, use an oiled 30cm (12in) non-stick frying pan. Cook for 5 minutes on each side or until golden brown and crisp.

These cabbage-based pancakes are a huge favourite in Japan, where they are known as okonomiyaki, which is basically translated as 'fried stuff you like'.

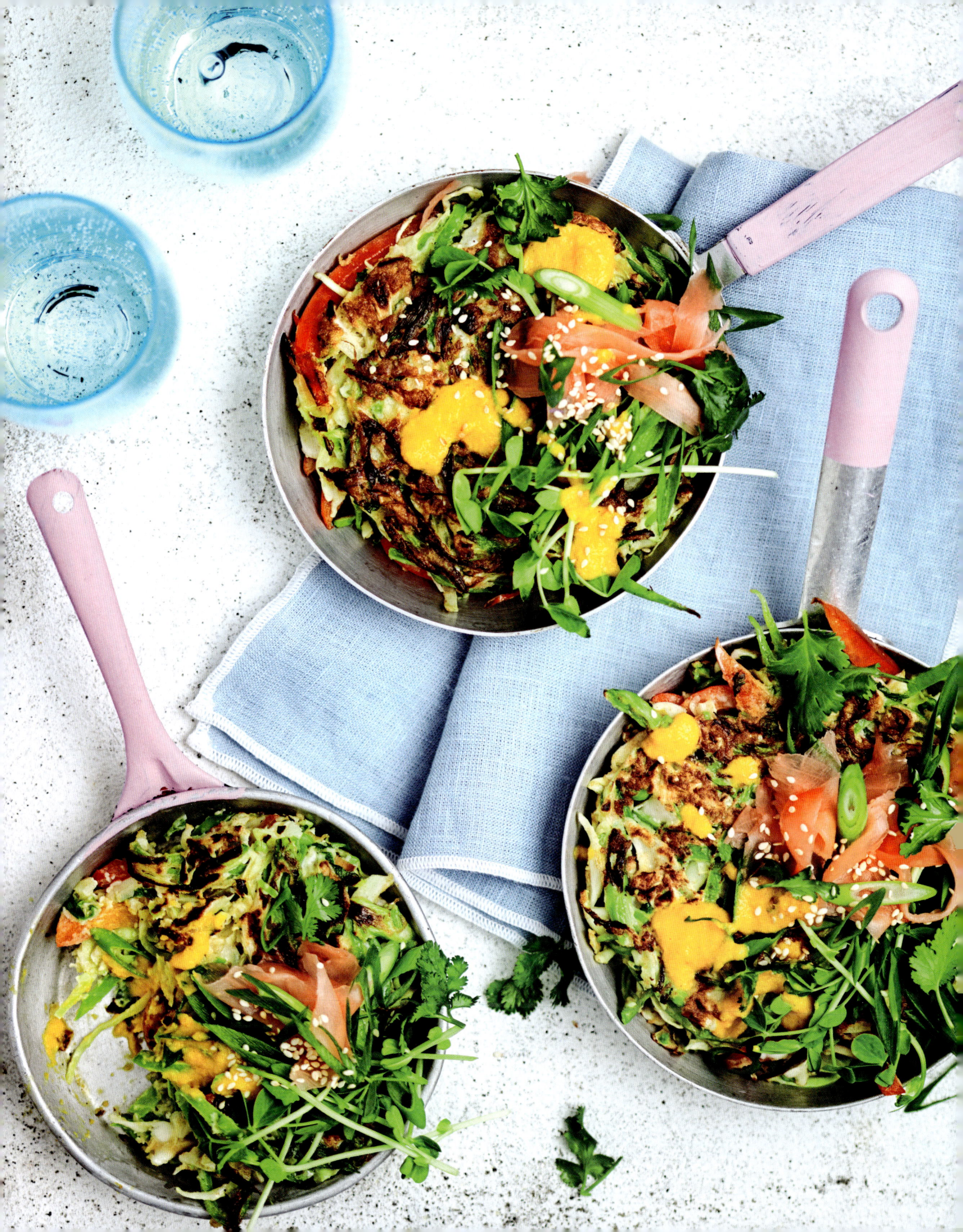

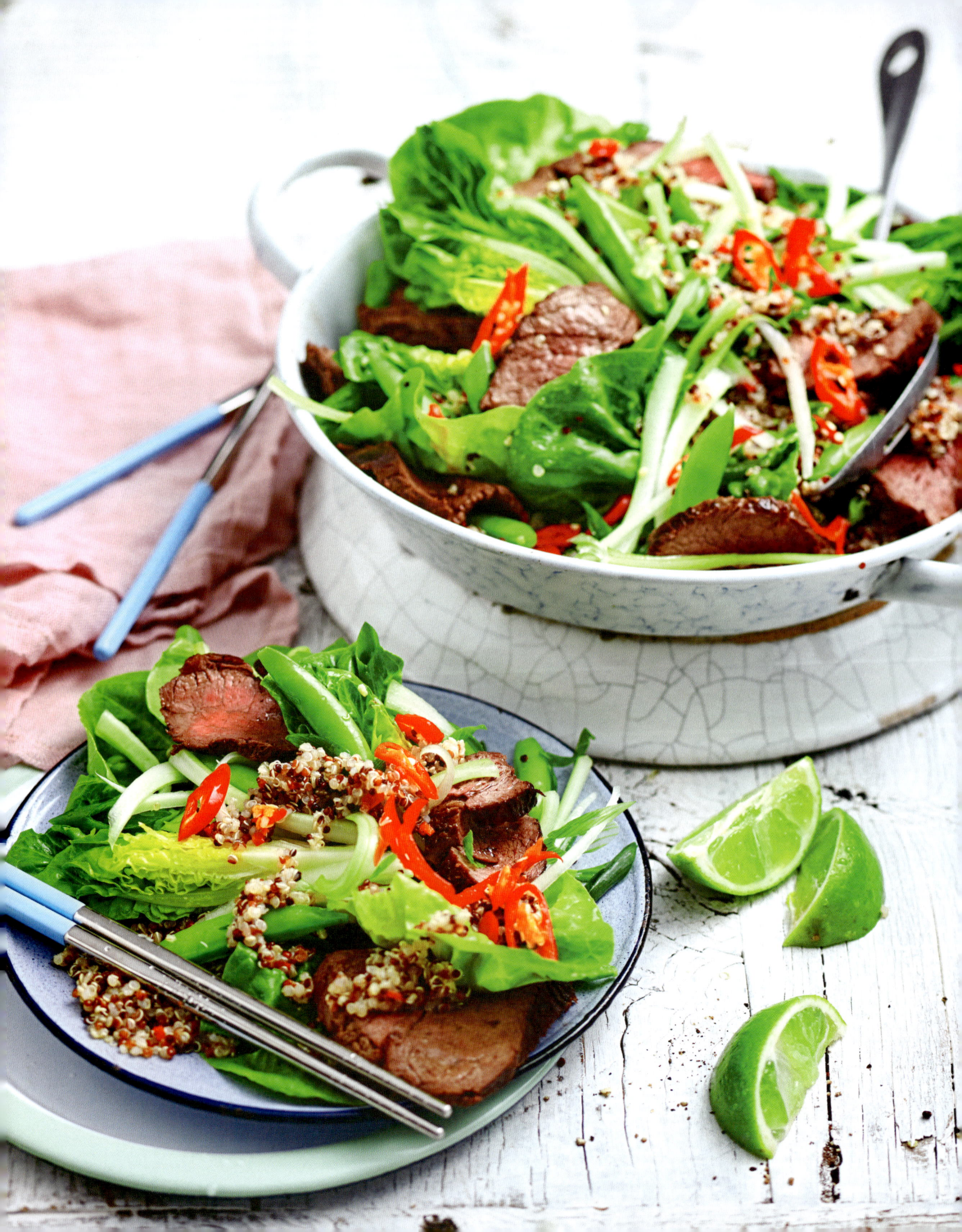

| | | | | | |
|---|---|---|---|---|---|
| ● 18.1g total fat (3.8g saturated fat) | ● 1659kJ (396 cal) | ● 23.8g carbohydrate | ● 30.2g protein | ● 7.2g fibre | ● 625mg sodium |

# Ginger beef & quinoa
# SALAD

**PREP + COOK TIME** 35 MINUTES **SERVES** 4

$2/3$ cup (135g) tri-coloured quinoa, rinsed well

$1\frac{1}{4}$ cups (310ml) water

1 tablespoon fish sauce

4cm ($1\frac{1}{2}$in) piece fresh ginger, grated finely

1 clove garlic, crushed

$\frac{1}{2}$ teaspoon freshly ground black pepper

400g ($12\frac{1}{2}$oz) piece beef fillet

200g ($6\frac{1}{2}$oz) sugar snap peas, trimmed

1 butter (boston) lettuce (195g), leaves separated

2 baby gem lettuce, quartered

2 celery stalks (300g), trimmed, cut into matchsticks

3 green onions (scallions), sliced thinly

1 fresh long red chilli, sliced thinly

1 medium lime (90g), cut into wedges

**LIME, GINGER & CHILLI DRESSING**

2 tablespoons lime juice

2 tablespoons extra virgin olive oil

2cm ($3/4$in) piece fresh ginger, grated finely

1 fresh long red chilli, seeded, chopped finely

**1** Place quinoa and the water in a medium saucepan over high heat, cover; bring to the boil. Reduce heat to low; cook, covered, for 10 minutes. Stand, covered, for 10 minutes.

**2** Meanwhile, place fish sauce, ginger, garlic and pepper in a small bowl; stir to combine. Coat beef with ginger mixture. Sear beef all over in a heated oiled large heavy-based frying pan; cook over high heat for 4 minutes for medium or until cooked to your liking. Remove from heat; stand, covered loosely with foil, for 5 minutes. Slice thinly.

**3** Boil, steam or microwave sugar snap peas until just tender; drain.

**4** Make lime, ginger and chilli dressing.

**5** Place quinoa, lettuce, celery, peas and dressing in a large bowl; toss to combine.

**6** Divide quinoa mixture among four plates or bowls; top evenly with beef. Sprinkle with green onion and chilli; serve with lime wedges.

**LIME, GINGER & CHILLI DRESSING** Place ingredients in a small bowl; stir to combine.

**TIP** This recipe can be prepared a day ahead; store portions in airtight containers in the fridge, ready for lunch the next day.

# Satisfying TOASTED & OPEN SANDWICHES

## BROAD BEAN, APPLE & WALNUT

**PREP TIME** 20 MINUTES **SERVES** 2

Place 1 cup thawed frozen broad (fava) beans in a large heatproof bowl, cover with boiling water; stand for 3 minutes. Rinse under cold water; drain, then peel. Combine beans, 1 teaspoon finely grated lemon rind, 1 tablespoon lemon juice, 1 tablespoon each coarsely chopped fresh dill and mint, 2 trimmed thinly sliced celery stalks (200g), ½ small thinly sliced red apple (65g) and ¼ cup coarsely chopped walnuts in a large bowl. Season with pepper. Spread 2 thick slices toasted multigrain sourdough bread (140g) with 1 tablespoon cashew spread each. Top each with 2 cos (romaine) lettuce leaves and half of the bean mixture. Sprinkle each with 5g (¼oz) baby rocket (arugula) and top with extra lemon rind.

**TIP** Cashew spread can be found in the health food section of the supermarket and in health food stores.

**NUTRITIONAL COUNT PER SERVING** 18.7g total fat (1.8g saturated fat); 1724kJ (411 cal); 41.9g carbohydrate; 13.8g protein; 9.1g fibre; 401mg sodium

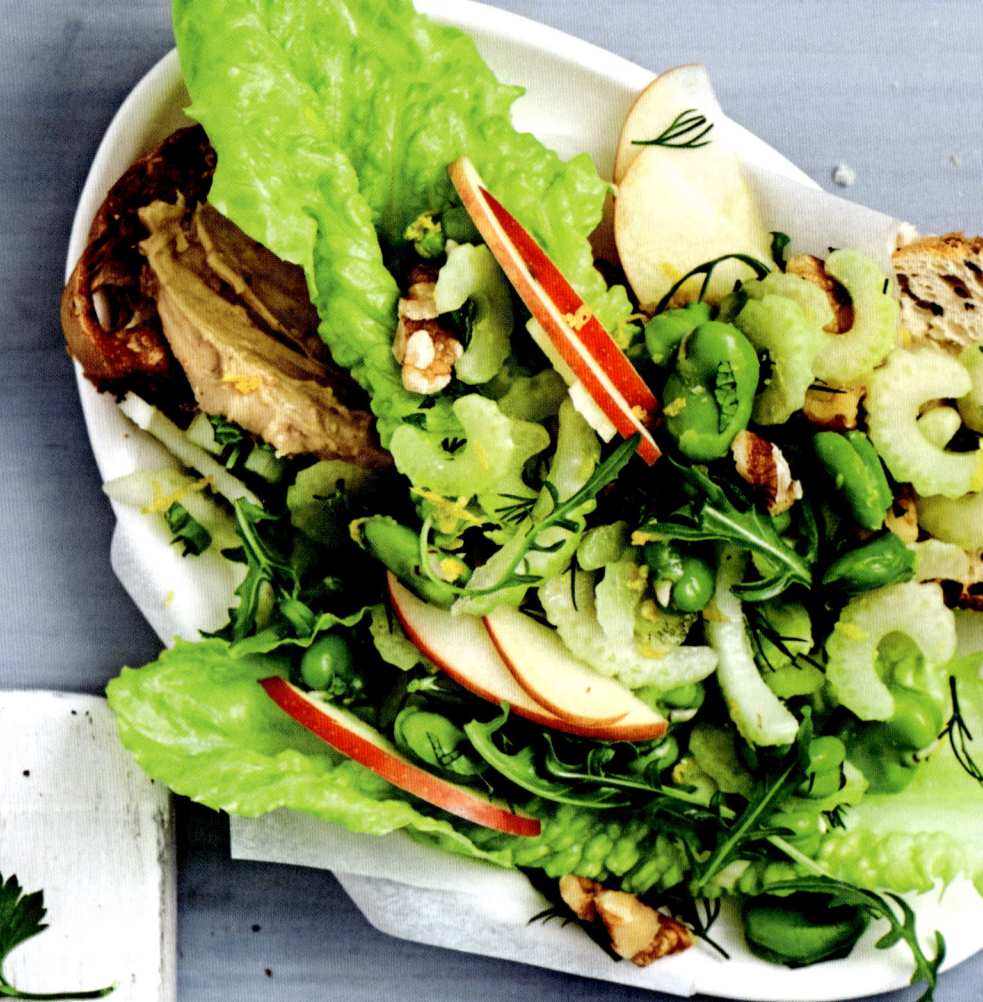

## AVOCADO, TAHINI & SUMAC TOMATOES

**PREP + COOK TIME** 40 MINUTES **SERVES** 2

Preheat oven to 180°C/350°F. Halve 3 medium roma (egg) tomatoes lengthways, place skin-side down on a small oven tray lined with baking paper; sprinkle with ½ teaspoon sumac and spray lightly with olive oil. Roast for 30 minutes or until tomato is collapsed slightly. Place ½ clove crushed garlic, ¼ cup low-fat plain yoghurt, 1 tablespoon tahini and 1 teaspoon lemon juice in a small bowl; whisk to combine. Top 2 slices toasted wholegrain sourdough bread (120g) evenly with ¼ sliced small avocado. Spoon tahini mixture over avocado; top with tomatoes and fresh flat-leaf parsley leaves.

**TIP** Cook extra sumac tomatoes and store in an airtight container in the fridge for up to 4 days to use in pastas, salads and sandwiches.

**NUTRITIONAL COUNT PER SERVING** 26.9g total fat (5g saturated fat); 1785kJ (426 cal); 28.4g carbohydrate; 13.2g protein; 8.8g fibre; 431mg sodium

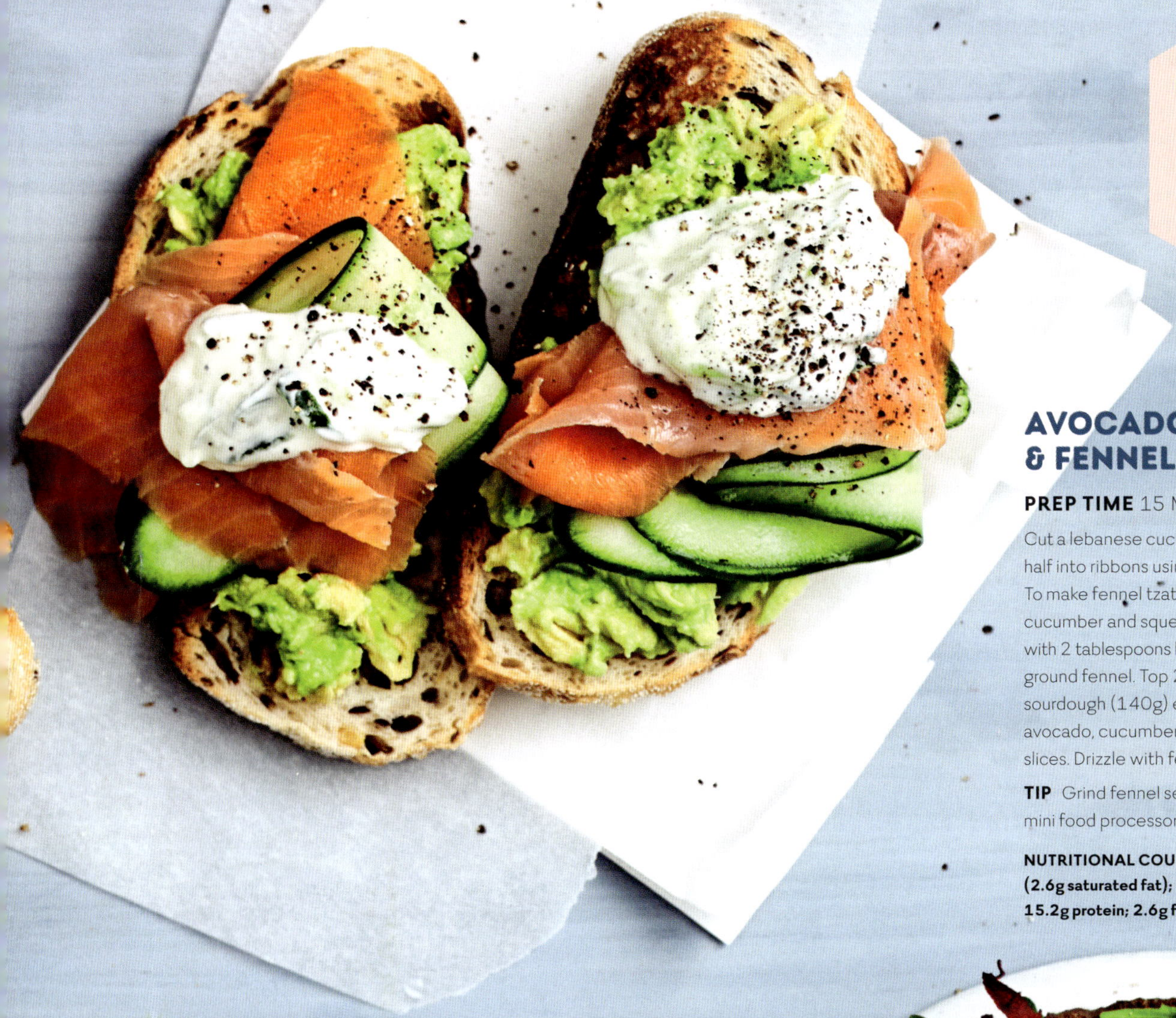

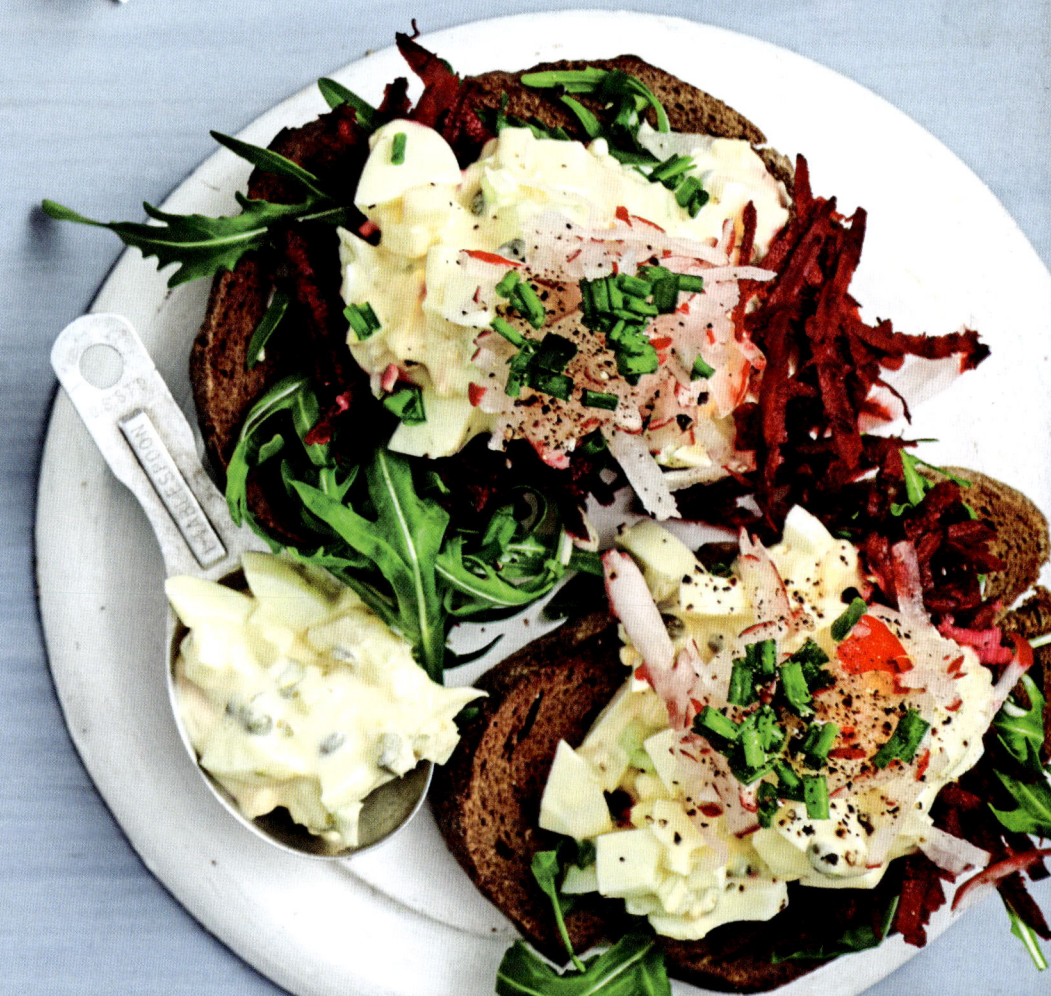

**DR JO SAYS**
Broad beans deliver protein and several nutrients, including folate, iron and magnesium. They are also fantastic for fibre, with 1 cup adding 12g fibre to the meal.

## AVOCADO, TROUT & FENNEL TZATZIKI

**PREP TIME** 15 MINUTES **SERVES** 2

Cut a lebanese cucumber in half lengthways; cut one half into ribbons using a vegetable peeler or mandoline. To make fennel tzatziki, coarsely grate remaining cucumber and squeeze out excess moisture; combine with 2 tablespoons low-fat plain yoghurt and ½ teaspoon ground fennel. Top 2 slices of toasted soy and linseed sourdough (140g) evenly with half a small mashed avocado, cucumber ribbons and 60g (2oz) smoked trout slices. Drizzle with fennel tzatziki.

**TIP** Grind fennel seeds in a mortar and pestle or a mini food processor, if ground fennel is unavailable.

**NUTRITIONAL COUNT PER SERVING 11.7g total fat (2.6g saturated fat); 1098kJ (262 cal); 22.8g carbohydrate; 15.2g protein; 2.6g fibre; 268mg sodium**

## CREAMY EGG & SALAD

**PREP + COOK TIME** 15 MINUTES **SERVES** 2

Place 3 small room-temperature eggs in a small saucepan; cover with cold water. Bring to the boil, covered, then remove lid. Boil for 5 minutes; drain. When cool enough to handle, peel eggs. Roughly mash eggs in a medium bowl with 2 tablespoons low-fat natural Greek-style yoghurt, 1 tablespoon low-fat mayonnaise, 2 teaspoons dijon mustard, 2 teaspoons extra virgin olive oil, 2 teaspoons drained, rinsed and chopped baby capers and 1 trimmed and finely chopped celery stalk (100g). Combine 1 small peeled and coarsely grated beetroot (beet) (100g) and 2 coarsely grated red radishes (70g) in a small bowl. Top 2 thin slices toasted rye bread (90g) with ½ cup each of rocket (arugula) and half each of the beetroot and egg mixtures. Sprinkle with 1 tablespoon finely chopped chives; season with pepper.

**TIP** You can make the egg mixture a day ahead. Store in an airtight container in the fridge and assemble sandwiches just before serving.

**NUTRITIONAL COUNT PER SERVING 14.4g total fat (3.6g saturated fat); 1490kJ (356 cal); 34.1g carbohydrate; 18.8g protein; 6.8g fibre; 771mg sodium**

**NUTRITIONAL COUNT PER SERVING**

| ● 18.4g total fat (2.6g saturated fat) | ● 1912kJ (456 cal) | ● 34.4g carbohydrate | ● 30.6g protein | ● 11.8g fibre | ● 663mg sodium |

# Rawslaw with
# POACHED CHICKEN

**PREP + COOK TIME** 40 MINUTES **SERVES** 4

400g (12½oz) chicken breasts, halved horizontally

3 cups (750ml) salt-reduced chicken stock

2 teaspoons fennel seeds, toasted

1 medium fennel bulb (300g), sliced thinly (see tip), fronds and stalks reserved

½ cup (100g) tri-coloured quinoa, rinsed well

2 cups (160g) finely shredded red cabbage

150g (4½oz) celeriac (celery root), peeled, cut into matchsticks

1 bunch mixed baby carrots (400g), peeled, sliced thinly (see tip)

1 medium firm pear (230g), unpeeled, cut into matchsticks

¼ cup (30g) coarsely chopped walnuts, toasted

**MUSTARD-CURRANT DRESSING**

2 tablespoons extra virgin olive oil

1 tablespoon apple cider vinegar

1 tablespoon lemon juice

1 tablespoon wholegrain mustard (seeded mustard)

1 tablespoon currants

2 teaspoons honey

2 teaspoons finely grated lemon rind

**1** Place chicken, the stock, 1 teaspoon fennel seeds and fennel stalks in a medium saucepan; bring to a simmer. Cook, covered, over medium heat for 15 minutes or until chicken is cooked through. Using tongs, carefully transfer chicken to a plate or tray; leave to cool slightly. Reserve ¼ cup strained poaching liquid; discard remaining liquid and solids.

**2** Meanwhile, cook quinoa following packet directions; cool.

**3** Make mustard-currant dressing.

**4** Place quinoa, fennel, cabbage, celeriac, carrot, pear, remaining fennel seeds and reserved fennel fronds in a large bowl. Drizzle with dressing.

**5** Slice chicken; add to salad. Sprinkle with walnuts to serve.

**MUSTARD-CURRANT DRESSING** Place ingredients, including reserved poaching liquid, in a screw-top jar; shake well. Season to taste.

**DID YOU KNOW?** It's important you read the ingredient panel on any processed food before buying, so you know what you're getting. Unfortunately, many commercially produced gluten-free foods on supermarket shelves are made with potato and rice flours, so they're high in refined carbohydrates, which are quick to digest.

**TIP** Use a V-slicer or mandoline, if you have one, to cut the fennel and carrots thinly.

**DR JO SAYS**
Many people with type 1 diabetes also have coeliac disease. However, many commercial gluten-free products have a high GI. Skip these and opt for gluten-free wholegrains, such as quinoa, brown basmati rice, buckwheat or teff.

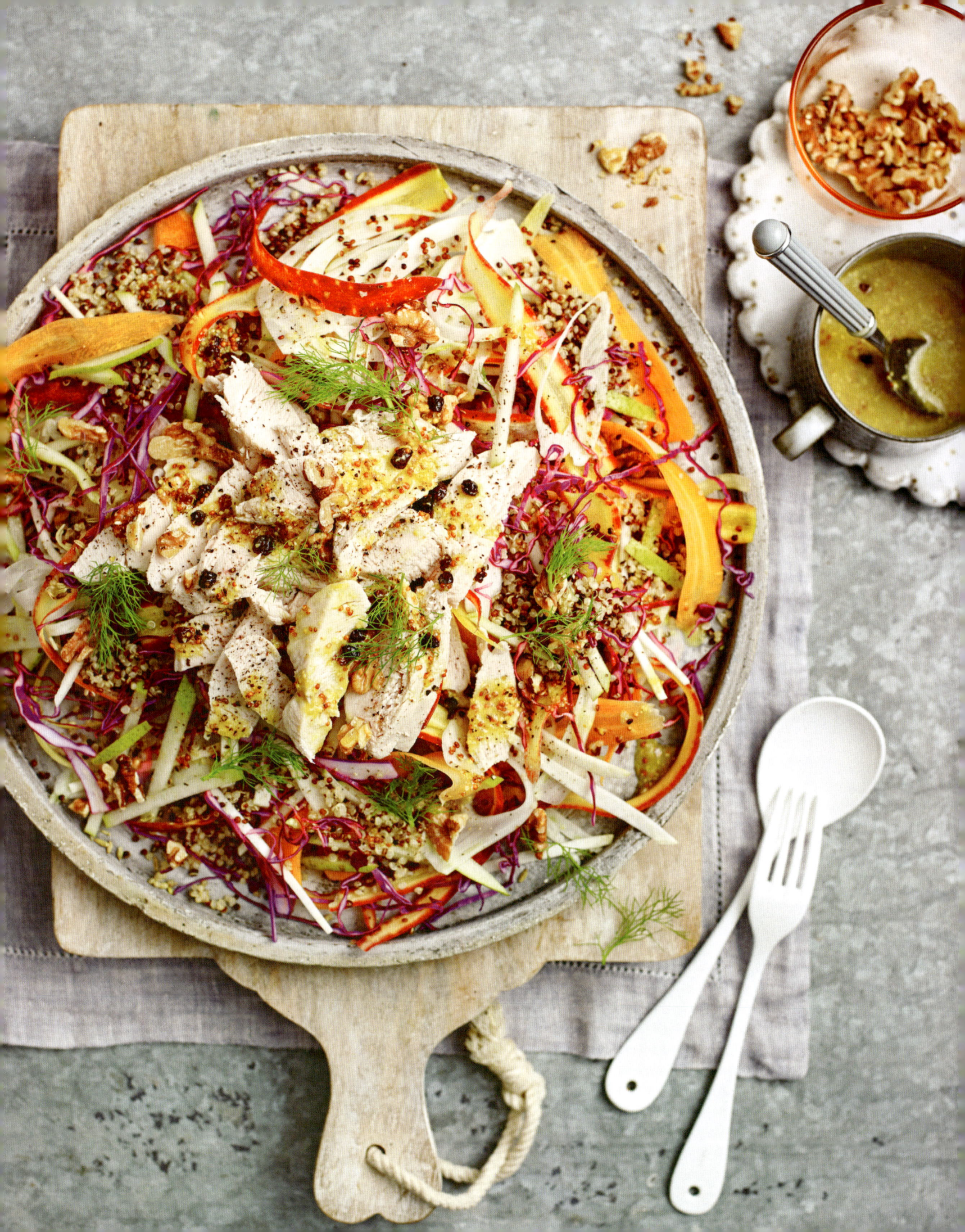

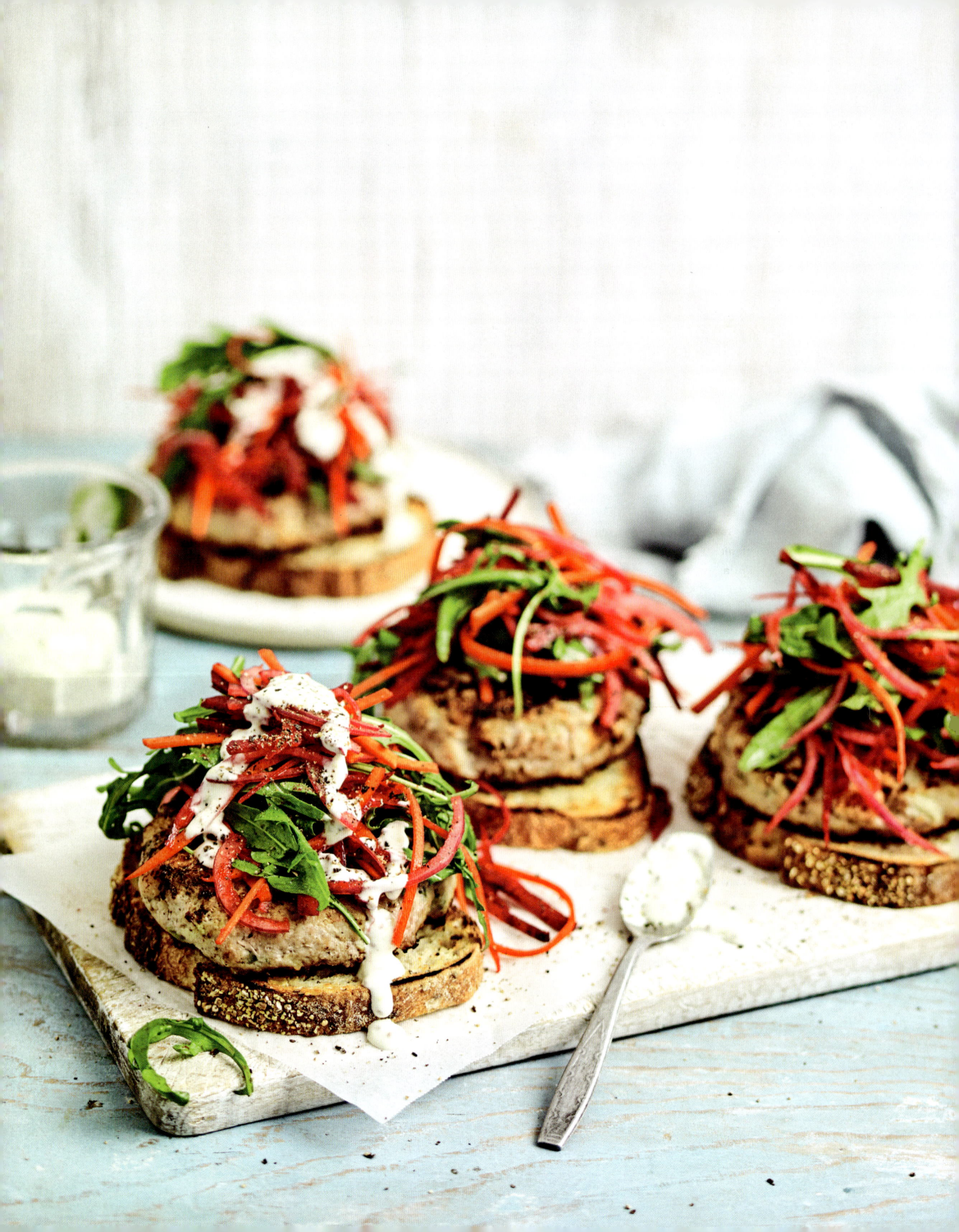

| | | | | | |
|---|---|---|---|---|---|
| ● 17.9g total fat (5.7g saturated fat) | ● 1804kJ (431 cal) | ● 30.5g carbohydrate | ● 31.2g protein | ● 9.9g fibre | ● 348mg sodium |

# OPEN PORK BURGERS
## *with mustard yoghurt*

**PREP + COOK TIME** 40 MINUTES (+ REFRIGERATION) **SERVES** 4

400g (12½oz) extra lean minced (ground) pork
1 tablespoon fresh thyme leaves, chopped finely
1½ teaspoons ground cumin
1½ teaspoons ground coriander
1 clove garlic, crushed
1 egg
1 small green apple (130g), grated coarsely
400g (12½oz) can no-added-salt cannellini beans,
  drained, rinsed
olive-oil spray
1 cup (15g) baby rocket (arugula)
1 medium carrot (120g), cut into matchsticks (see tip)
1 medium beetroot (beet) (175g), cut into matchsticks
  (see tip)
½ small red onion (50g), sliced thinly
2 teaspoons apple cider vinegar
¼ teaspoon finely grated orange rind
2 teaspoons orange juice
2 teaspoons extra virgin olive oil
4 slices wholegrain bread (120g)
**MUSTARD YOGHURT**
⅓ cup (95g) natural Greek-style yoghurt
3 teaspoons wholegrain mustard (seeded mustard)

**1** Combine pork, thyme, cumin, coriander, garlic, egg, apple and beans in a large bowl; mix well. Season with pepper. Using wet hands, shape mixture into 4 patties. Cover; refrigerate for 20 minutes to firm.

**2** Heat a medium non-stick frying pan over medium heat; spray lightly with oil. Cook burgers for 6 minutes each side or until cooked through.

**3** Meanwhile, make mustard yoghurt.

**4** Toss rocket, carrot, beetroot and onion in a bowl; drizzle with combined vinegar, orange rind, juice and oil.

**5** Lightly toast bread. Top each slice with a pork pattie, a quarter of the salad and a quarter of the mustard yoghurt.

**MUSTARD YOGHURT** Combine ingredients in a small bowl.

**TIP** To save time, coarsely grate the carrot and beetroot instead of cutting them into matchsticks.

| ● 13.4g total fat (5.2g saturated fat) | ● 1236kJ (295 cal) | ● 24.3g carbohydrate | ● 16.6g protein | ● 4.8g fibre | ● 780mg sodium |

# Spanakopita
# QUESADILLAS

**PREP + COOK TIME** 35 MINUTES **SERVES** 4

2 teaspoons olive oil

1 small red onion (100g), chopped finely

1 clove garlic, crushed

200g (6½oz) baby spinach leaves, chopped coarsely (see tip)

2 eggs, beaten lightly

100g (3oz) reduced-fat fetta, crumbled

1½ tablespoons finely grated parmesan

2 teaspoons finely grated lemon rind

⅓ cup coarsely chopped fresh dill

4 wholegrain tortillas (160g)

1 lebanese cucumber (130g), chopped coarsely

250g (8oz) cherry tomatoes, halved

⅓ cup (95g) tzatziki

1 medium lemon (140g), cut into wedges

**1** Heat oil in a large heavy-based non-stick frying pan over medium heat. Cook onion, garlic and spinach, stirring, for 2 minutes or until softened. Transfer to a large bowl; stand to cool slightly. Wipe pan clean with paper towel.

**2** Add egg, fetta, parmesan, lemon rind and 2 tablespoons of the dill to spinach mixture. Season with pepper; mix well to combine.

**3** Heat frying pan over low heat. Spread a quarter of the spinach mixture over one half of a tortilla; fold over to enclose. Repeat with remaining spinach mixture and tortillas. Cook quesadillas, in batches, for 3 minutes each side or until warmed through and golden.

**4** Combine cucumber, tomato and remaining dill in a medium bowl; season with pepper.

**5** Cut quesadillas into wedges. Serve with cucumber salad, tzatziki and lemon wedges.

**TIP** Instead of baby spinach leaves, you can use the larger spinach leaves, if you like.

**DID YOU KNOW?** This recipe is a twist on the popular Greek spinach pie known as spanakopita. Traditionally, spinach is combined with fetta, onions and dill, and wrapped in a crisp, flaky fillo pastry. Here we wrap the filling in tortillas, but it tastes just as delicious.

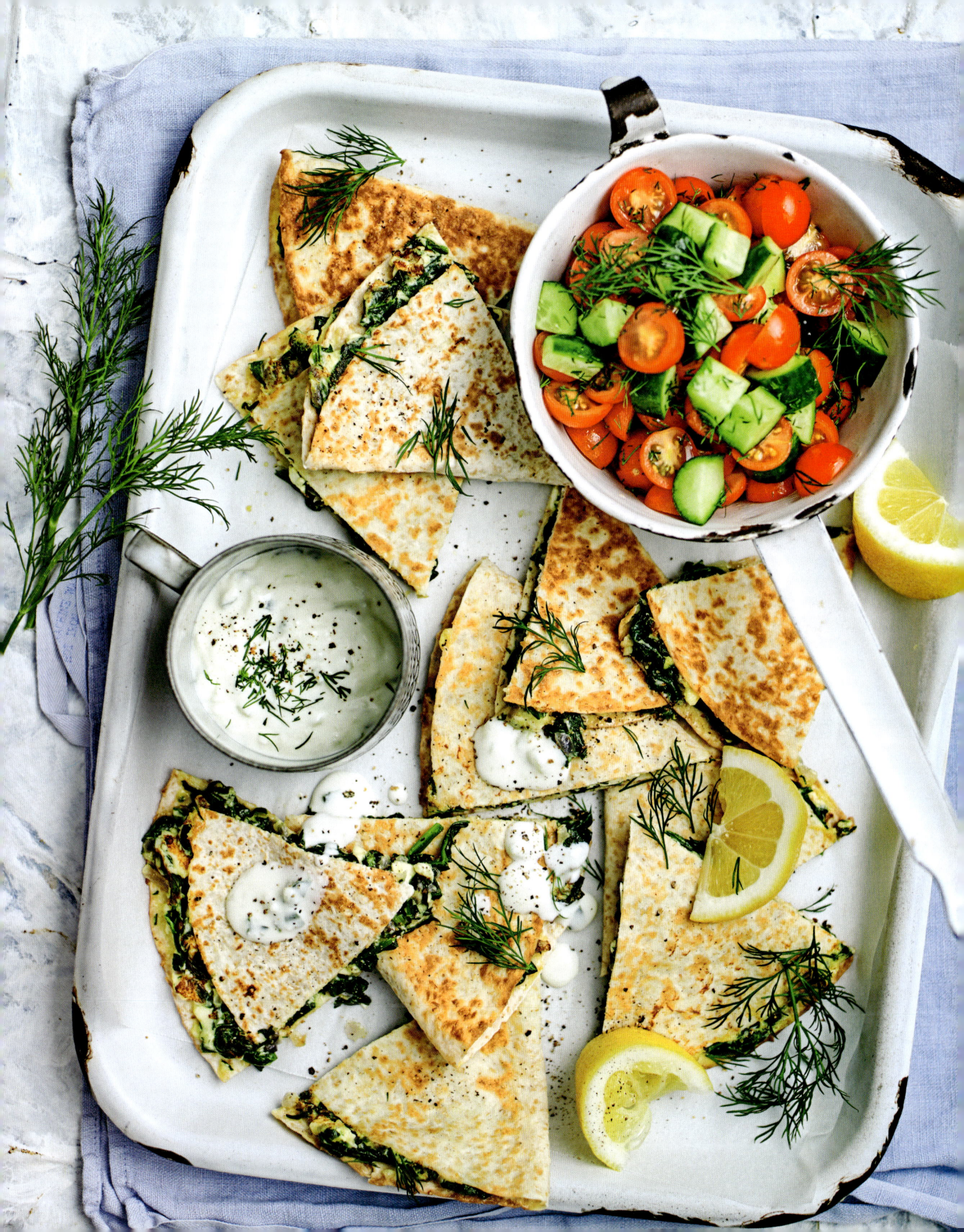

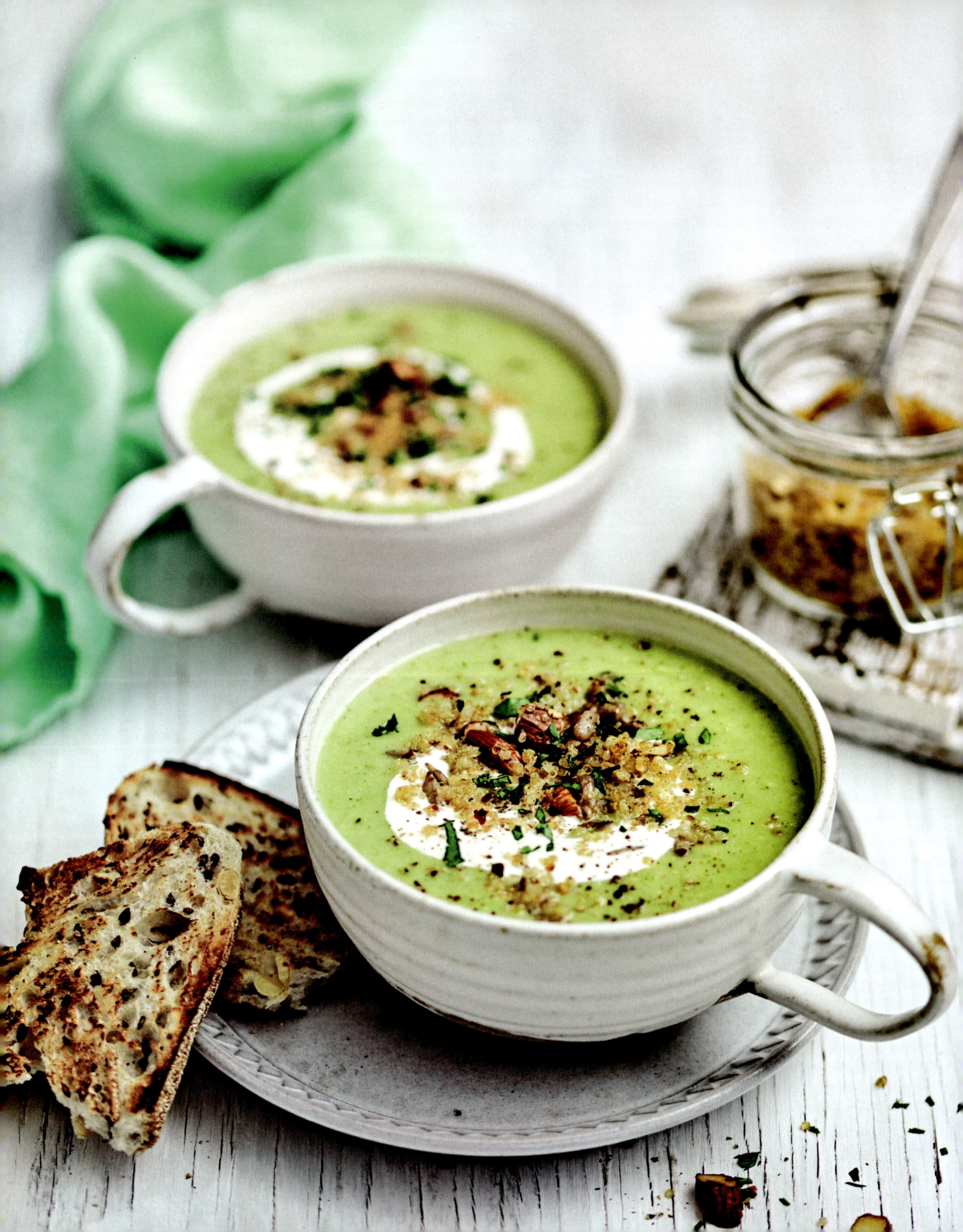

| 26.7g total fat (3.6g saturated fat) | 2145kJ (512 cal) | 41.9g carbohydrate | 19.4g protein | 13.2g fibre | 765mg sodium |
|---|---|---|---|---|---|

# CREAMY BROCCOLI SOUP
## with crispy quinoa

**PREP + COOK TIME** 40 MINUTES **SERVES** 4

1 tablespoon olive oil
1 medium leek (350g), sliced thinly
2 sticks celery (300g), trimmed, chopped finely
2 cloves garlic, crushed
1 large head broccoli (400g), cut into florets
2 medium zucchini (240g), chopped coarsely
1 large potato (300g), peeled, chopped coarsely
2¼ cups (560ml) salt-reduced vegetable stock
2¾ cups (680ml) water
⅓ cup (95g) natural Greek-style yoghurt
2 slices soy and linseed bread (140g), toasted

**CRISPY QUINOA**
½ cup (100g) white quinoa, rinsed well
2 tablespoons olive oil
2 tablespoons sunflower seeds
2 tablespoons coarsely chopped roasted almonds
1 teaspoon chilli flakes
2 cloves garlic, crushed
2 tablespoons finely chopped fresh flat-leaf parsley

**1** Heat oil in a large heavy-based saucepan over medium–high heat. Add leek and celery; cook, stirring, for 3 minutes or until softened. Add garlic; cook for 1 minute or until fragrant.

**2** Add broccoli, zucchini, potato, stock and the water to pan; bring to the boil. Reduce heat to low–medium; simmer for 10 minutes or until vegetables are tender. Remove soup from heat; cool slightly.

**3** Meanwhile, make crispy quinoa.

**4** Blend or process soup until smooth. Season to taste with pepper.

**5** Divide soup among four bowls; top each with 1 tablespoon of the yoghurt and season with pepper. Sprinkle with crispy quinoa and serve with toast.

**CRISPY QUINOA** Cook quinoa according to packet directions; drain well. Heat oil in a medium frying pan over medium heat. Add quinoa, sunflower seeds, almonds and chilli flakes; cook, stirring, for 10 minutes or until quinoa browns lightly. Add garlic and parsley; cook, stirring, for 1 minute or until fragrant. Transfer to a plate to cool; it will crisp as it cools.

**TIPS** This recipe can be prepared up to the end of step 4 a day ahead; store soup in an airtight container in the fridge. Reheat the soup just before serving.
Store the crispy quinoa in an airtight container.

| ● 14.8g total fat (2.7g saturated fat) | ● 1176kJ (281 cal) | ● 6.9g carbohydrate | ● 24.5g protein | ● 11.3g fibre | ● 597mg sodium |

# Prawn & broccoli
# FRIED 'RICE'

**PREP + COOK TIME** 30 MINUTES **SERVES** 4

2 large eggs
2 medium heads broccoli (700g), broken into florets
2 tablespoons reduced–salt soy sauce
2 teaspoons sesame oil
2 tablespoons olive oil
1 medium onion (150g), sliced thinly
3 cloves garlic, crushed
4cm (1½in) piece fresh ginger, grated finely
2 fresh long red chillies, 1 seeded and chopped finely,
   1 sliced thinly
400g (12½oz) uncooked prawns (shrimp), peeled,
   cleaned, halved lengthways
2 tablespoons water
3 green onions (scallions), 2 chopped finely, 1 sliced
   thinly lengthways
1 cup (120g) frozen peas
150g (4½oz) sugar snap peas, sliced thinly
2 cups (160g) bean sprouts

**1** Cook eggs in a saucepan of boiling water for 6 minutes. Run under cold water until cool; peel.

**2** Meanwhile, process broccoli until chopped finely to form broccoli 'rice'.

**3** Combine soy sauce and sesame oil in a small bowl.

**4** Heat olive oil in a large wok over high heat. Add onion; stir–fry for 2 minutes. Add garlic, ginger and chopped chilli; stir–fry for 30 seconds. Add prawns; stir–fry for 1 minute or until cooked through. Add the water; bring to the boil. Add chopped green onion and broccoli; stir–fry for 2 minutes. Add peas and sugar snap peas; stir–fry for 2 minutes. Add soy sauce mixture; stir–fry until well combined.

**5** Remove from heat. Stir through bean sprouts.

**6** Divide broccoli 'rice' and prawn mixture among four bowls or plates; top with sliced chilli, sliced green onion and half a boiled egg each.

**TIPS** You can make this the night before and divide broccoli 'rice' and prawn mixture among four take–away containers or airtight containers. Refrigerate to take to work and reheat for lunch the next day.

If you don't have a wok, use a large frying pan instead.

**DR JO SAYS**
Going for a walk after a meal is a terrific way to help get blood glucose levels under control. When you move, muscles are stimulated to take up glucose from the blood.

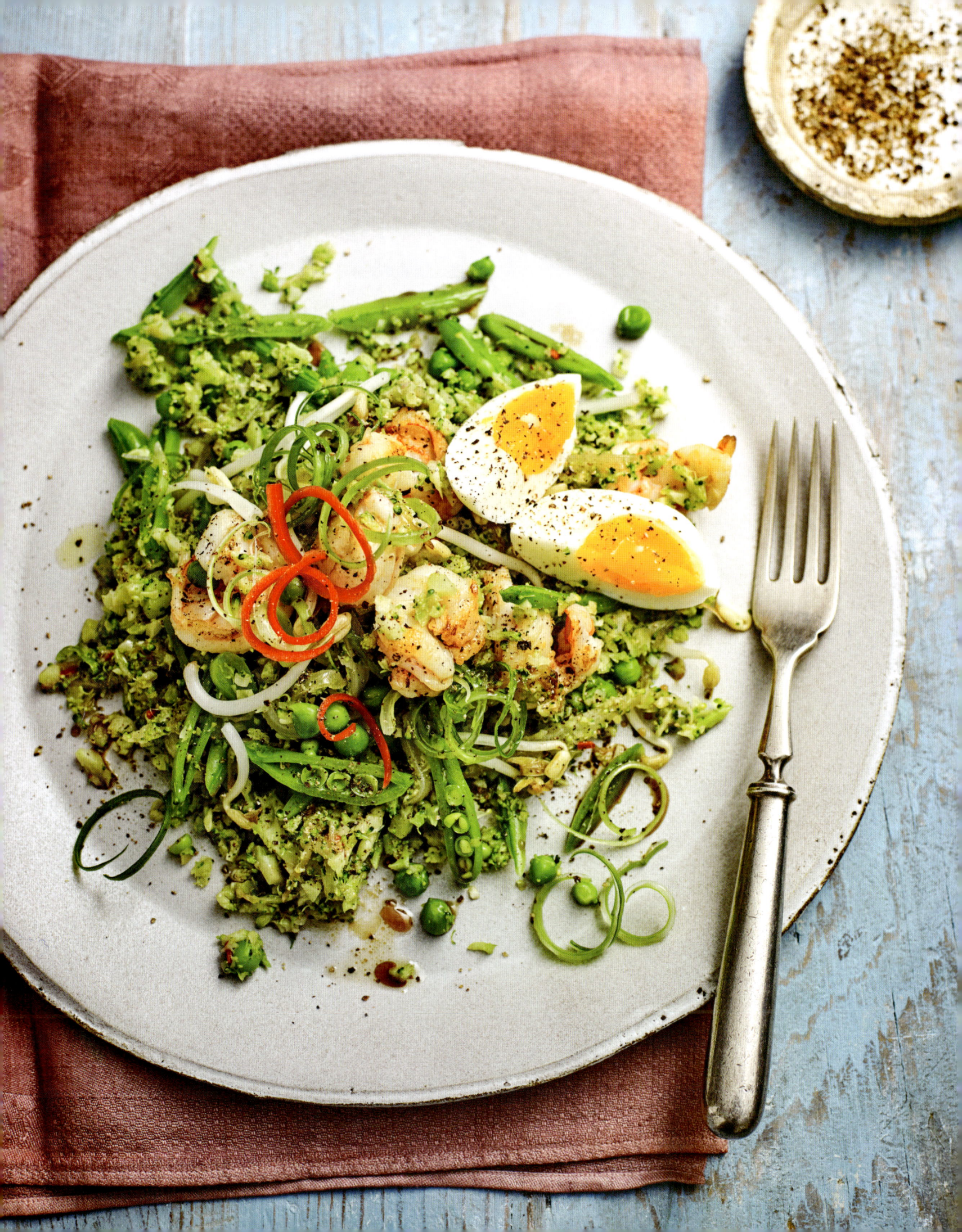

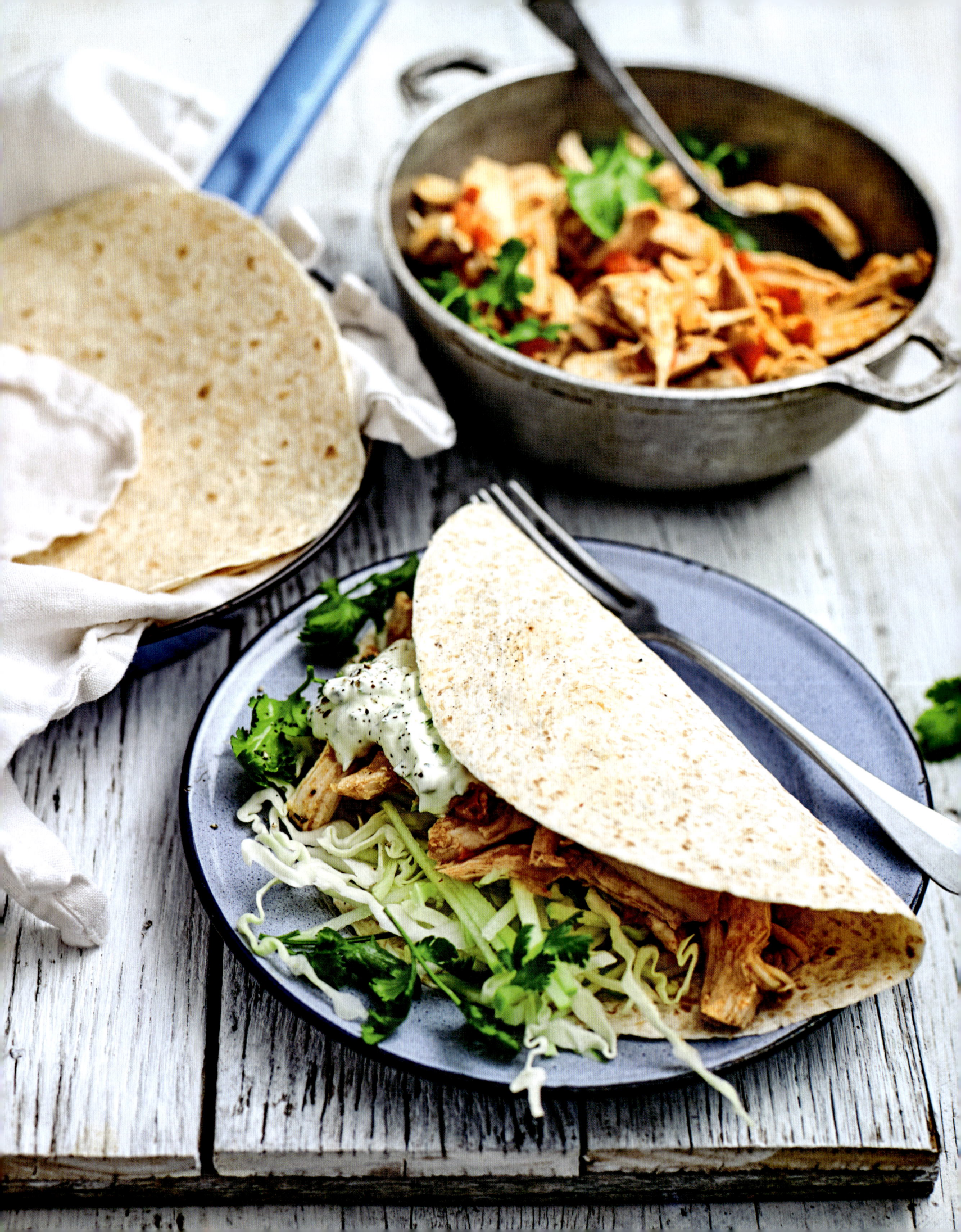

| ● 12.4g total fat (3.6g saturated fat) | ● 1434kJ (342 cal) | ● 27.6g carbohydrate | ● 28.1g protein | ● 4.5g fibre | ● 538mg sodium |
|---|---|---|---|---|---|

# Pulled chicken
# TORTILLAS

**PREP + COOK TIME** 45 MINUTES (+ COOLING) **SERVES** 4

400g (12½oz) chicken breast fillets
1 cup (250ml) salt-reduced chicken stock
1 teaspoon smoked paprika
1 teaspoon ground cumin
¼ teaspoon chilli powder
2 cloves garlic, crushed
1 small onion (80g), chopped finely
1 large ripe tomato (220g), diced finely
1 teaspoon brown sugar
4 wholegrain tortillas (160g)
2 tablespoons coarsely chopped fresh coriander
 (cilantro)
2 tablespoons light sour cream
2 tablespoons fresh coriander (cilantro) leaves

**CABBAGE & APPLE SALAD**

1 small green apple (130g)
2 cups (160g) shredded white cabbage
¼ cup fresh coriander (cilantro) leaves
1 tablespoon extra virgin olive oil
2 teaspoons apple cider vinegar

**1** Place chicken, the stock, paprika, cumin, chilli, garlic, onion, tomato and brown sugar in a medium heavy-based saucepan; bring to the boil over high heat. Reduce heat to low; cook, covered, for 10 minutes. Remove from heat; leave chicken to cool in sauce for 15 minutes.

**2** Remove chicken from pan; shred using two forks. Bring sauce to the boil; cook over medium-high heat for 20 minutes or until thickened and reduced by half. Return chicken to sauce.

**3** Meanwhile, make cabbage and apple salad.

**4** Warm tortillas following packet directions. Fill tortillas evenly with pulled chicken mixture and salad.

**5** Stir chopped coriander through sour cream; spoon evenly onto tortillas. Serve tortillas sprinkled with coriander leaves.

**CABBAGE & APPLE SALAD** Core and cut apple into matchsticks. Combine cabbage, apple and coriander in a large bowl. Add combined oil and vinegar, season with pepper; toss to combine.

| ● 16.5g total fat (4.6g saturated fat) | ● 1452kJ (346 cal) | ● 26.6g carbohydrate | ● 19.7g protein | ● 6.1g fibre | ● 276mg sodium |

# Zucchini, spinach &
# SWEET POTATO FRITTATA

**PREP + COOK TIME** 1 HOUR **SERVES** 4

1 tablespoon extra virgin olive oil
1 medium leek (350g), sliced thinly
2 cloves garlic, crushed
200g (6½oz) baby spinach leaves
6 eggs, beaten lightly
1 small orange sweet potato (250g), grated coarsely
1 cup (180g) cooked brown rice (see tip)
⅓ cup fresh basil leaves, chopped coarsely
100g (3oz) fresh ricotta, crumbled
30g (1oz) finely grated parmesan
2 large zucchini (300g), sliced thinly lengthways
   into ribbons
olive-oil spray
60g (2oz) rocket (arugula) leaves
2 tablespoons fresh basil leaves, extra, to serve

**1** Preheat oven to 180°C/350°F. Grease a 20cm x 30cm (8in x 12in) slice pan; line base with baking paper.
**2** Heat 2 teaspoons of the oil in a medium frying pan over medium heat; cook leek and garlic, stirring, for 5 minutes or until softened. Add spinach, stir until wilted; cool slightly.
**3** Blend or process spinach mixture and eggs until spinach is finely chopped but not pureed. Pour into a large bowl; stir in sweet potato, rice, basil, ricotta and ¼ cup of the parmesan. Season with pepper.
**4** Pour mixture into pan, top with overlapping zucchini slices, placing them lengthways; press in lightly. Spray lightly with oil; sprinkle with remaining parmesan.
**5** Bake for 30 minutes or until egg mixture is set. Stand in pan for 5 minutes to cool, before cutting evenly into eight slices.
**6** Drizzle remaining oil over rocket leaves. Serve two slices of frittata each, with rocket and extra basil leaves.

**TIP** You will need to cook about ⅓ cup raw low-GI doongarra brown rice to get the amount of cooked rice needed for this recipe. Or, you could use the leftover rice from the turkey & rice kofta recipe on page 94 if you have recently made that recipe.

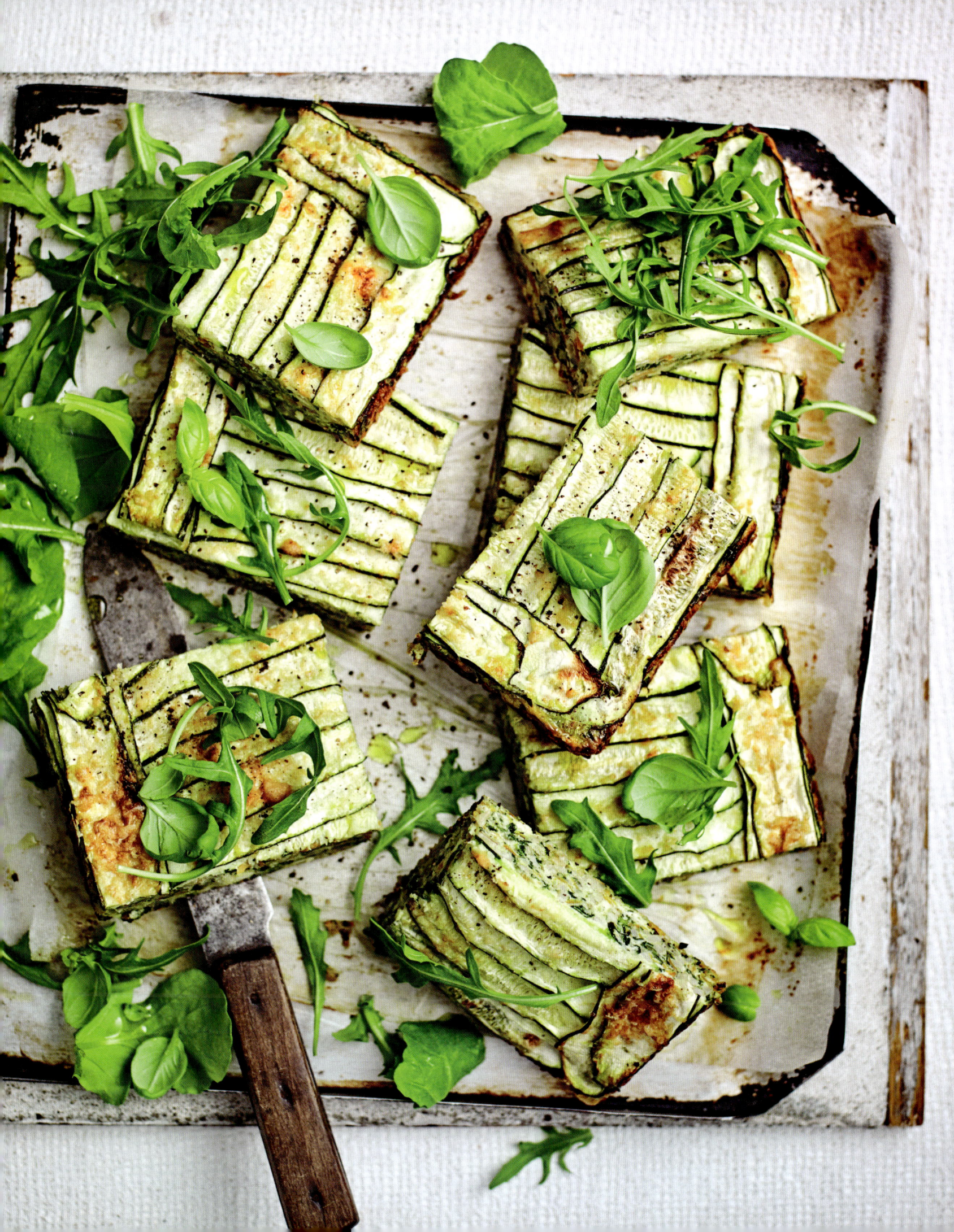

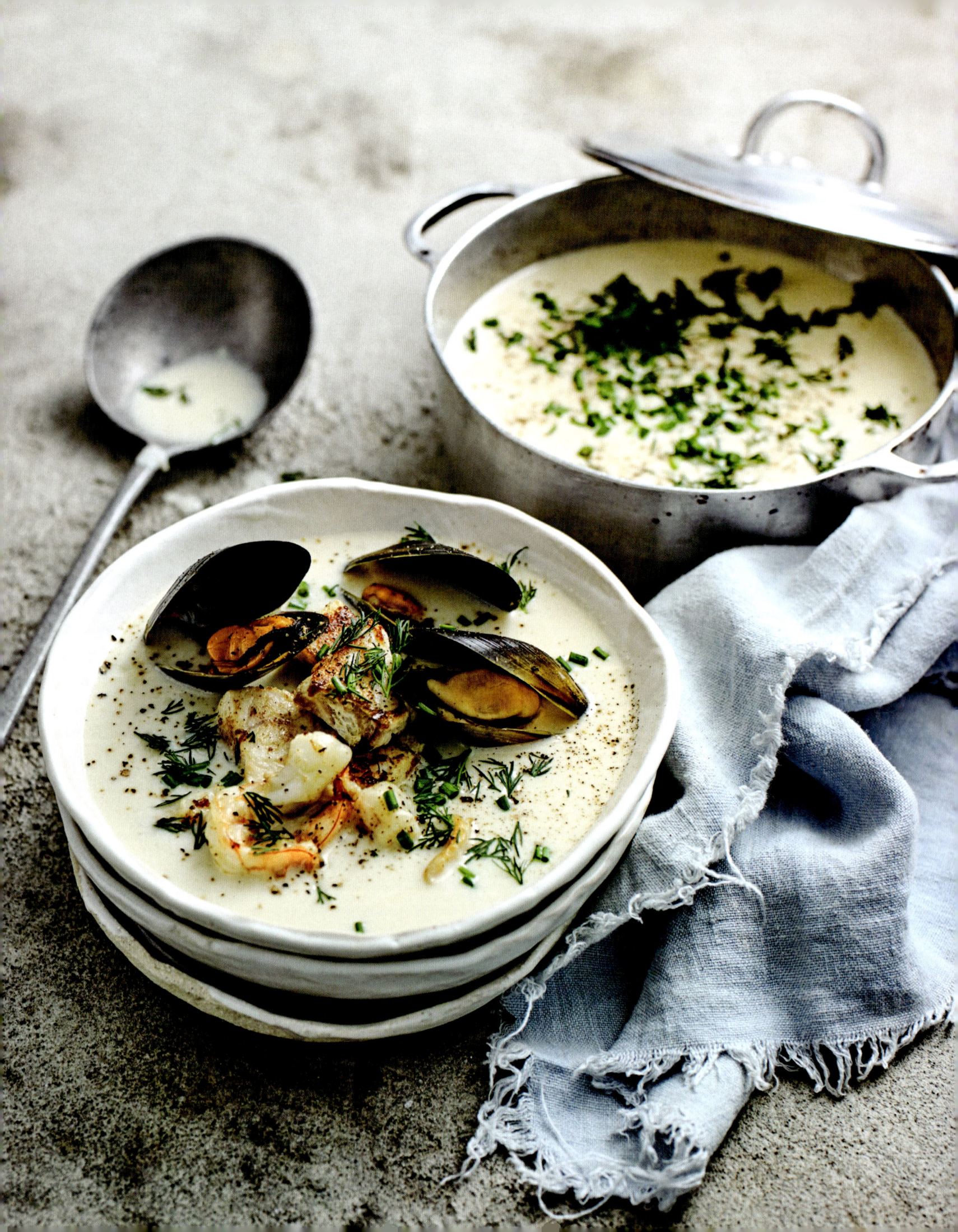

| | | | | | |
|---|---|---|---|---|---|
| ● 14.1g total fat (5g saturated fat) | ● 1477kJ (353 cal) | ● 21.9g carbohydrate | ● 31.7g protein | ● 5.4g fibre | ● 532mg sodium |

# Creamy
# SEAFOOD SOUP

**PREP + COOK TIME** 55 MINUTES **SERVES** 4

1 tablespoon extra virgin olive oil

2 celery stalks (300g), trimmed, chopped coarsely

1 medium leek (350g), sliced thinly

1 teaspoon ground nutmeg

250g (8oz) desiree potatoes, cut into
2cm (¾in) pieces

300g (9½oz) cauliflower, cut into small florets

1 cup (250ml) salt-reduced chicken stock

3 cups (750ml) milk

2¼ cups (560ml) water

olive-oil spray

300g (9½oz) firm white fish fillets, cut into
3cm (1¼in) pieces (see tip)

150g (4½oz) uncooked king prawns (shrimp),
peeled, deveined, halved lengthways

12 black mussels, cleaned

2 tablespoons coarsely chopped fresh dill tips

2 tablespoons finely chopped fresh chives

**1** Heat oil in a large heavy-based saucepan over medium heat. Add celery, leek and nutmeg; cook, covered, stirring frequently, for 10 minutes or until softened.

**2** Add potato, cauliflower, stock, milk and 2 cups of the water to pan; bring to the boil. Reduce heat to low; simmer, partially covered, for 25 minutes or until potato breaks down and starts to thicken the soup. Cool slightly, then blend or process until smooth.

**3** Meanwhile, heat a non-stick frying pan over medium-high heat; spray with oil. Add fish; cook, turning halfway through cooking time, for 4 minutes or until cooked through. Transfer to a plate. Add prawns to pan; cook for 2 minutes or until cooked through. Transfer to plate with fish. Add mussels and remaining water to pan; cook, covered, shaking pan occasionally, for 2 minutes or until mussels open.

**4** Divide soup among four bowls; top with seafood. Sprinkle with dill and chives; season with pepper.

**TIP** We used ling here, but any firm white fish fillet, such as snapper, blue-eye trevalla or whiting, would work equally as well.

**DID YOU KNOW?** Mussels must be tightly closed when bought, indicating they are alive. Not all mussels will open, even after extended cooking. For more information, see 'mussels' under 'seafood' in the glossary, page 236.

| ● 16.1g total fat (3.2g saturated fat) | ● 1983kJ (473 cal) | ● 46.1g carbohydrate | ● 35.3g protein | ● 5.2g fibre | ● 160mg sodium |

# CHICKEN NOODLE SALAD
## with dill & olive yoghurt

**PREP + COOK TIME** 30 MINUTES **SERVES** 4

2 chicken breast fillets (400g)

2 teaspoons olive oil

2 medium zucchini (240g)

180g (5½oz) green tea soba noodles

½ cup (20g) snow pea sprouts

1 tablespoon pine nuts, toasted

2 tablespoons chopped fresh dill

**DILL & OLIVE YOGHURT**

1 cup (280g) natural yoghurt

2 tablespoons tahini

2 tablespoons seeded green olives, sliced thinly

¼ cup fresh dill, chopped finely

1 tablespoon lemon juice

1 clove garlic, crushed

**1** Preheat oven to 180°C/350°F.

**2** Season chicken with pepper. Heat oil in a medium ovenproof frying pan over medium–high heat; cook chicken for 2 minutes each side or until golden. Transfer to oven; bake for 10 minutes or until chicken is cooked through. Transfer chicken to a plate; cool slightly.

**3** Meanwhile, make dill and olive yoghurt.

**4** Using a vegetable spiraliser, cut zucchini into spirals (see tip).

**5** Cook soba noodles in a large saucepan of boiling water according to packet directions. Meanwhile, place zucchini in a large colander in the sink. When noodles are tender, reserve 2 tablespoons of cooking water, then drain noodles into the colander over zucchini (this will be enough to soften the zucchini 'noodles'). Drain well; transfer to a large bowl.

**6** Cut chicken into 1cm (½in) thick slices. Add yoghurt mixture and reserved cooking water to noodle mixture; toss gently to coat well.

**7** Divide noodle mixture, chicken and sprouts evenly among four bowls. Sprinkle with pine nuts and dill to serve.

**DILL & OLIVE YOGHURT** Combine ingredients in a medium bowl; season to taste with pepper.

**TIP** To cut the zucchini, use a spiraliser, a kitchen gadget that cuts vegetables into long, thin spirals. If you don't have one, you can use a mandoline or V-slicer. In a pinch, use a vegetable peeler to slice the zucchini into long ribbons, then slice lengthways into thin strips using a sharp knife.

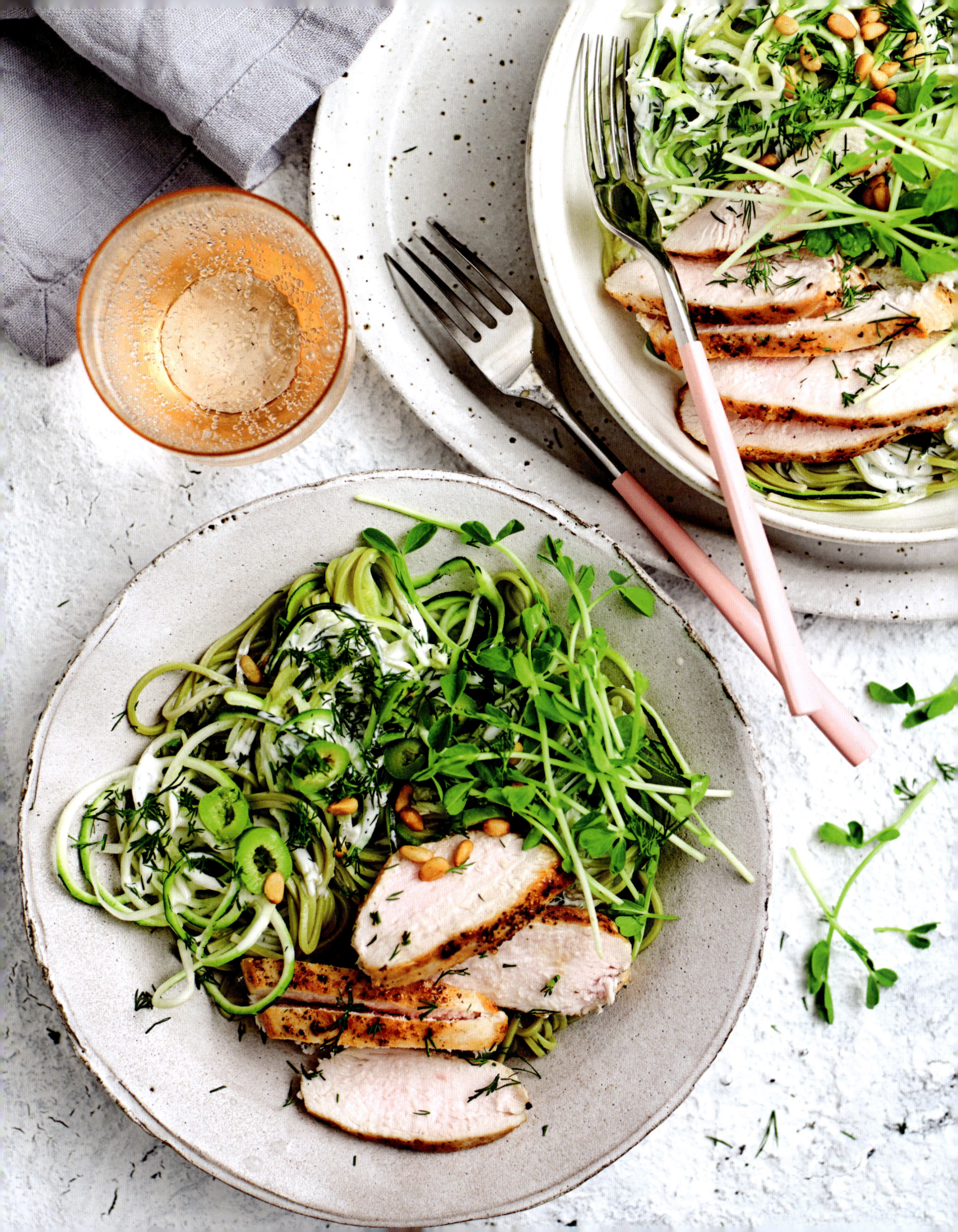

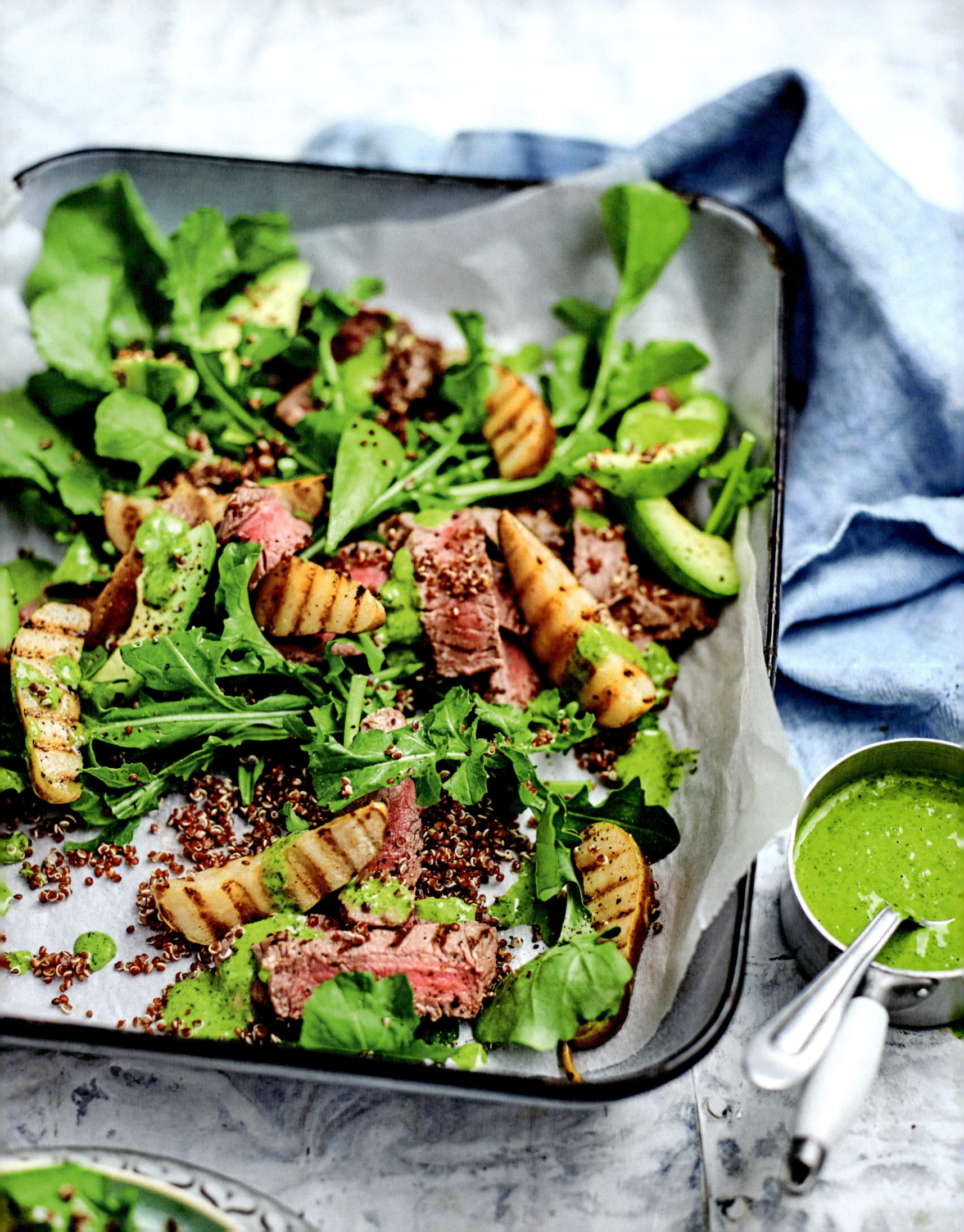

**NUTRITIONAL COUNT PER SERVING**

| • 29g total fat (6.1g saturated fat) | • 1805kJ (431 cal) | • 12.1g carbohydrate | • 27.6g protein | • 4.8g fibre | • 129mg sodium |
| --- | --- | --- | --- | --- | --- |

# GRILLED BEEF
## pear, rocket & avocado salad

**PREP + COOK TIME** 40 MINUTES **SERVES** 4

$\frac{1}{3}$ **cup (65g) red quinoa, rinsed well (see tip)**
$\frac{2}{3}$ **cup (160ml) water**
**1 small corella pear (100g), cored, cut into 8 wedges**
**olive-oil spray**
**4 x 100g (3oz) beef fillet steaks**
**2 bunches rocket (arugula) (250g), washed, trimmed**
**1 small avocado (200g), sliced**

**HERB DIJON DRESSING**
**$\frac{1}{4}$ cup (60ml) extra virgin olive oil**
**2 tablespoons white wine vinegar**
**3 teaspoons dijon mustard**
**2 tablespoons coarsely chopped fresh tarragon**
**2 tablespoons fresh dill tips**
**2 tablespoons fresh mint leaves**
**1 tablespoon water**

**1** Place quinoa and the water in a small saucepan over high heat; bring to the boil. Reduce heat to low; cook, covered, for 10 minutes or until all liquid is absorbed. Fluff with a fork.

**2** Meanwhile, heat a grill plate (or grill pan) over medium-high heat. Spray pear slices with oil; cook pear for 1 minute on each side or until grill marks appear. Transfer to a plate.

**3** Spray steaks with oil; cook on hot grill plate for 3 minutes each side for medium or until cooked to your liking. Transfer to a plate. Cover loosely with foil; rest for 10 minutes, then cut into thick slices across the grain.

**4** Meanwhile, make herb dijon dressing.

**5** Place quinoa, pear, steak, rocket and avocado on a platter or divide among four plates. Drizzle with dressing to serve.

**HERB DIJON DRESSING** Process ingredients until smooth; season to taste with pepper.

**DR JO SAYS**
Once a trendy health food, quinoa has been welcomed into the mainstream and we now have some of our own crops here in Australia. It's a good source of protein, low GI and great for fibre, making it an excellent choice for people with diabetes.

**TIP** Swap red quinoa for white or tri-coloured quinoa, if you like. While all colours of quinoa are nutritionally equal, red quinoa holds its shape better when cooked, and has a more crunchy texture.

**DID YOU KNOW?** Quinoa seeds should be washed before cooking as they contain a bitter coating, known as saponins, which requires rinsing. Simply rinse under running water until the water runs clear.

| ● 10.4g total fat (3.2g saturated fat) | ● 1211kJ (289 cal) | ● 26.9g carbohydrate | ● 14g protein | ● 15g fibre | ● 616mg sodium |
|---|---|---|---|---|---|

# SPICED CAULIFLOWER SOUP
## *with chickpea croûtons*

**PREP + COOK TIME** 40 MINUTES **SERVES** 4

**3 teaspoons extra virgin olive oil**

**1 tablespoon madras curry paste**

**1 medium onion (150g), sliced thinly**

**2 cloves garlic, crushed**

**1½ teaspoons cumin seeds**

**1 teaspoon coriander seeds**

**750g (1½lb) cauliflower florets**

**2 medium tomatoes (300g), peeled, seeded, chopped finely**

**2½ cups (625ml) salt–reduced vegetable stock**

**1½ cups (375ml) water**

**400g (12½oz) can no–added–salt chickpeas (garbanzo beans), drained, rinsed**

**⅓ cup (80ml) canned light coconut milk**

**¼ cup fresh coriander (cilantro) leaves**

**1 fresh long red chilli, sliced thinly**

**1 lime (65g), cut into wedges**

**CHICKPEA CROÛTONS**

**400g (12½oz) can no–added–salt chickpeas (garbanzo beans), drained, rinsed**

**1 teaspoon extra virgin olive oil**

**½ teaspoon ground cumin**

**1** Heat oil in a large heavy–based saucepan over medium heat. Add curry paste, onion, garlic, cumin seeds, coriander seeds and cauliflower. Cook, stirring, for 5 minutes or until cauliflower starts to soften. Add tomato, stock and the water; bring to the boil. Reduce heat to low; cook, covered, for 20 minutes or until vegetables are very soft. Add chickpeas; cook for 2 minutes or until warmed through.

**2** Meanwhile, preheat oven to 220°C/425°F.

**3** Make chickpea croûtons.

**4** Cool cauliflower mixture slightly; blend or process until smooth. Return to pan, add coconut milk; stir over low heat until heated through.

**5** Divide soup among four bowls; top with chickpea croûtons, coriander leaves and chilli. Season with pepper; serve with lime wedges.

**CHICKPEA CROÛTONS** Grease and line a small oven tray with baking paper. Toss chickpeas with oil and cumin to coat; spread over tray. Bake for 15 minutes or until chickpeas are crisp and golden.

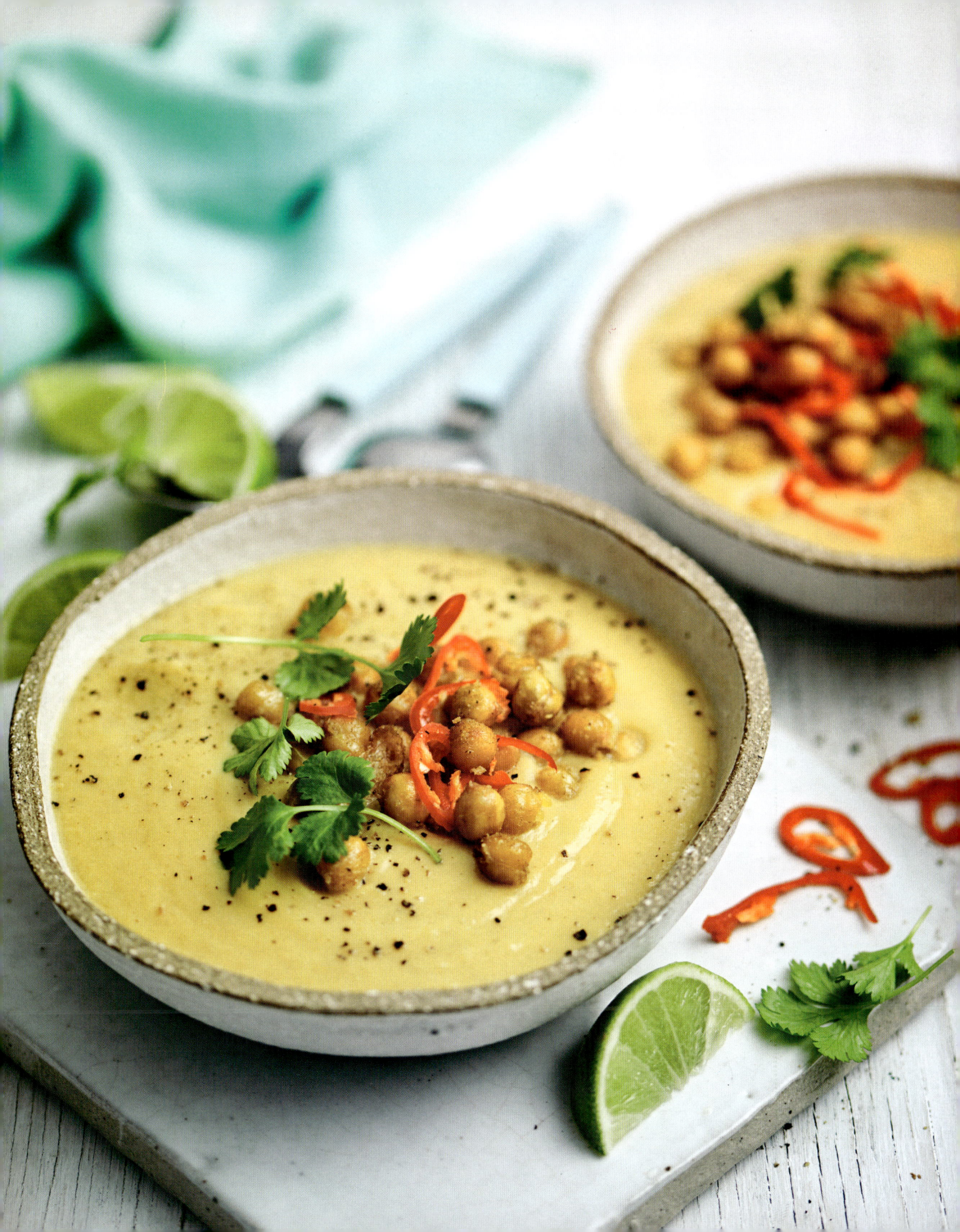

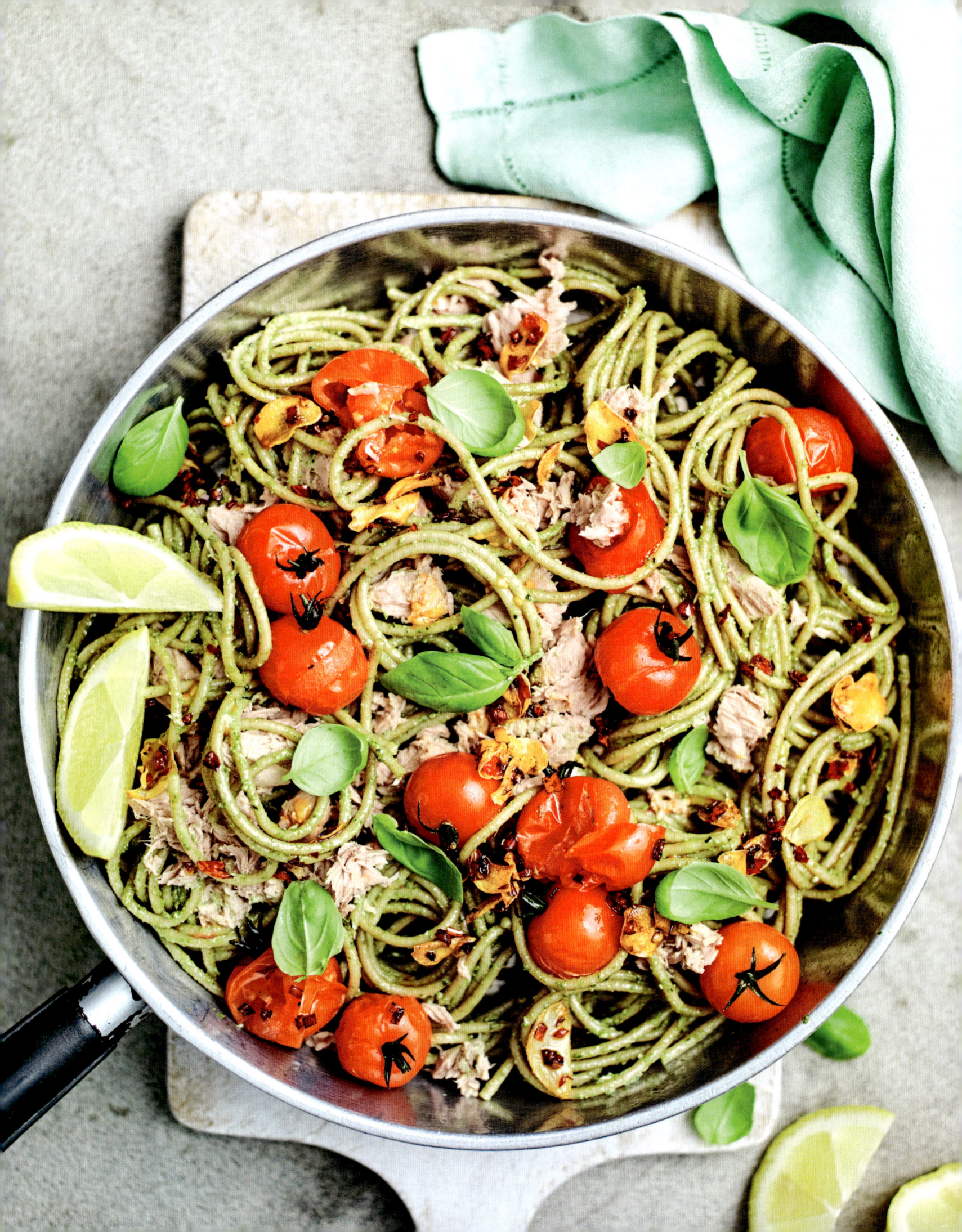

**NUTRITIONAL COUNT PER SERVING**

| | | | | | |
|---|---|---|---|---|---|
| ● 17.9g total fat (3.6g saturated fat) | ● 1983kJ (473 cal) | ● 48.8g carbohydrate | ● 22.8g protein | ● 11.1g fibre | ● 183mg sodium |

# TUNA PASTA
## with pesto & tomatoes

**PREP + COOK TIME** 25 MINUTES **SERVES** 4

300g (9½oz) wholemeal spaghetti
2 tablespoons extra virgin olive oil
2 cloves garlic, sliced thinly
2 fresh long red chillies, chopped finely
400g (12½oz) cherry truss tomatoes
185g (6oz) canned tuna in springwater, drained, flaked
⅓ cup fresh basil leaves
1 medium lemon (140g), cut into wedges

**PESTO**

⅔ cup fresh basil leaves
⅓ cup (25g) finely grated parmesan
1½ tablespoons pine nuts
1 clove garlic, crushed
⅓ cup (80ml) water

**1** Cook pasta in a large saucepan of boiling water following packet directions until tender.

**2** Meanwhile, make pesto (see tip).

**3** Reserve ¼ cup of cooking water, then drain pasta.

**4** Heat a large non-stick frying pan over medium heat. Add oil, garlic and chilli; cook, stirring, for 30 seconds or until fragrant. Add tomatoes; cook, stirring, for 2 minutes or until blistered.

**5** Add pasta to pan with pesto and reserved cooking water. Increase heat to high; cook, stirring, for 2 minutes or until sauce is thickened. Stir through tuna; season with pepper.

**6** Sprinkle pasta with basil leaves; serve with lemon wedges.

**PESTO** Blend or process ingredients until smooth.

---

**DO AHEAD** You can make the pesto a day ahead and store, covered, in the fridge.

| | | | | | |
|---|---|---|---|---|---|
| ● 15g total fat (5g saturated fat) | ● 1571kJ (375 cal) | ● 33.3g carbohydrate | ● 17.7g protein | ● 14.6g fibre | ● 306mg sodium |

# BLACK BEAN CHILLI
## with guacamole & corn 'chips'

PREP + COOK TIME 40 MINUTES **SERVES** 4

olive-oil spray

1 large red onion (300g), diced finely

1 medium red capsicum (bell pepper) (200g),
   seeded, diced finely

1 large carrot (180g), chopped finely

3 celery stalks (450g), trimmed, chopped finely

2 cloves garlic, crushed

2 teaspoons ground cumin

2 teaspoons mexican chilli powder

1 teaspoon smoked paprika

1 teaspoon dried oregano

1 tablespoon tomato paste

400g (12½oz) can diced tomatoes

400g (12½oz) can black beans, drained, rinsed

1 cup (250ml) water

3 slices corn mountain bread (75g), cut into
   12 triangles each (see tip)

⅓ cup (40g) grated reduced-fat tasty cheese

½ cup (140g) plain yoghurt

½ cup fresh coriander (cilantro) leaves

1 lime (65g), cut into wedges

**GUACAMOLE**

1 small avocado (200g)

¼ cup (70g) natural yoghurt

3 teaspoons lime juice

**1** Spray a large heavy-based saucepan with oil; heat over medium heat. Add onion, capsicum, carrot and celery; cook, stirring, for 5 minutes or until onion softens.

**2** Add garlic, spices and oregano to pan; cook, stirring, for 1 minute. Add tomato paste; cook, stirring, for a further minute. Add tomatoes, black beans and the water; bring to the boil. Reduce heat to low; cook, covered, stirring occasionally, for 20 minutes or until vegetables soften.

**3** Meanwhile, preheat oven to 200°C/400°F.

**4** Make guacamole.

**5** Place mountain bread triangles on an oven tray. Place in oven for 5 minutes or until light golden and crisp.

**6** Evenly divide black bean chilli, guacamole, corn 'chips', cheese and yoghurt among four bowls; sprinkle with coriander and season with pepper. Serve with lime wedges.

**GUACAMOLE** Mash ingredients in a small bowl until smooth.

**TIP** Making your own corn 'chips' from corn mountain bread makes this a healthier option than using regular corn chips. Each mountain bread slice will yield 12 triangles, (36 in total), which is 9 'chips' per serve.

**DR JO SAYS**

Don't be scared of including good fats, such as avocado, nuts, seeds and extra virgin olive oil in your daily diet. These foods are beneficial for blood glucose and insulin control, while helping you to control your appetite.

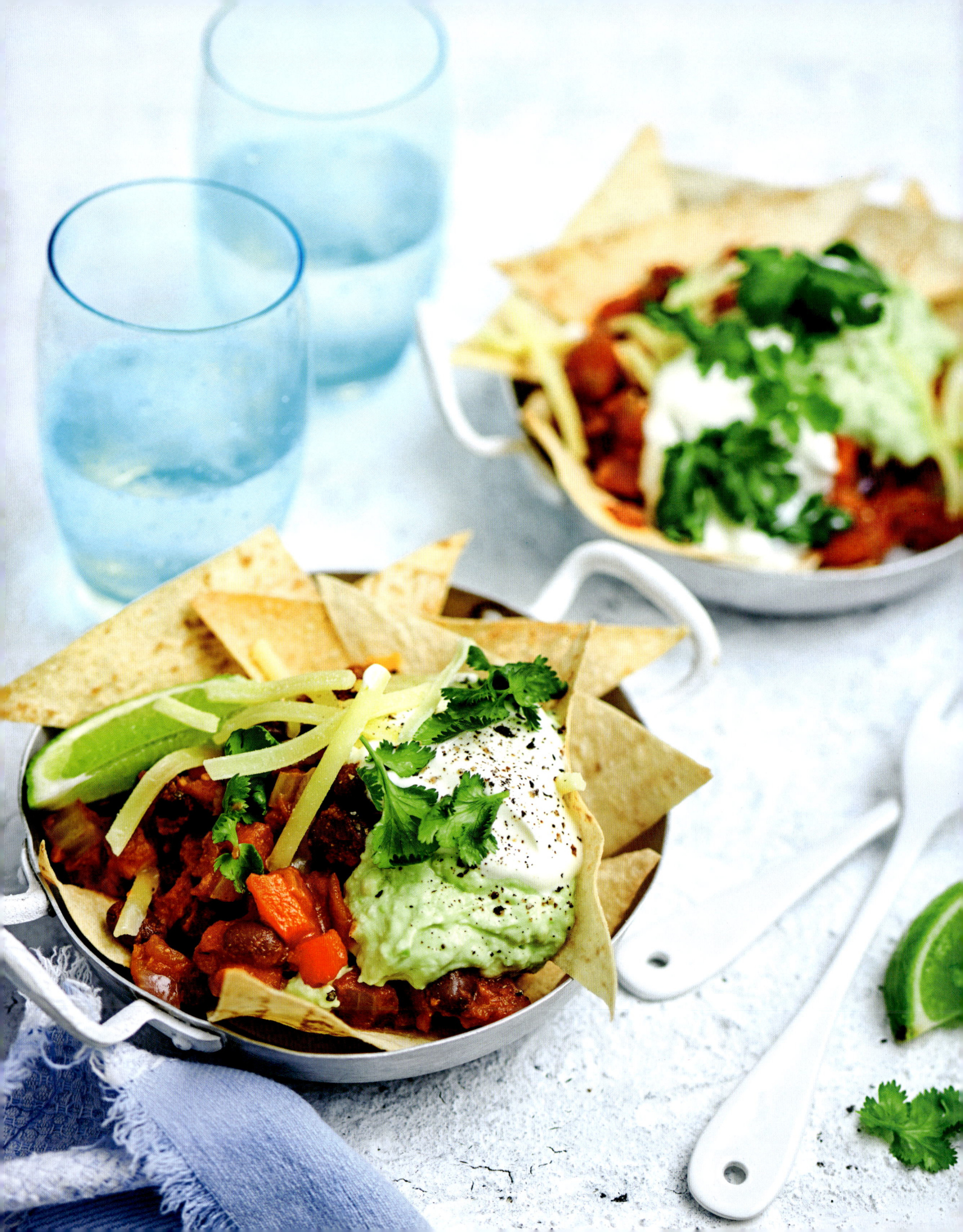

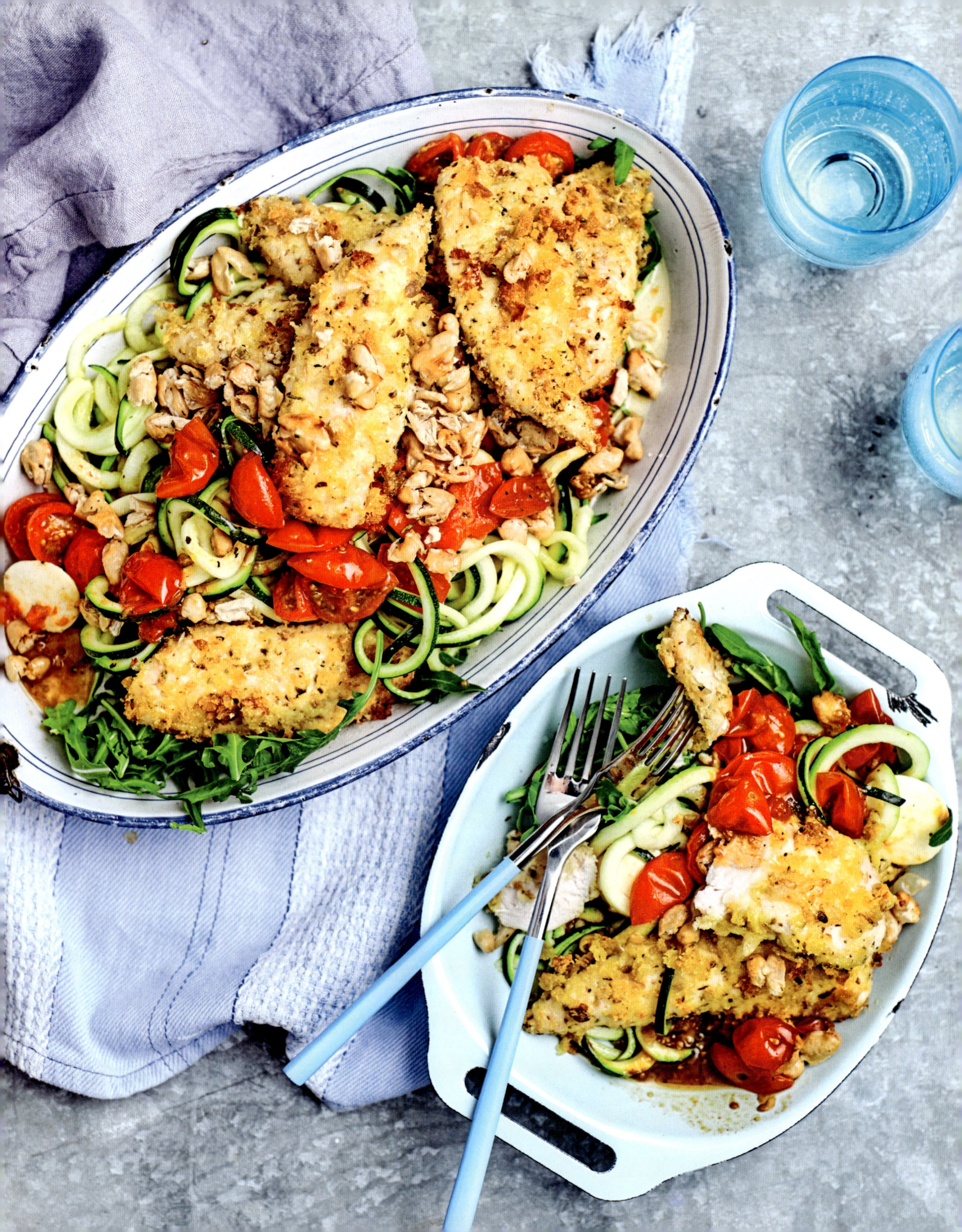

| | | | | | |
|---|---|---|---|---|---|
| ● 14.2g total fat (4.8g saturated fat) | ● 1700kJ (406 cal) | ● 27.7g carbohydrate | ● 36.6g protein | ● 8.4g fibre | ● 488mg sodium |

# Chicken parmigiana
# SALAD

**PREP + COOK TIME** 45 MINUTES **SERVES** 4

400g (12½oz) can no-added-salt cannellini beans, drained, rinsed
2 teaspoons finely chopped fresh rosemary leaves
olive-oil spray
500g (1lb) cherry tomatoes, halved
¾ cup (75g) wholegrain breadcrumbs
⅓ cup (25g) finely grated parmesan
1 teaspoon dried oregano
400g (12½oz) chicken tenderloins
1 egg, beaten lightly
2 large zucchini (300g)
50g (1½oz) cherry bocconcini, drained, halved
125g (4oz) rocket (arugula)

**BALSAMIC DRESSING**
1 tablespoon extra virgin olive oil
1 tablespoon balsamic vinegar
2 teaspoons honey
1 small clove garlic, crushed

**1** Preheat oven to 200°C/400°F.

**2** Pat beans dry with paper towel. Spread over a large oven tray. Sprinkle with rosemary and spray with oil; roast for 20 minutes or until golden brown and crisp.

**3** Meanwhile, spread tomatoes over another large oven tray. Spray with olive oil, season with pepper; roast for 10 minutes or until skins begin to blister.

**4** Combine breadcrumbs, parmesan and oregano in a medium bowl. Use tongs to move tomatoes to one side of oven tray. Place chicken on tray next to tomatoes, brush with egg; press on breadcrumb mixture to cover. Spray with oil; bake for 15 minutes or until crumb coating is golden brown and chicken is cooked through. Transfer chicken to a plate.

**5** Using a vegetable spiraliser, cut zucchini into spirals (see tip).

**6** Remove and reserve half the tomatoes to a plate. Add zucchini and bocconcini to tray of remaining tomatoes; toss to coat in pan juices.

**7** Make balsamic dressing.

**8** Divide rocket among four bowls or plates. Top with vegetable mixture, crisp beans and chicken. Drizzle over balsamic dressing to serve.

**BALSAMIC DRESSING** Place ingredients plus reserved tomatoes in a large screw-top jar; shake well to combine.

**TIP** To cut the zucchini, use a spiraliser, a kitchen gadget that cuts vegetables into long, thin spirals. If you don't have one, you can use a mandoline or V-slicer.

In a pinch, use a vegetable peeler to slice the zucchini into long ribbons, then slice lengthways into thin strips using a sharp knife.

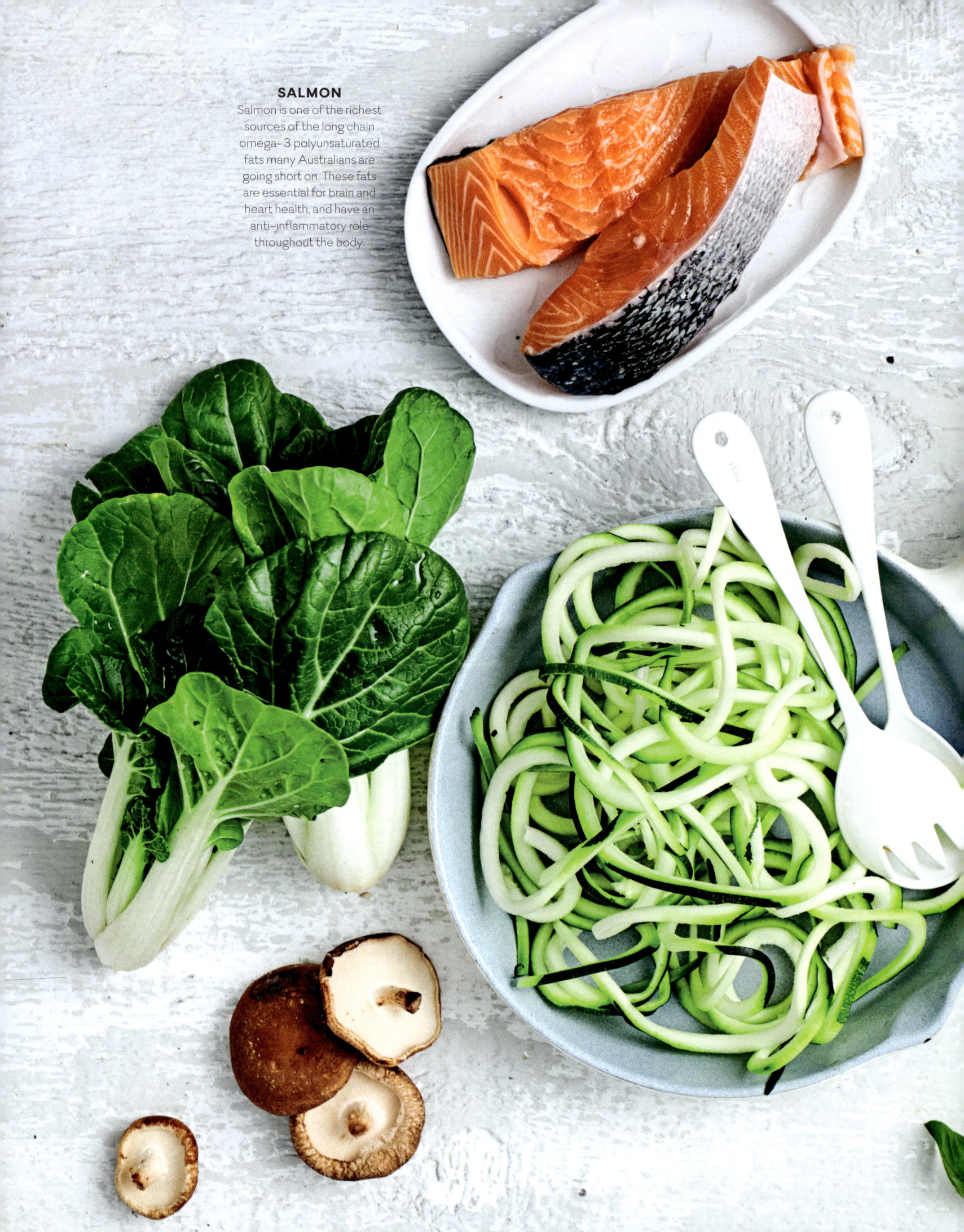

**SALMON**
Salmon is one of the richest sources of the long chain omega-3 polyunsaturated fats many Australians are going short on. These fats are essential for brain and heart health, and have an anti-inflammatory role throughout the body.

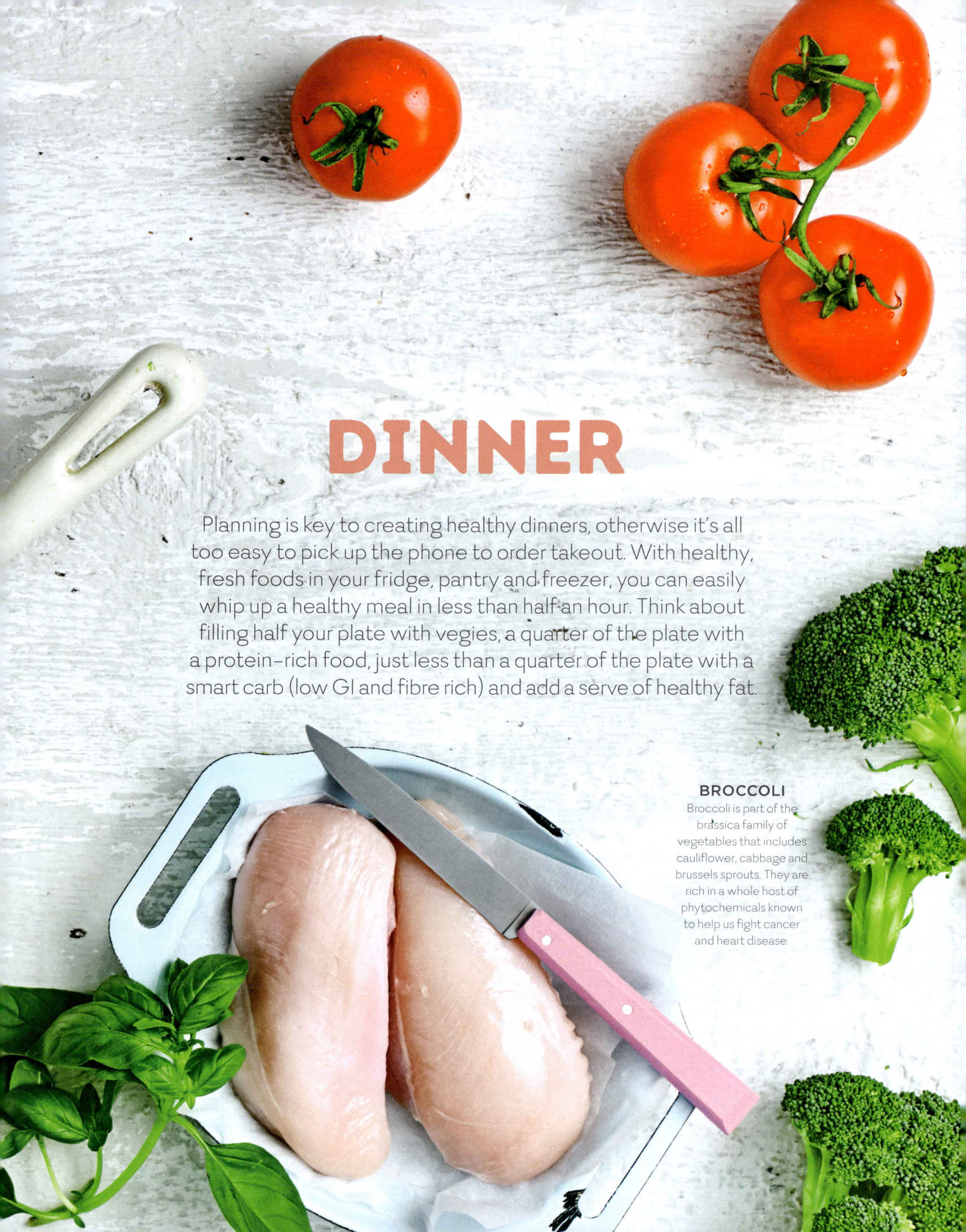

# DINNER

Planning is key to creating healthy dinners, otherwise it's all too easy to pick up the phone to order takeout. With healthy, fresh foods in your fridge, pantry and freezer, you can easily whip up a healthy meal in less than half an hour. Think about filling half your plate with vegies, a quarter of the plate with a protein–rich food, just less than a quarter of the plate with a smart carb (low GI and fibre rich) and add a serve of healthy fat.

**BROCCOLI**
Broccoli is part of the brassica family of vegetables that includes cauliflower, cabbage and brussels sprouts. They are rich in a whole host of phytochemicals known to help us fight cancer and heart disease.

| • 11.3g total fat (1.9g saturated fat) | • 1440kJ (344 cal) | • 38.4g carbohydrate | • 19.9g protein | • 4.5g fibre | • 435mg sodium |

# Fast pipi & squid
# PAELLA

**PREP + COOK TIME** 30 MINUTES **SERVES** 4

300g (9½oz) squid hoods, cleaned
2 teaspoons finely grated lemon rind
1 tablespoon lemon juice
2 tablespoons extra virgin olive oil
1 cup (250ml) salt-reduced fish stock
1 cup (250ml) water
¾ cup (150g) doongara low-GI white rice
1 pinch saffron threads
2 teaspoons smoked paprika
1 medium leek (350g), trimmed, chopped finely
3 cloves garlic, crushed
1 large red capsicum (bell pepper) (350g),
  chopped coarsely
500g (1lb) pipis
2 tablespoons water, extra
⅓ cup small fresh basil leaves
1 medium lemon (140g), extra, cut into wedges

**1** Cut squid hoods down centre and open out; score the inside in a diagonal pattern, then cut into thin strips. Place squid, lemon rind and juice, and 2 teaspoons of the oil in a medium bowl. Cover; refrigerate until required.

**2** Meanwhile, place stock and the water in a medium saucepan; bring to the boil over high heat. Add rice, saffron and smoked paprika, reduce heat to low; cook, covered, for 10 minutes or until water is absorbed. Stand, covered, for 5 minutes then fluff with a fork.

**3** Heat remaining oil in a 30cm (12in) paella pan or heavy-based frying pan over medium heat. Cook leek and garlic, stirring, for 5 minutes. Add capsicum; cook for 2 minutes. Transfer vegetables to a plate. Reheat pan over medium heat, add squid; cook for 1 minute or until just cooked through. Transfer squid to a plate. Add pipis and the extra water to pan; cook, covered, shaking pan gently, for 4 minutes or until pipis open. Add rice and leek mixture to pan; stir to combine.

**4** Top paella with squid and basil leaves; serve with lemon.

**TIP** This cheat's version of paella involves cooking the rice and seafood separately, making this more foolproof than the traditional cooking method, but still delivering a tasty dish.

**PIPIS**, a variety of clam, are sold live. Due to their sandy habitat, they may contain a bit of grit, so ask the fishmonger if they have been purged (stored in aerated saltwater for at least 24 hours to eliminate sand). If not, place them in a solution of cool water and sea salt (30g salt per litre of water/1oz per 4 cups) for several hours, or overnight, in a cool part of the house (if you refrigerate them they'll close up and won't 'spit out' the sand).

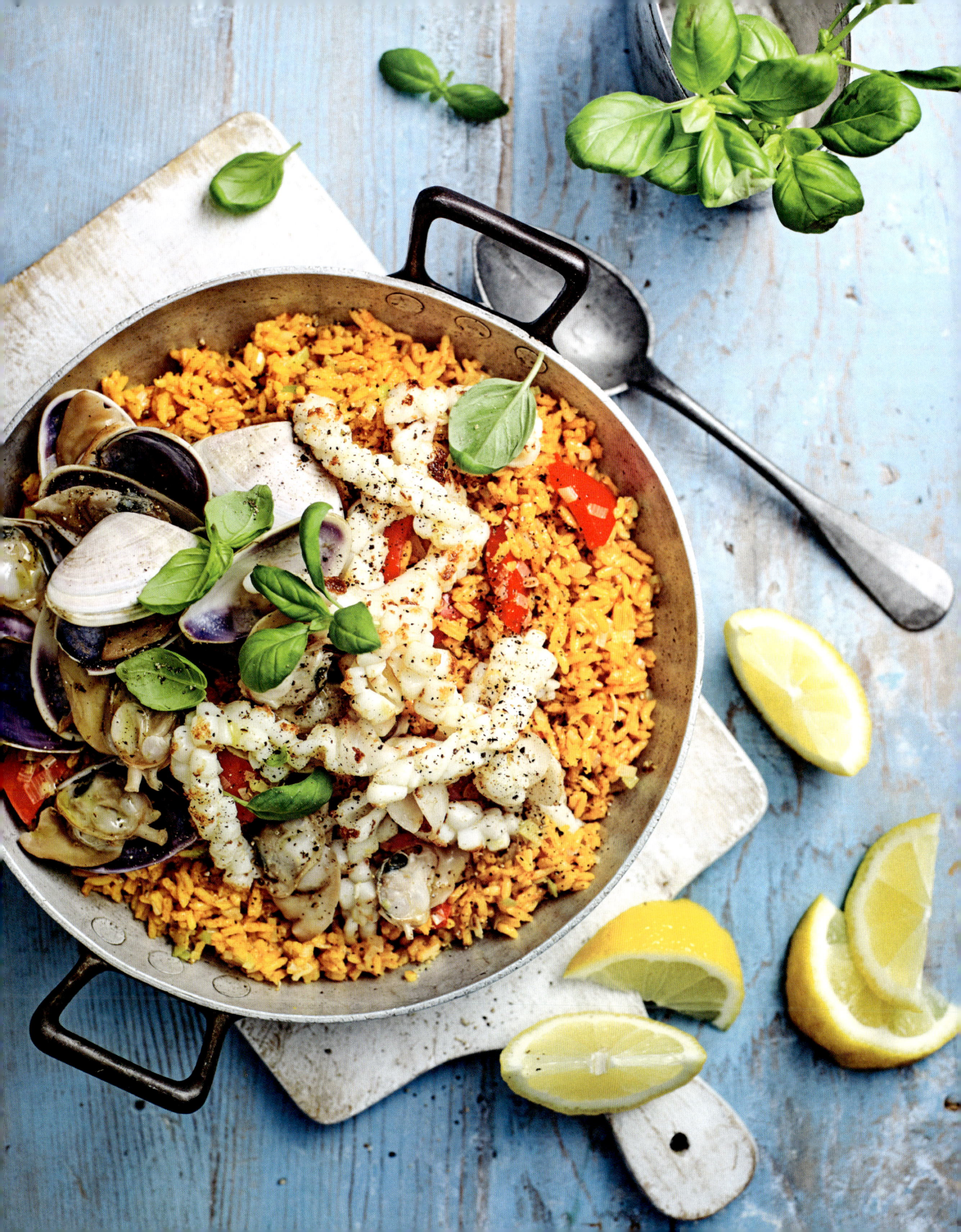

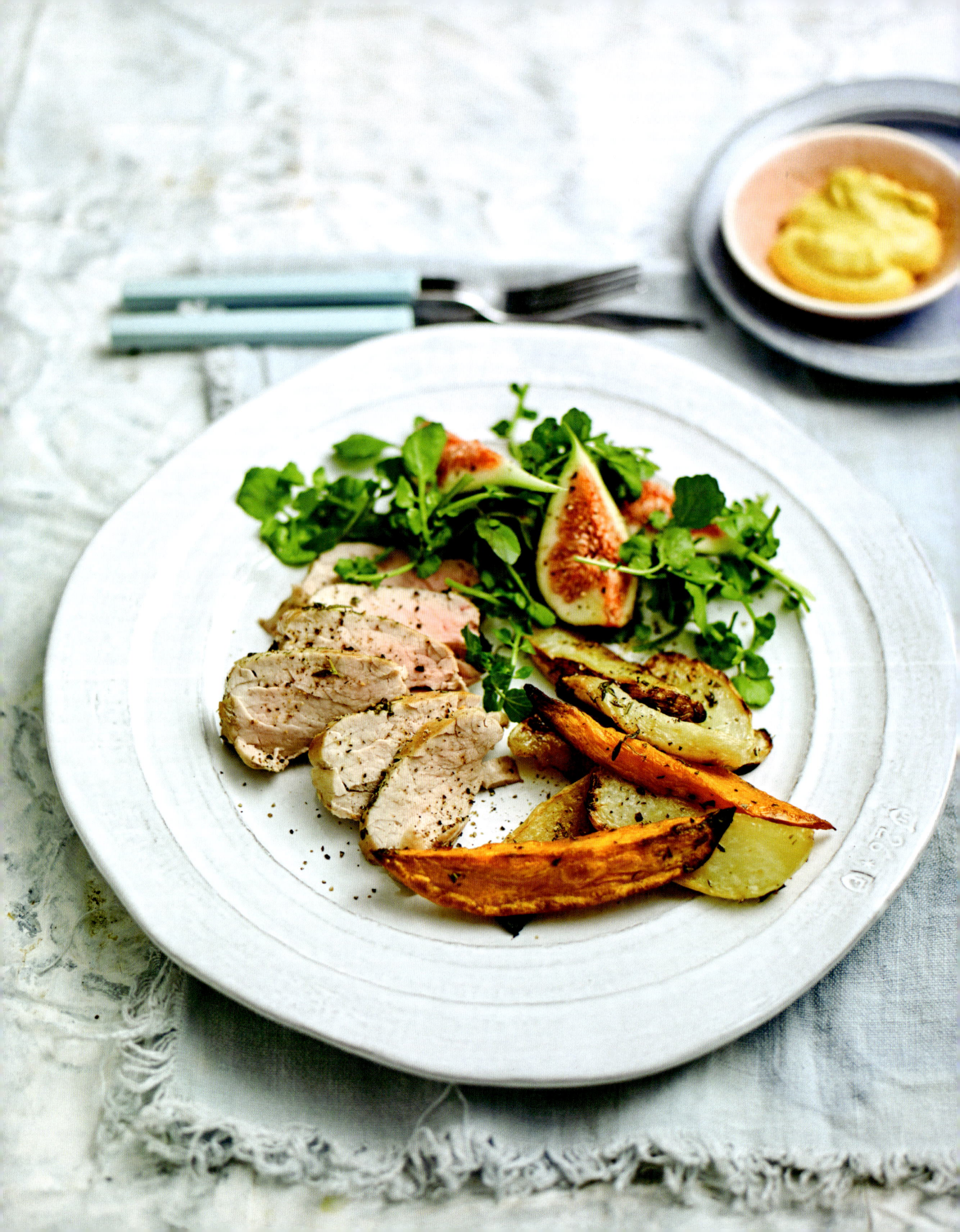

**NUTRITIONAL COUNT PER SERVING**

| ● 17.9g total fat (3g saturated fat) | ● 1828kJ (436 cal) | ● 29.6g carbohydrate | ● 33.7g protein | ● 11g fibre | ● 419mg sodium |

# HERB-ROASTED PORK
## with sweet potato & turnip fries

**PREP + COOK TIME** 40 MINUTES **SERVES** 4

2 tablespoons finely chopped fresh rosemary leaves

2 tablespoons fresh thyme leaves

2 cloves garlic, crushed

¼ cup (60ml) olive oil

4 medium turnips (920g), peeled, cut into thin wedges

1 small orange sweet potato (250g), peeled,
    cut into thin wedges

500g (1lb) pork fillets

6 medium fresh figs (360g), quartered

100g (3oz) trimmed watercress sprigs

1 medium lemon (140g), juiced

2 tablespoons dijon mustard

**1** Preheat oven to 240°C/475°F. Line two large oven trays with baking paper.

**2** Combine rosemary, thyme, garlic and oil in a large bowl; season with pepper. Add turnip, sweet potato and pork to bowl; toss to coat in marinade. Spread turnip and sweet potato over one tray; roast for 10 minutes.

**3** Place pork on remaining tray; roast with vegetables for a further 20 minutes for medium or until pork is cooked to your liking. Remove pork from tray, cover loosely with foil; rest for 10 minutes, then slice pork thinly.

**4** Place figs and watercress in a small bowl; drizzle with lemon juice.

**5** Serve pork with roast vegetables, figs and watercress, and accompany with mustard.

**TIP** Try other woody herbs such as sage or tarragon in this marinade.

| ● 19.1g total fat (4.4g saturated fat) | ● 1668kJ (398 cal) | ● 25.5g carbohydrate | ● 25.5g protein | ● 9.2g fibre | ● 64mg sodium |

# Spicy roast salmon
# BURRITO BOWLS

**PREP + COOK TIME** 40 MINUTES **SERVES** 4

½ cup (100g) red quinoa, rinsed well (see tip)
1 cup (250ml) water
400g (12½oz) can no-added-salt kidney beans, drained, rinsed
300g (9½oz) skinless boneless salmon fillets
1½ teaspoons mexican chilli powder
3 medium roma (egg) tomatoes (180g), chopped coarsely
1 small red onion (100g), sliced thinly
½ cup fresh coriander (cilantro), chopped coarsely
2 tablespoons lime juice
3 teaspoons olive oil
1 small clove garlic, crushed
80g (2½oz) mixed salad leaves
½ small avocado (100g), sliced into thin wedges
1 lime (65g), cut into wedges

**1** Preheat oven to 220°C/425°F. Line a small oven tray with baking paper.

**2** Place quinoa and the water in a small saucepan; bring to the boil. Reduce heat to low; cook, covered, for 20 minutes or until water is absorbed. Remove from heat; fluff grains with a fork and stir through beans.

**3** Meanwhile, place salmon on oven tray; sprinkle with chilli powder. Roast salmon for 12 minutes for medium or until cooked to your liking.

**4** Place tomato, onion and coriander in a medium bowl, season with pepper; mix well.

**5** Combine lime juice, oil and garlic in a small bowl. Flake salmon into large pieces. Divide quinoa mixture, tomato salad, salad leaves, avocado and salmon evenly among four bowls. Drizzle with lime dressing; season with pepper and serve with lime wedges.

**TIP** If you like, use white or tri-coloured quinoa instead of red quinoa. Quinoa seeds should be washed before cooking as they contain a bitter coating, known as saponins, which requires rinsing. Simply rinse under running water until the water runs clear.

**DR JO SAYS**
Salmon is one of the richest sources of the long-chain omega-3 fats. These fats help to reduce inflammation in the body, and are essential for heart and brain health.

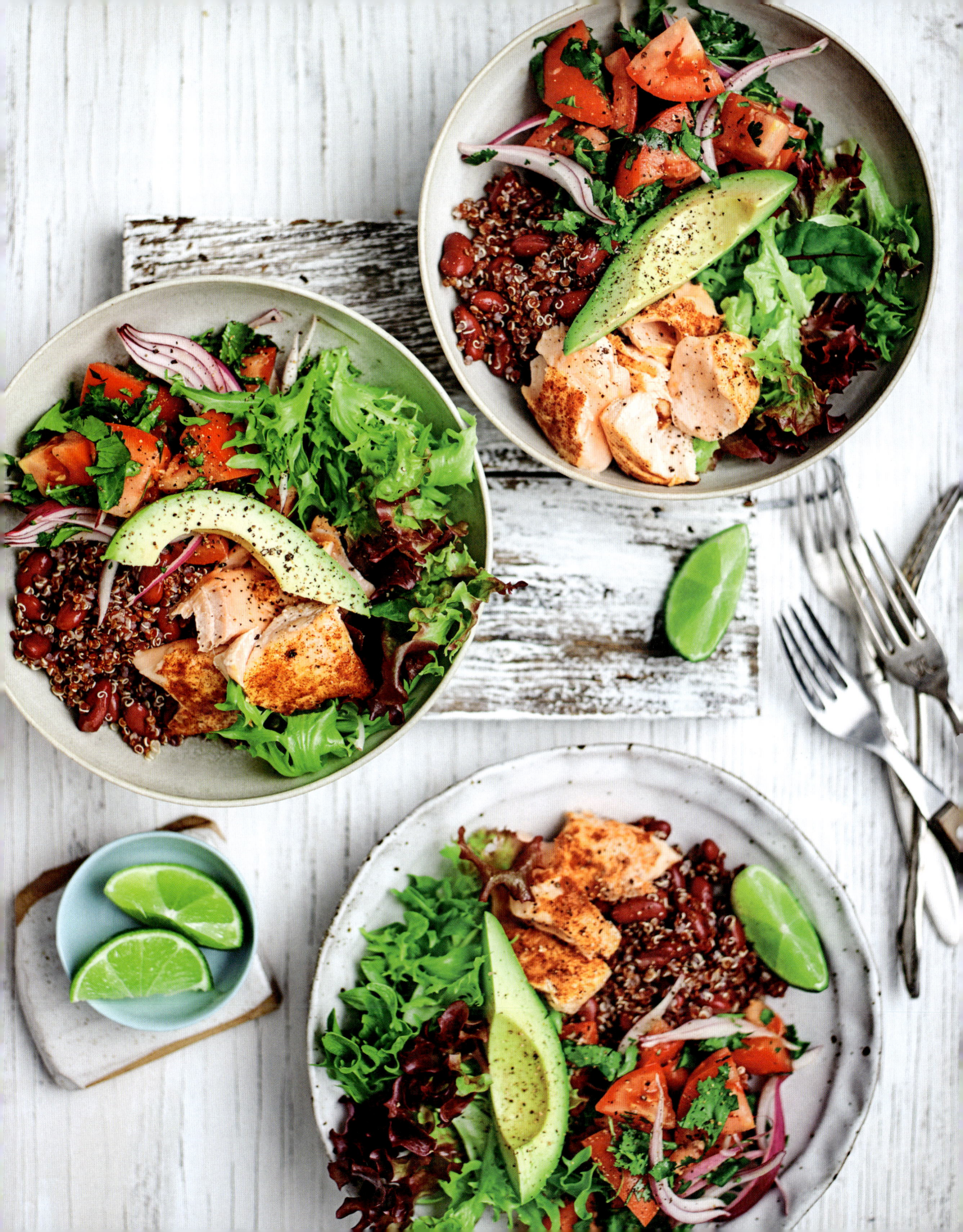

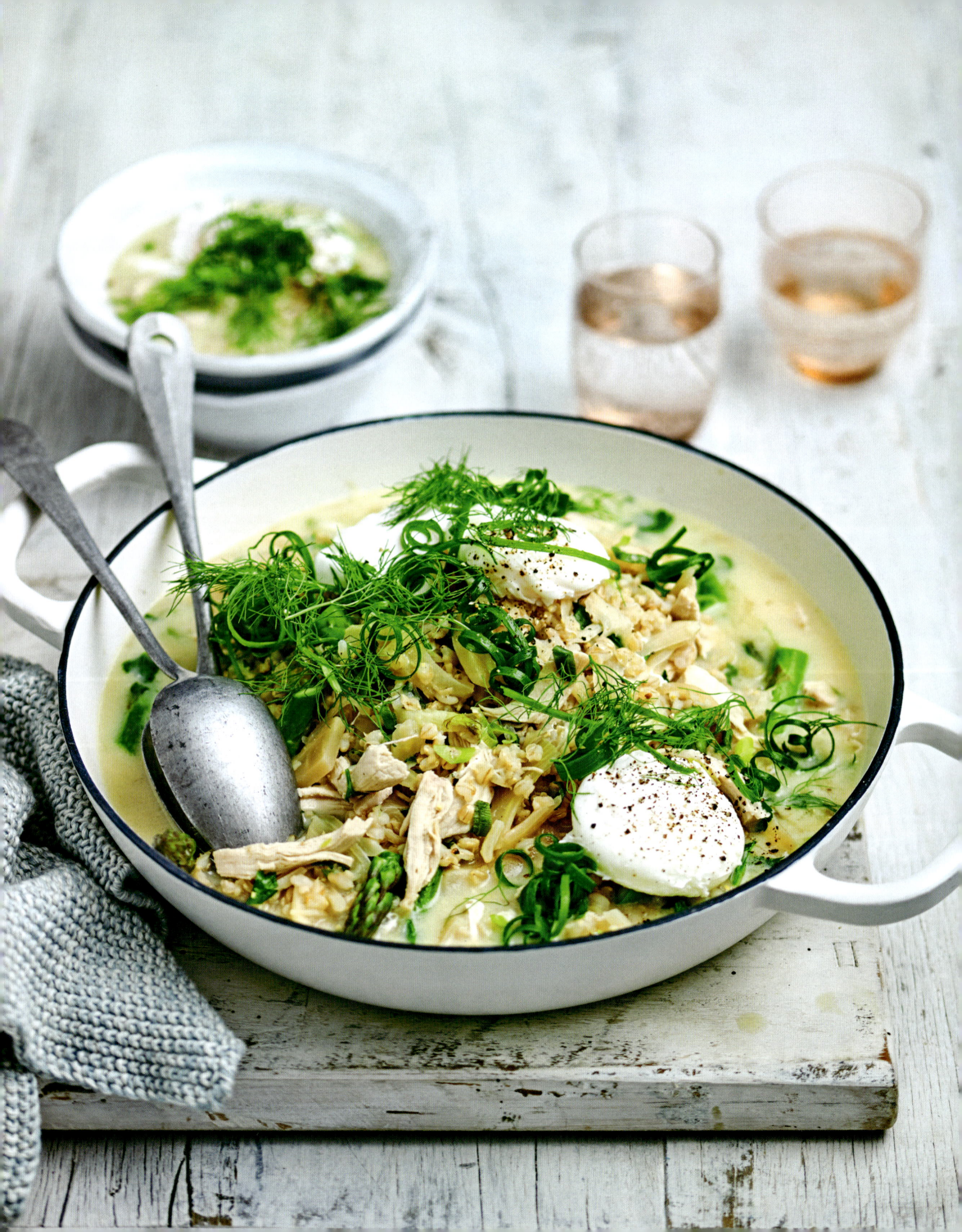

## NUTRITIONAL COUNT PER SERVING

| ● 17.4g total fat (4.4g saturated fat) | ● 2004kJ (478 cal) | ● 36.4g carbohydrate | ● 38.4g protein | ● 9.9g fibre | ● 554mg sodium |
|---|---|---|---|---|---|

# Chicken & barley
# AVGOLEMONO STEW

**PREP + COOK TIME** 1 HOUR **SERVES** 4

3 green onions (scallions)
1 litre (4 cups) water
2 cups (500ml) salt-reduced chicken stock
1 cup (200g) pearl barley
2 chicken breast fillets (400g)
6 large eggs
¼ cup (60ml) lemon juice
2 teaspoons white vinegar
1 tablespoon extra virgin olive oil
1 medium onion (150g), sliced thinly
1 large fennel bulb (550g), sliced thinly, fronds reserved
1 bunch asparagus (170g), trimmed, cut into
   4cm (1½in) lengths
½ cup fresh flat-leaf parsley leaves, chopped coarsely

**1** Slice two green onions thinly crossways. Slice one green onion thinly lengthways; place in a bowl of iced water to curl.

**2** Place the water and stock in a large heavy-based saucepan, cover; bring to the boil. Add barley and chicken, reduce heat to low; simmer, covered, for 10 minutes or until chicken is cooked through. Remove chicken; transfer to a plate to cool. Continue to cook barley, covered, for a further 30 minutes or until tender. Once chicken is cool enough to handle, shred into bite-sized pieces.

**3** Whisk 2 of the eggs and lemon juice in a medium bowl; refrigerate until required.

**4** Meanwhile, poach remaining eggs, one at a time, in a deep saucepan of simmering water combined with vinegar for 2 minutes. Remove with a slotted spoon; drain on paper towel. Stand until required.

**5** Heat oil in a large heavy-based frying pan over high heat. Add onion and fennel; cook, stirring occasionally, for 10 minutes or until softened. Add to barley mixture with chicken and asparagus; bring to the boil. Reduce heat to low-medium; whisk in egg and lemon mixture. Cook, stirring gently, until barley mixture thickens slightly; do not boil (see tip). Stir through sliced green onion and parsley.

**6** Top chicken mixture with poached eggs; sprinkle with curly green onion and fennel fronds to serve.

**DR JO SAYS**
Like oats, barley contains a soluble fibre called beta-glucan that can help with blood glucose and cholesterol management. It also has a low GI, making it a good grain choice.

**AVGOLEMONO** is the Greek version of chicken soup; it is thickened with an egg and lemon sauce that gives the dish a silky, rich flavour. The sauce can also be added to stews, as we do here, or served with vegetables.

**TIP** When adding the egg and lemon mixture, it is important to not let the chicken mixture boil, as this will curdle the egg; the egg will cook in the heat of the chicken and barley mixture.

**NUTRITIONAL COUNT PER SERVING**

| ● 19.3g total fat (2.9g saturated fat) | ● 1338kJ (319 cal) | ● 10.6g carbohydrate | ● 21.7g protein | ● 8.2g fibre | ● 451mg sodium |
| --- | --- | --- | --- | --- | --- |

# SARDINES WITH
## roast broccoli & almond 'gremolata'

**PREP + COOK TIME** 30 MINUTES **SERVES** 4

500g (1lb) broccoli, cut into small florets
2 tablespoons extra virgin olive oil
1 small onion (80g), chopped finely
1 teaspoon finely chopped fresh rosemary leaves
400g (12½oz) can no-added-salt cannellini beans, drained, rinsed
175g (5½oz) vine sweet mini capsicums (bell peppers), trimmed, halved lengthways
12 butterflied fresh sardines (360g)

**ALMOND 'GREMOLATA'**
¼ cup finely chopped fresh flat-leaf parsley
2 tablespoons slivered almonds, toasted, chopped coarsely
1 tablespoon extra virgin olive oil
½ teaspoon finely grated lemon rind
1 tablespoon lemon juice

**1** Preheat oven to 200°C/400°F. Line an oven tray with baking paper.

**2** Toss broccoli with 1 tablespoon of the oil, place onto tray; roast for 8 minutes or until browned. Turn; roast for a further 3 minutes or until browned evenly.

**3** Heat another 2 teaspoons of the oil in a small saucepan over medium heat. Cook onion and rosemary, stirring, for 5 minutes or until onion softens. Add beans; stir until warmed through.

**4** Make almond 'gremolata'.

**5** Preheat a grill pan (or grill plate or barbecue) on high heat. Toss capsicum with remaining oil; grill for 3 minutes on each side or until softened and light grill marks appear; transfer to a plate.

**6** Season sardines with pepper. Barbecue sardines, skin-side down, for 2 minutes; turn, cook for a further 1 minute or until cooked through.

**7** Serve sardines with broccoli, capsicum and bean mixture, topped with 'gremolata'.

**ALMOND 'GREMOLATA'** Combine ingredients in a small bowl.

**DR JO SAYS**
A Mediterranean-style diet, with extra virgin olive oil in a starring role, has been shown to improve cholesterol, blood glucose control and lower other cardiovascular disease risk factors.

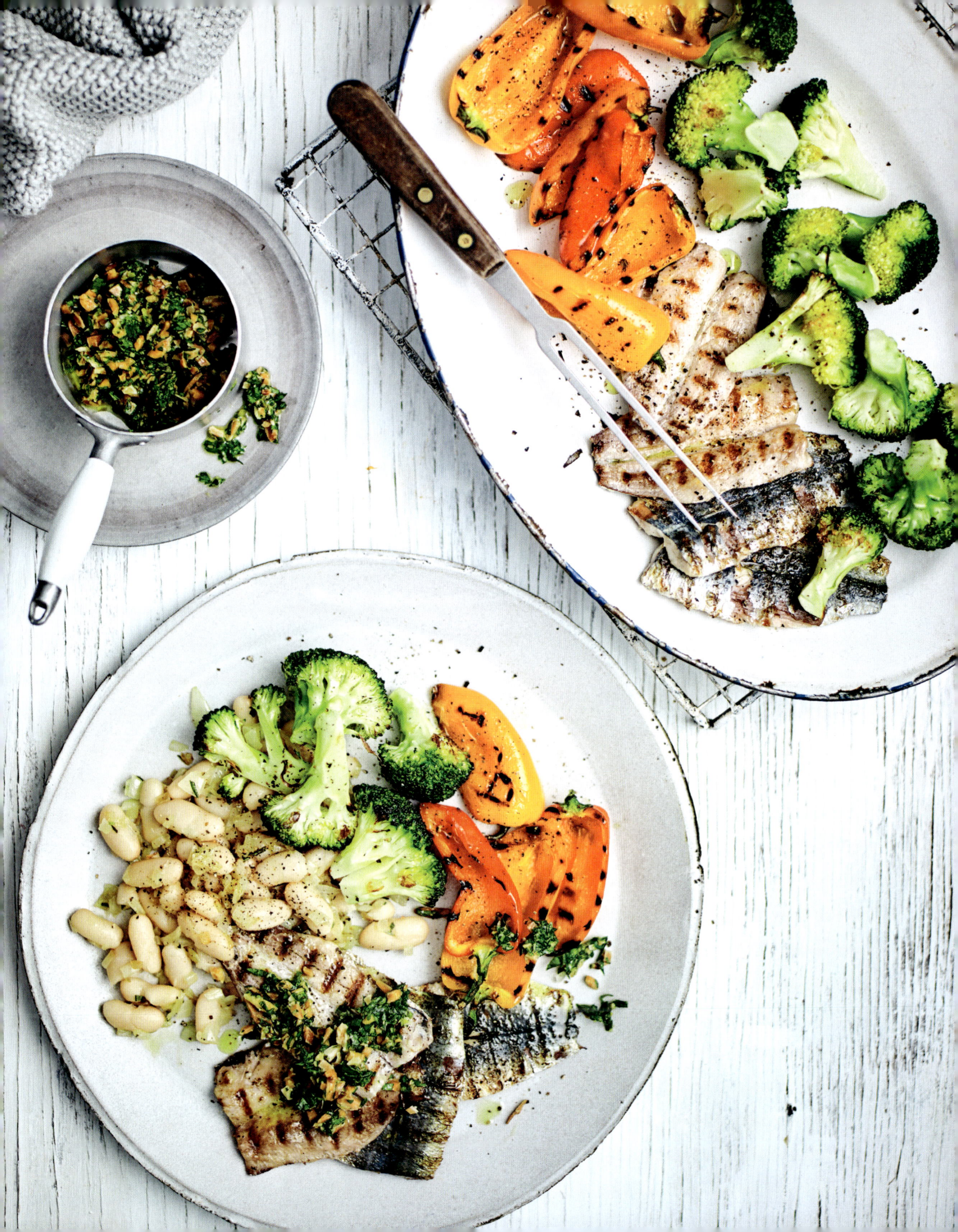

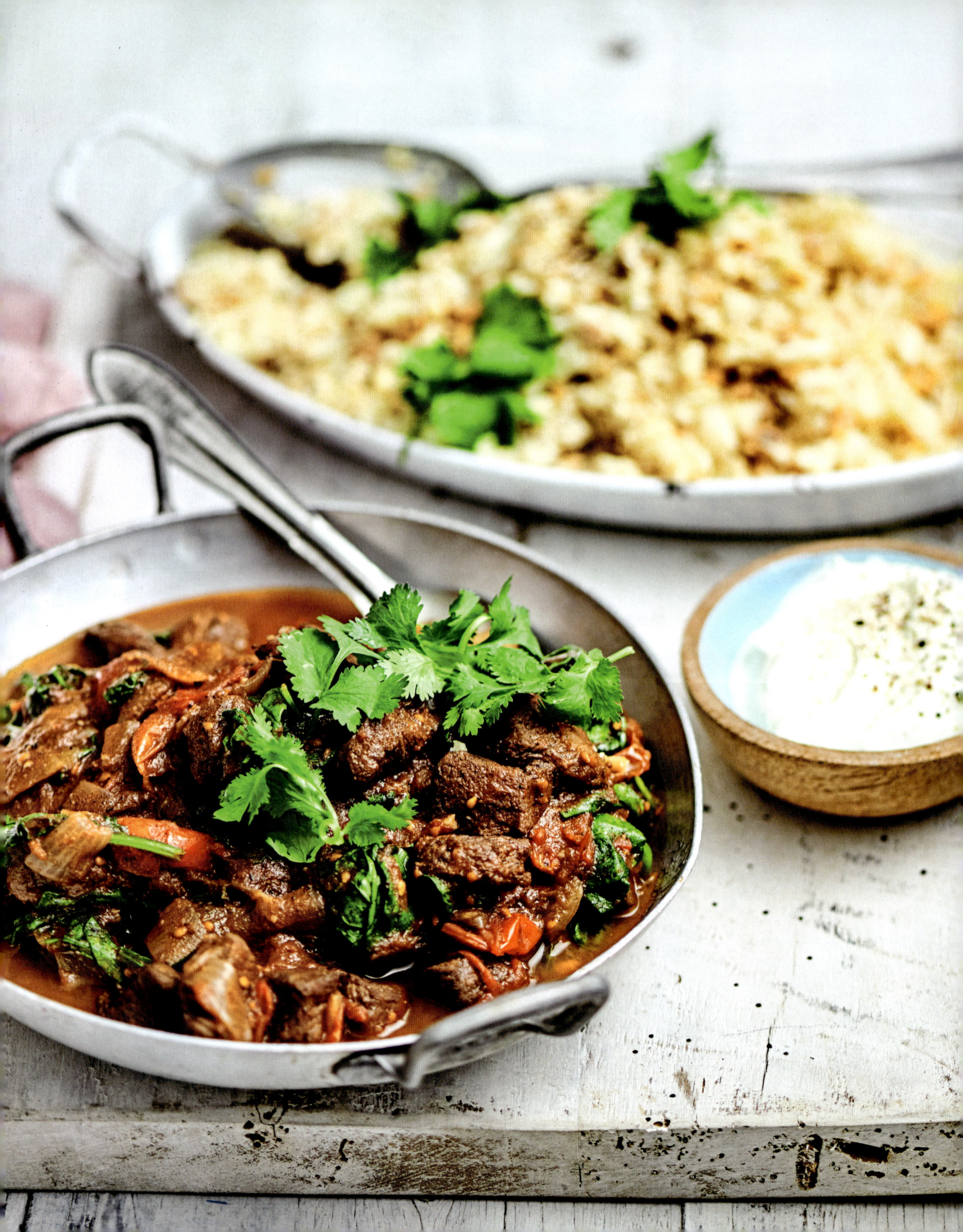

| ● 13.9g total fat (4.2g saturated fat) | ● 1535kJ (366 cal) | ● 22.3g carbohydrate | ● 32.2g protein | ● 10.9g fibre | ● 162mg sodium |

# FAST LAMB CURRY WITH
## sticky chickpea & cauliflower rice

**PREP + COOK TIME** 45 MINUTES **SERVES** 4

400g (12½oz) lamb loin steaks, cut into
  2cm (¾in) pieces
1 teaspoon ground cumin
1 teaspoon chilli powder
½ teaspoon ground cardamom
¼ teaspoon ground cloves
¼ teaspoon cracked black pepper
1 small onion (80g), chopped coarsely
2 teaspoons extra virgin olive oil
400g (12½oz) can cherry tomatoes
1 cup (250ml) water
100g (3oz) baby spinach leaves
⅓ cup fresh coriander (cilantro) leaves
¼ cup (70g) natural Greek-style yoghurt

**STICKY CHICKPEA & CAULIFLOWER RICE**
½ medium cauliflower (750g), broken into florets
400g (12½oz) can salt-reduced chickpeas
  (garbanzo beans), drained, rinsed
2 teaspoons extra virgin olive oil
3½ teaspoons ground cumin
¼ cup (70g) natural Greek-style yoghurt

**1** Place lamb, cumin, chilli, cardamom, cloves, pepper and onion in a bowl; stir well to combine.

**2** Heat oil in a large heavy-based saucepan over high heat. Add lamb mixture; cook, stirring occasionally, for 10 minutes or until lamb is browned and onion is soft. Add tomatoes and the water; bring to the boil. Reduce heat to low; cook, covered, for 25 minutes or until sauce thickens slightly. Add spinach; stir until wilted.

**3** Meanwhile, make sticky chickpea and cauliflower rice.

**4** Divide chickpea and cauliflower rice and lamb curry among four bowls; sprinkle with coriander leaves. Place yoghurt in a small bowl, season with pepper.

**STICKY CHICKPEA & CAULIFLOWER RICE** Process cauliflower and chickpeas until chopped coarsely. Heat oil in a large non-stick frying pan over high heat. Cook cauliflower mixture and cumin, stirring frequently, for 3 minutes or until just warmed through. Add yoghurt; stir to combine.

**DR JO SAYS**
Cauliflower is a highly nutritious non-starchy vegetable with anti-cancer and anti-inflammatory properties. Use it to replace half the potato in mash to lower the carbohydrate and glycaemic load.

**TIP** Coat the lamb in the spice mixture and refrigerate overnight, to save time when preparing it the next day.

**CAULIFLOWER** is such a versatile vegetable. You can use it as a 'pizza' base, or use it to replace rice in other recipes. Simply grate or finely chop the cauliflower in a food processor, then use it to make 'cauliflower rice' in place of regular rice.

| ● 20.6g total fat (4.6g saturated fat) | ● 1652kJ (394 cal) | ● 17.4g carbohydrate | ● 31.5g protein | ● 8.6g fibre | ● 566mg sodium |
|---|---|---|---|---|---|

# Lamb & pumpkin
# SHEPHERD'S PIE

**PREP + COOK TIME** 1 HOUR 30 MINUTES **SERVES** 4

2 tablespoons extra virgin olive oil
400g (12½oz) minced (ground) lamb
400g (12½oz) button mushrooms, trimmed
4 small cloves garlic
1 medium leek (350g), chopped finely
2 medium carrots (240g), chopped finely
2 tablespoons tomato paste
2 tablespoons wholemeal spelt flour
2 cups (500ml) salt-reduced beef stock
1 tablespoon worcestershire sauce
⅓ cup fresh tarragon leaves, chopped
700g (1½lb) jap pumpkin, peeled,
  chopped coarsely (see tip)
¼ cup (60ml) skim milk
2 tablespoons pepitas (pumpkin seed kernels)
1 tablespoon fresh flat-leaf parsley leaves

**1** Preheat oven to 200°C/400°F.

**2** Heat half the oil in a large heavy-based ovenproof frying pan over high heat. Add lamb; cook, stirring with a wooden spoon to break up any clumps, for 5 minutes. Transfer to a large heatproof bowl using a slotted spoon; taking care to leave fat in the pan.

**3** Add mushrooms and garlic to pan; cook for 5 minutes or until golden. Transfer mushrooms to bowl with lamb using a slotted spoon. Add leek and carrot; cook for 2 minutes or until softened. Add tomato paste; cook, stirring, for 1 minute. Stir in flour, stock, worcestershire sauce and tarragon; bring mixture to the boil. Reduce heat to medium; cook, stirring occasionally, for 20 minutes or until sauce thickens slightly. Return lamb and mushroom mixture to pan.

**4** Meanwhile, steam, boil or microwave pumpkin until tender. Drain; transfer to a bowl. Add milk; mash until smooth; season to taste with pepper.

**5** Spoon mashed pumpkin over lamb mixture; brush with remaining oil. Transfer to the oven; cook for 40 minutes or until golden, adding pepitas for last 15 minutes of cooking time. Sprinkle with parsley to serve.

**TIP** Use a sharp serrated bread knife to slice the pumpkin.

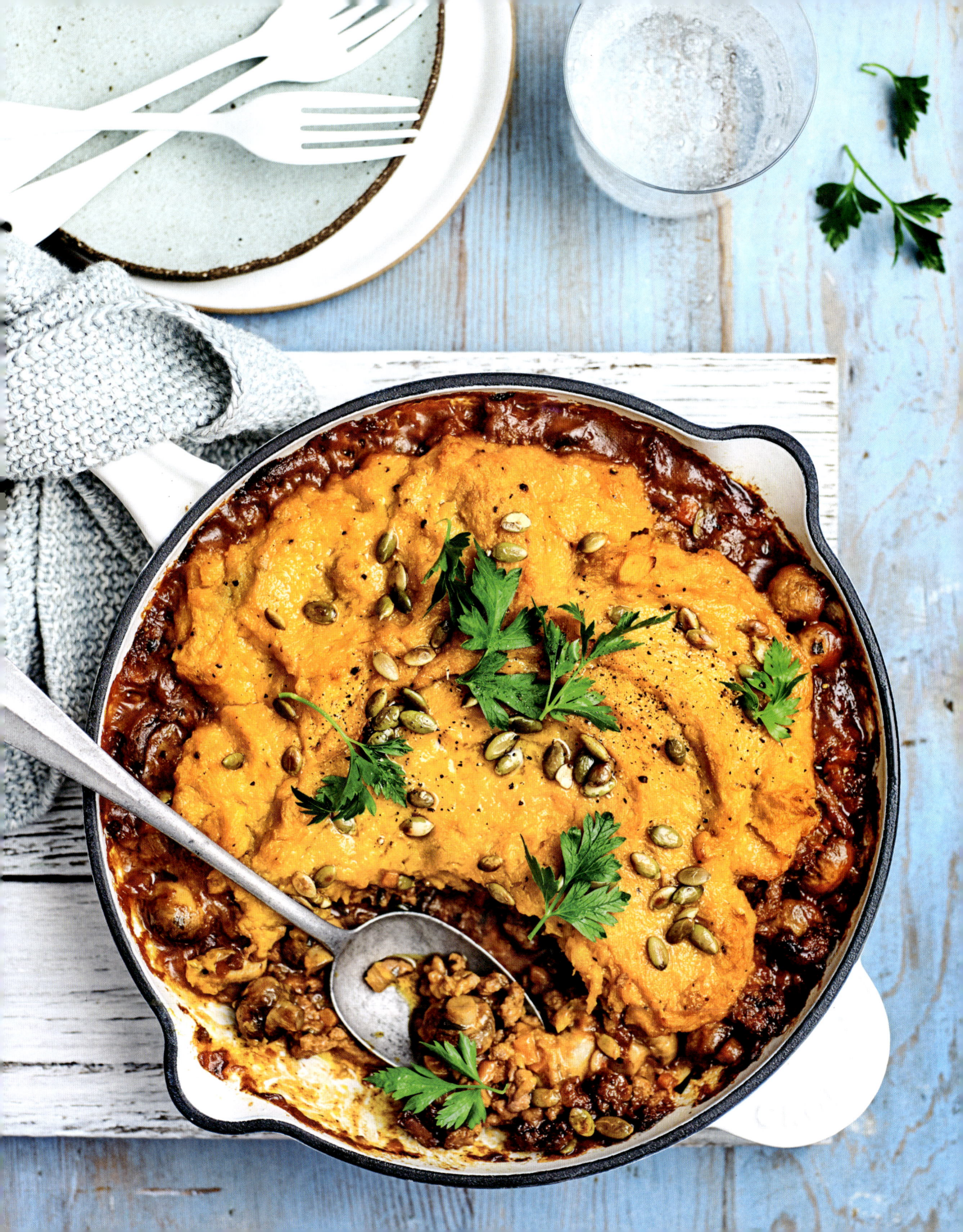

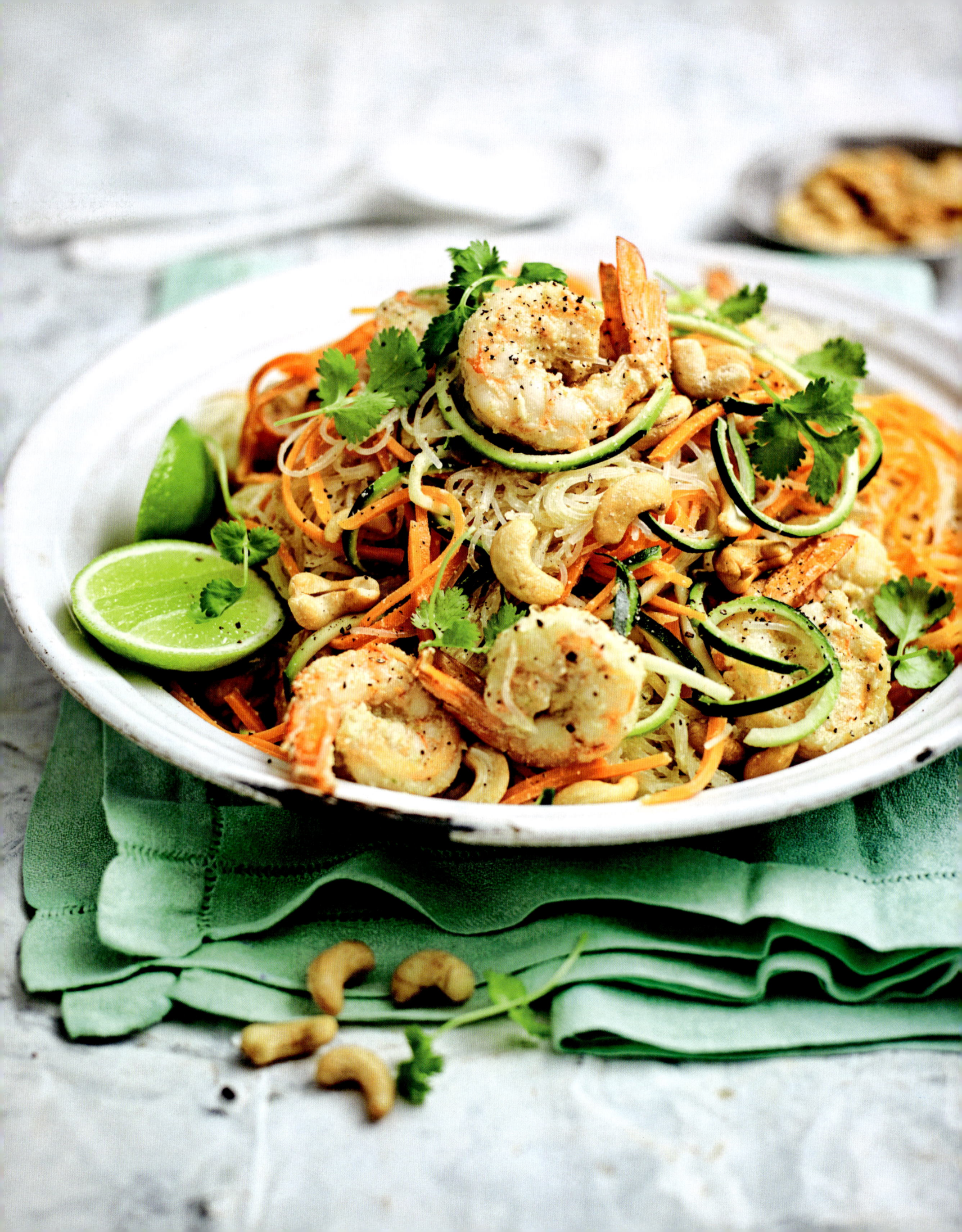

| ● 18.9g total fat (3g saturated fat) | ● 1988kJ (475 cal) | ● 44.2g carbohydrate | ● 28.6g protein | ● 6.2g fibre | ● 392mg sodium |

# Prawn & zucchini 'noodle' PAD THAI

**PREP + COOK TIME** 30 MINUTES **SERVES** 4

30g (1oz) coarsely chopped seeded dates
$2/3$ cup (100g) roasted cashews, 1 tablespoon reserved
$2/3$ cup (160ml) water
2 tablespoons lime juice
1 teaspoon cayenne pepper
1 tablespoon coarsely chopped fresh ginger
2 cloves garlic, crushed
$1/2$ bunch fresh coriander (cilantro), roots and stems
washed and chopped finely, leaves picked
1 large zucchini (150g)
150g ($4\frac{1}{2}$oz) mung bean vermicelli
1 tablespoon extra virgin olive oil
800g ($1\frac{1}{2}$lb) uncooked king prawns (shrimp), peeled,
deveined, with tails intact
2 medium carrots (240g), cut into matchsticks
2 limes (130g), cut into cheeks

**1** Process dates, cashews, the water, lime juice, cayenne, ginger, garlic and coriander roots and stems in a small food processor until mixture forms a smooth paste.

**2** Using a vegetable spiraliser, cut zucchini into spirals (see tip). Blanch zucchini noodles in a saucepan of boiling water; drain, rinse under cold water.

**3** Cook vermicelli according to packet directions until tender; drain.

**4** Heat oil in a large wok or heavy-based frying pan over high heat. Add prawns and carrot; stir-fry for 2 minutes or until prawns are just cooked through. Add cashew paste; stir to combine and warm through.

**5** Add vermicelli, zucchini and half the coriander leaves to wok; stir-fry for 1 minute or until heated through, season to taste with pepper.

**6** Top pad thai with remaining coriander leaves and reserved cashews, serve with lime cheeks.

**TIP** If you have a vegetable spiraliser, making vegetable noodles is a cinch. If not, slice the zucchini using a julienne peeler, mandoline or V-slicer. In a pinch, use a vegetable peeler to slice the zucchini into long ribbons, then slice lengthways into thin strips using a sharp knife. You can also grate the zucchini on the coarse side of a box grater.

**DID YOU KNOW?** To blanch something is to cook it in boiling water for a few minutes and then refresh it in cold (or iced) water to stop the cooking process. This keeps the ingredients fresh, colourful, crisp and full of flavour.

| ● 20.7g total fat (5g saturated fat) | ● 1561kJ (372 cal) | ● 10.6g carbohydrate | ● 31.5g protein | ● 10.1g fibre | ● 407mg sodium |

# MUSTARD-ROASTED LAMB,
## roast cauliflower & minted greens

**PREP + COOK TIME** 45 MINUTES **SERVES** 4

800g (1½lb) cauliflower, cut into florets
¼ cup (60ml) extra virgin olive oil
2 cloves garlic, crushed
1 tablespoon fresh rosemary leaves, chopped finely
2 tablespoons dijon mustard
600g (1¼lb) french-trimmed lamb rack,
    all visible fat removed
200g (6½oz) baby green beans, trimmed
200g (6½oz) sugar snap peas, trimmed
½ cup fresh mint leaves, chopped finely

**1** Preheat oven to 200°C/400°F. Line two oven trays with baking paper.
**2** Place cauliflower on one tray, sprinkle with 2 teaspoons of the oil; roast for 25 minutes or until light golden and tender.
**3** Meanwhile, combine garlic, rosemary and mustard in a small bowl; mix well.
**4** Heat 1 tablespoon of the oil in a medium frying pan over medium–high heat. Cook lamb, turning, for 3 minutes or until seared on all sides. Transfer to a plate; stand for 5 minutes. Spread top of lamb with mustard mixture; place on second tray. Roast lamb for 15 minutes for medium or until cooked to your liking. Cover loosely with foil; rest for 5 minutes.
**5** Cook beans and sugar snap peas in a saucepan of boiling water for 3 minutes; drain, transfer to a bowl.
**6** Combine mint and remaining oil in a small bowl. Add mint mixture to beans and sugar snap peas; toss to coat.
**7** Drizzle lamb with pan juices. Serve with cauliflower and minted greens.

**DR JO SAYS**
Try to fill at least half of your plate at most meals with vegies. This boosts the nutrient density, while lowering the energy density. This means more nutrition and fewer kilojoules in every bite.

**OUR CLASSIC ROAST** is adapted to modern times, but retains the perfect match of lamb and mint, offering all the comforting flavour of a traditional roast dinner, but in a fraction of the time.

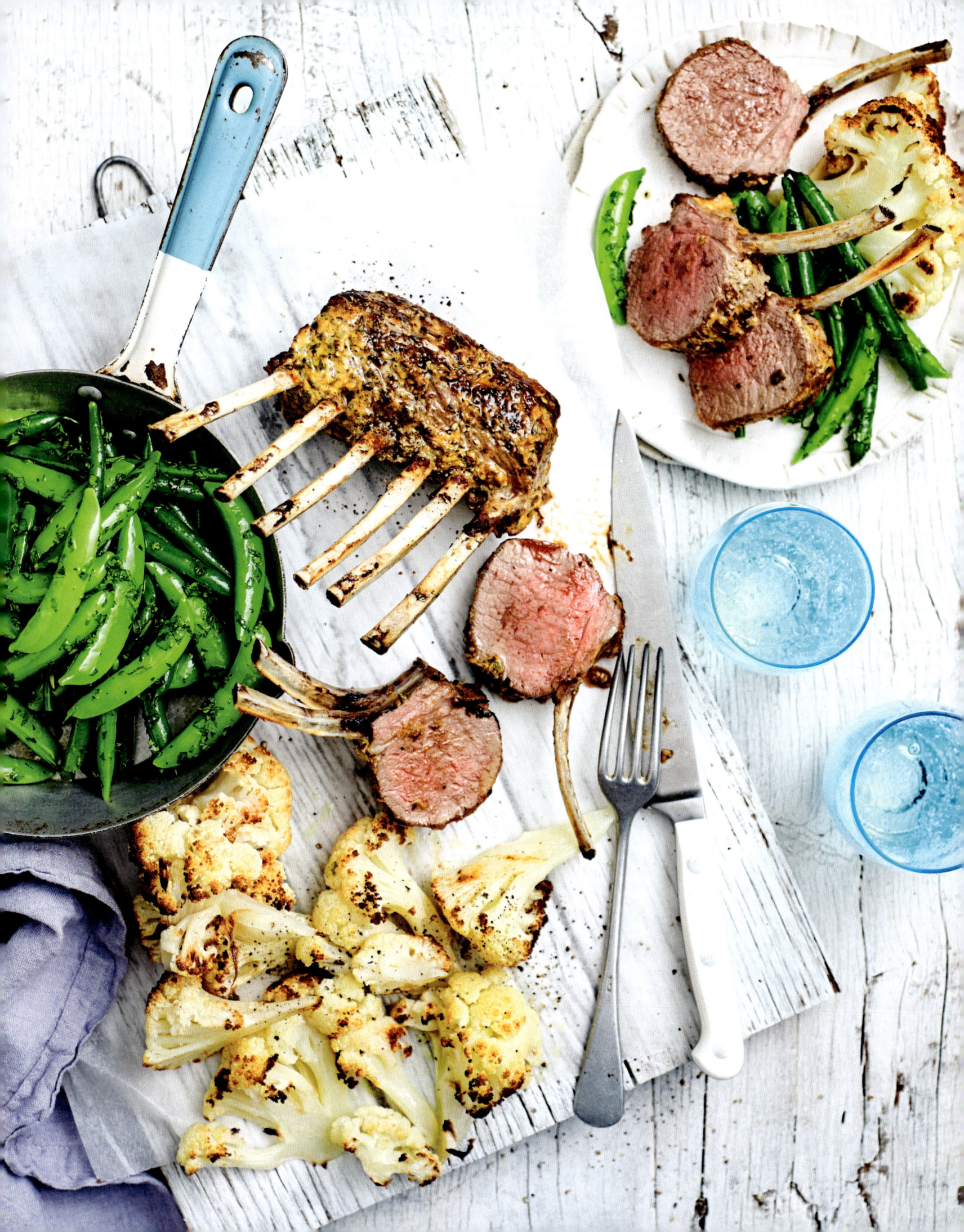

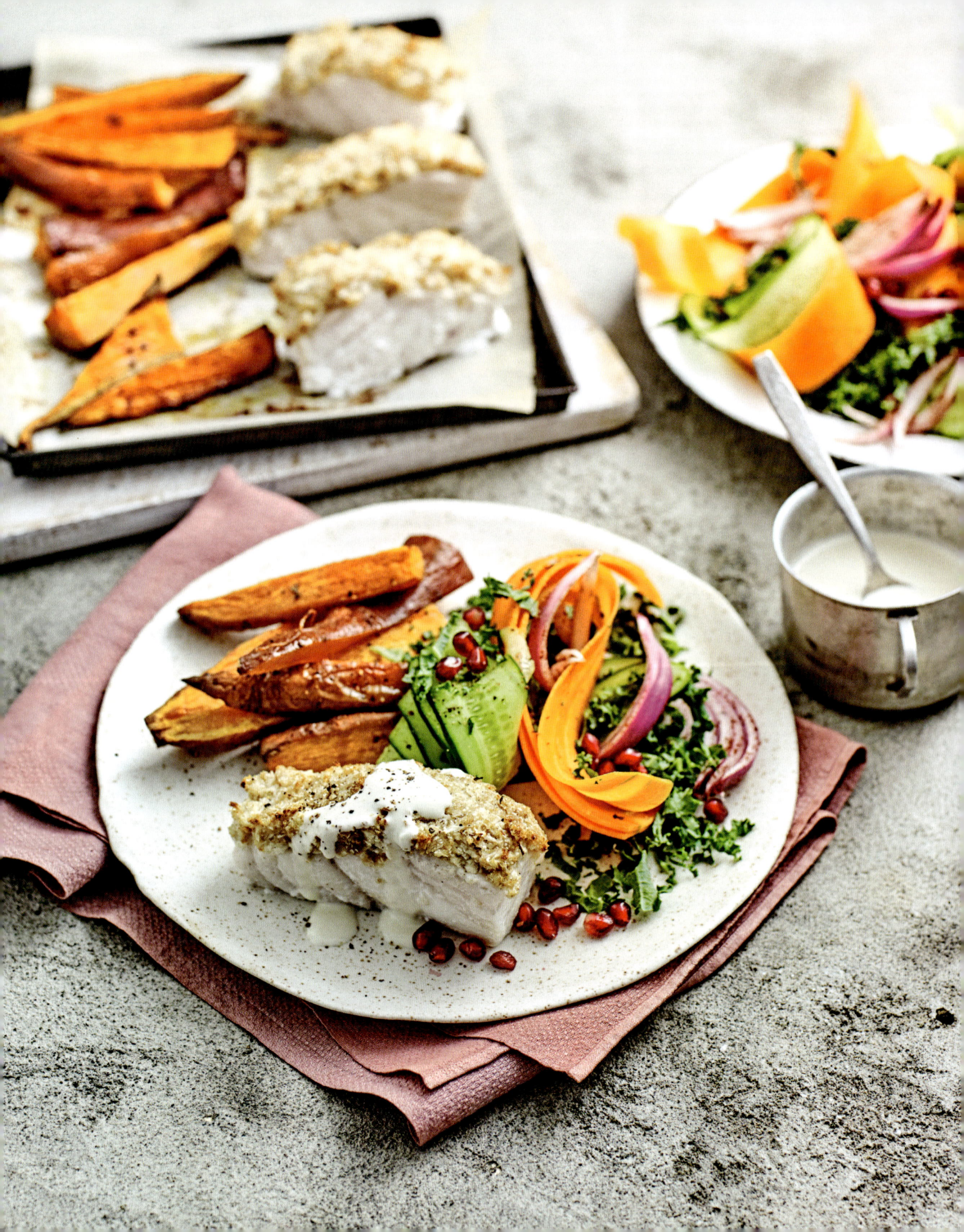

| | | | | | |
|---|---|---|---|---|---|
| ● 17.1g total fat (2.9g saturated fat) | ● 1961kJ (468 cal) | ● 42.2g carbohydrate | ● 31.3g protein | ● 10.6g fibre | ● 247mg sodium |

# BAKED FISH
## with cauliflower crumble

**PREP + COOK TIME** 45 MINUTES **SERVES** 4

2 medium orange sweet potatoes (800g), unpeeled,
  cut into thin wedges lengthways
2 tablespoons extra virgin olive oil
75g (2½oz) cauliflower florets
¼ cup (25g) wholegrain breadcrumbs
2 tablespoons chopped fresh chives
1 tablespoon finely chopped walnuts
¼ teaspoon ground cumin
4 x 120g (4oz) firm white fish fillets (see tips)
1 medium carrot (120g), sliced thinly lengthways into
  ribbons (see tips)
1 lebanese cucumber (130g), sliced thinly lengthways
  into ribbons (see tips)
2 cups (80g) kale, sliced thinly
½ small red onion (50g), sliced thinly
1 teaspoon ground sumac
2 tablespoons pomegranate seeds

**TAHINI-YOGHURT DRESSING**
1 tablespoon unhulled tahini
⅓ cup (95g) natural Greek-style yoghurt
1 tablespoon lemon juice
1 clove garlic, crushed
¼ cup (60ml) water

**1** Preheat oven to 200°C/400°F. Line two oven trays with baking paper.

**2** Place sweet potato on one tray; drizzle with 2 teaspoons of the oil. Roast for 10 minutes.

**3** Meanwhile, process cauliflower until chopped finely. Transfer to a large bowl; stir in breadcrumbs, chives, walnuts, cumin and 1 tablespoon of the oil.

**4** Place fish in a single layer on second tray; season with pepper. Press cauliflower mixture firmly and evenly over top of fish; drizzle with remaining oil. Place in oven with sweet potato. Bake for 20 minutes (depending on thickness of fish) or until fish is cooked through, crumb mixture is golden and sweet potato is golden and tender.

**5** Meanwhile, place carrot, cucumber and kale in a large bowl; toss to combine. Place onion and sumac in a small bowl, rub to coat onion with sumac; add to salad.

**6** Make tahini-yoghurt dressing.

**7** Divide fish, sweet potato and salad evenly among four plates; drizzle each with a quarter of the dressing. Sprinkle with pomegranate seeds to serve.

**TAHINI-YOGHURT DRESSING** Combine ingredients in a small bowl, adding a little water, if necessary, to reach the consistency of thickened cream (see tips).

**TIPS** We used 4cm (1½in) thick ling fillets here, but any firm white fish fillet, such as blue-eye trevalla, kingfish or snapper would work well. Use a vegetable peeler, V-slicer or mandoline to thinly slice the carrot and cucumber.

The dressing will thicken if left standing; simply stir in a little extra water to return it to the consistency of thickened cream.

| 18g total fat (3g saturated fat) | 2023kJ (484 cal) | 40g carbohydrate | 36g protein | 8g fibre | 68mg sodium |

# HARISSA CHICKEN
## with barley & chickpea salad

**PREP + COOK TIME** 50 MINUTES (+ REFRIGERATION) **SERVES** 4

2 chicken breast fillets (400g), halved horizontally, then halved lengthways on the diagonal (see tips)
3 teaspoons harissa paste (see tips)
600g (1¼lb) jap pumpkin, unpeeled, cut into thin wedges
1 teaspoon ground cinnamon
1 teaspoon ground cumin
1½ tablespoons extra virgin olive oil
260g (8½oz) cherry truss tomatoes
½ cup (100g) pearl barley
1½ cups (375ml) water
400g (12½oz) can no-added-salt chickpeas (garbanzo beans), drained, rinsed
¼ cup (50g) pepitas (pumpkin seed kernels), toasted
½ cup coarsely chopped fresh flat-leaf parsley
2 tablespoons lemon juice

**1** Preheat oven to 220°C/425°F. Line a large oven tray with baking paper.

**2** Combine chicken and harissa in a medium bowl. Cover; refrigerate for 1 hour.

**3** Combine pumpkin, cinnamon, cumin and 3 teaspoons of the oil on tray; roast for 15 minutes. Add tomatoes to tray; roast for a further 15 minutes or until pumpkin is tender and browned and tomatoes are softened.

**4** Meanwhile, place barley and the water in a medium saucepan; bring to the boil over medium heat. Cook for 25 minutes or until tender. Drain; rinse under cold water until cold. Transfer to a large bowl.

**5** Thread chicken onto skewers. Cook chicken on a heated oiled grill plate (or grill pan or barbecue) for 5 minutes each side or until cooked through.

**6** Add chickpeas, pepitas and parsley to barley. Whisk juice and remaining oil in a small jug; season to taste with pepper. Add dressing to salad; toss gently to combine.

**7** Serve chicken with barley salad, roasted pumpkin and tomatoes; sprinkle with extra parsley leaves, if you like.

**DR JO SAYS**

Adding an extra virgin olive oil-based dressing to a salad adds flavour, so you are likely to eat more vegies, but it also increases the absorption of antioxidants found in both the oil and the vegies.

**TIPS** Use 8 chicken tenderloins instead of cutting the breast fillets, if preferred.
Harissa is a very hot paste; there are many different brands available on the market, and the strengths vary enormously. However, if you have a low heat-level tolerance, you may find this, and any other recipe containing harissa, too hot to tolerate, even if you reduce the amount used. Substitute with a mild chilli sauce, or sprinkle the chicken with a pinch of chilli flakes, if you like.

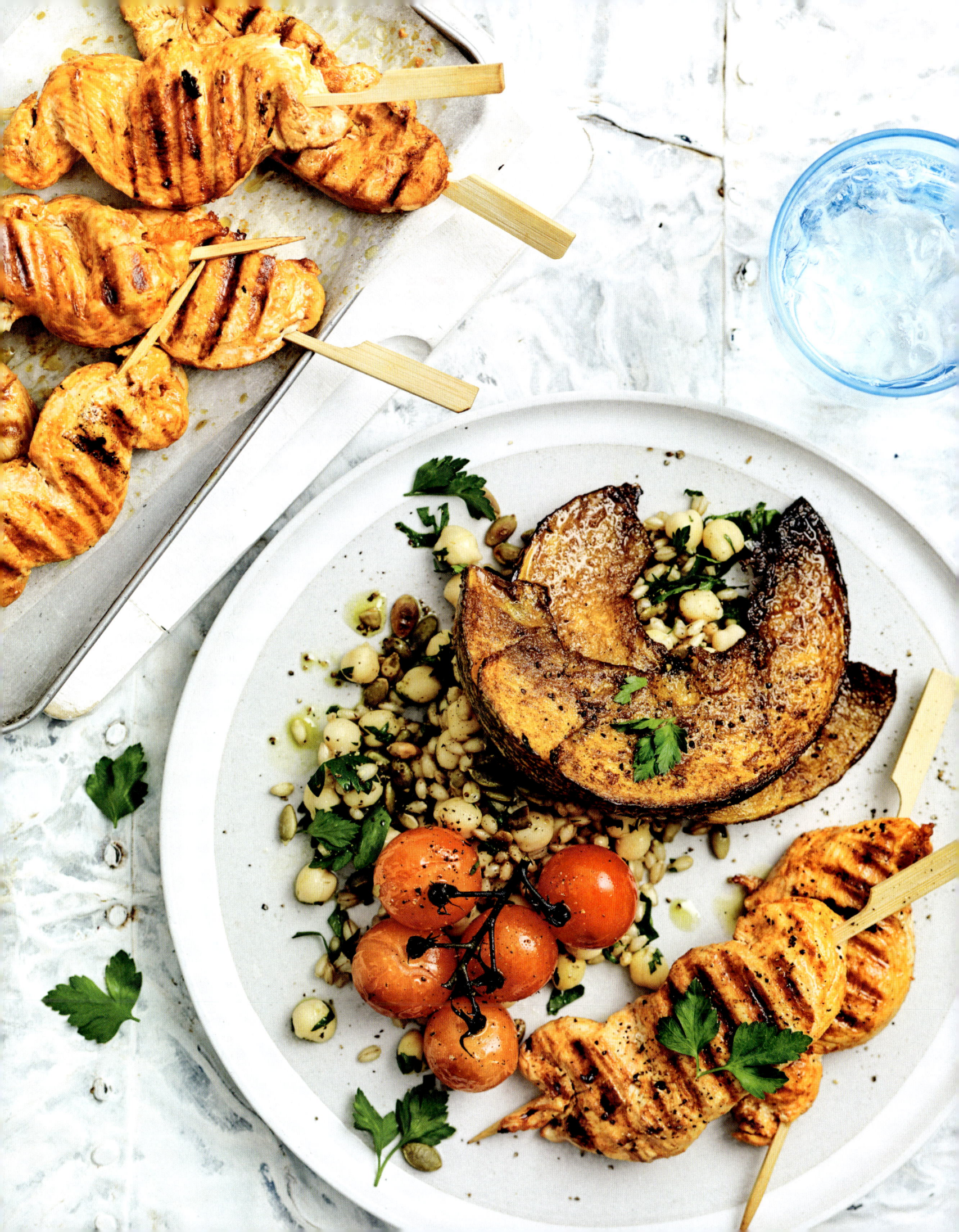

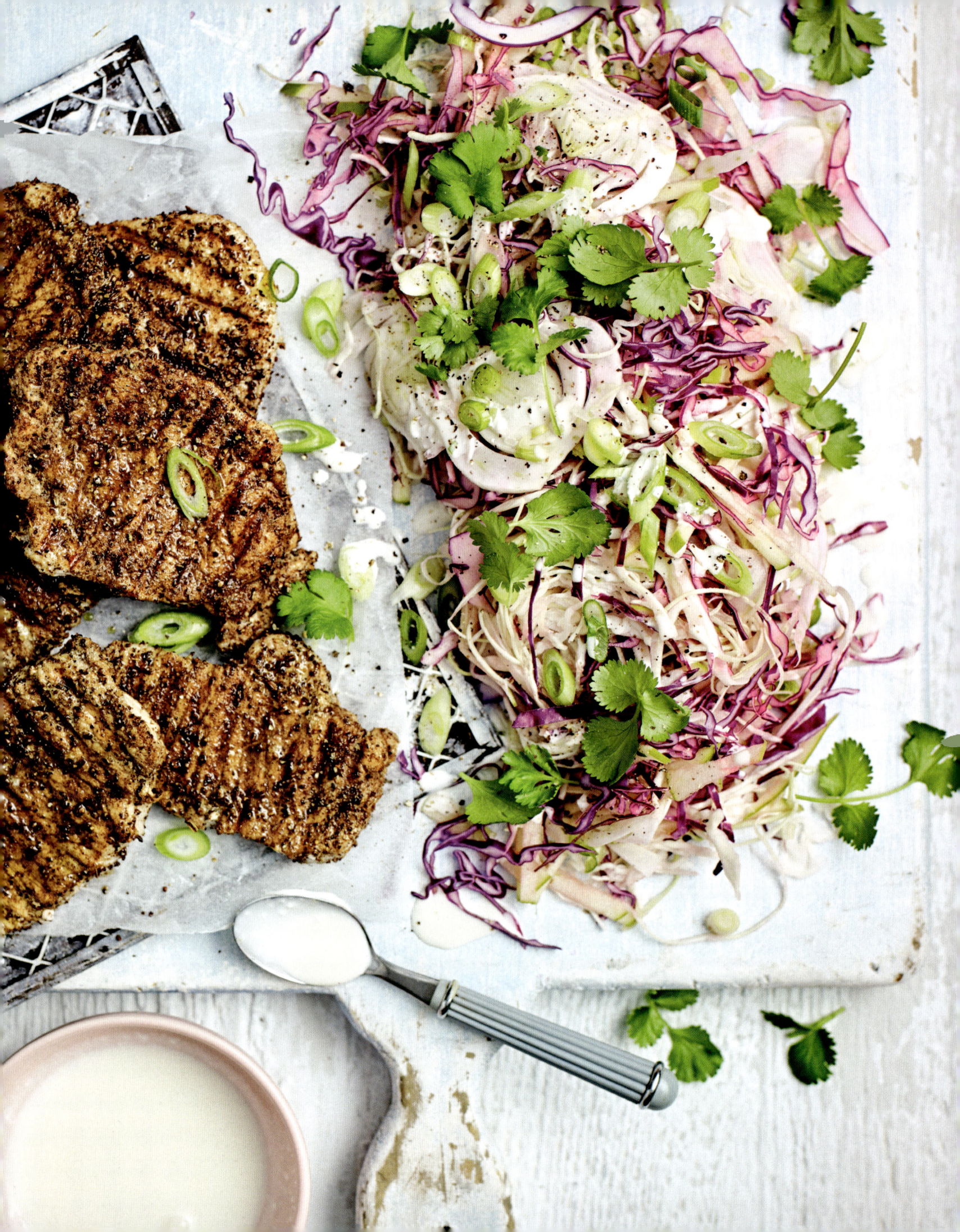

**NUTRITIONAL COUNT PER SERVING**

| | | | | | |
|---|---|---|---|---|---|
| 6.4g total fat (1.2g saturated fat) | 943kJ (225 cal) | 10.6g carbohydrate | 29g protein | 3.6g fibre | 156mg sodium |

# FENNEL-RUBBED PORK
## with fennel & apple slaw

**PREP + COOK TIME** 30 MINUTES **SERVES** 4

2 tablespoons fennel seeds

600g (1¼lb) pork loin steaks, fat trimmed, flattened into a 1cm (½in) thickness

**FENNEL & APPLE SLAW**

1 medium green apple (150g)

1 cup (80g) finely shredded red cabbage

1 cup (80g) finely shredded green cabbage

1 baby fennel bulb (130g), sliced thinly (see tip)

4 green onions (scallions), chopped finely

½ cup fresh coriander (cilantro) leaves

2 tablespoons whole-egg mayonnaise with olive oil

2 tablespoons apple cider vinegar

**1** Heat a small frying pan over high heat. Dry-fry fennel seeds for 2 minutes or until aromatic. Finely crush with a mortar and pestle or a spice grinder.

**2** Coat pork in fennel; season with pepper. Heat an oiled grill pan (or grill plate or barbecue) over high heat. Cook pork for 5 minutes each side or until golden and cooked through. Cover loosely with foil; rest for 5 minutes.

**3** Meanwhile, make fennel and apple slaw.

**4** Serve pork with fennel and apple slaw.

**FENNEL & APPLE SLAW** Core and cut apple into matchsticks. Combine cabbage, fennel, apple, onion and coriander in a large bowl. Toss through combined mayonnaise and vinegar; season with pepper.

**TIP** Use a mandoline or V-slicer, if you have one, to shave the fennel as thinly as possible.

**DR JO SAYS**

Eating an apple a day is good for heart health, with research showing a positive effect on blood cholesterol control. Apples have also been shown to reduce the risk of type 2 diabetes.

NUTRITIONAL COUNT PER SERVING

| 13.2g total fat (3.5g saturated fat) | 1378kJ (329 cal) | 10.3g carbohydrate | 35.7g protein | 7.8g fibre | 110mg sodium |

# CUMIN-SPICED STEAK
## with white bean hummus

**PREP + COOK TIME** 35 MINUTES **SERVES** 4

1½ tablespoons sunflower seeds

2 teaspoons pepitas (pumpkin seed kernels)

1 tablespoon cumin seeds

500g (1lb) beef fillet steaks

olive–oil spray

2 bunches broccolini (350g)

**WHITE BEAN HUMMUS**

400g (12½oz) can cannellini beans, drained, rinsed

1 clove garlic, crushed

2 teaspoons ground cumin

1 tablespoon tahini

½ cup fresh flat–leaf parsley leaves

2 tablespoons lemon juice

2 tablespoons water

**1** Make white bean hummus.

**2** Dry–fry sunflower seeds, pepitas and cumin seeds in a small heavy–based frying pan over medium heat for 2 minutes or until golden and aromatic. Using a mortar and pestle or spice grinder, coarsely grind seed mixture. Reserve 1 tablespoon for serving.

**3** Heat a grill plate (or grill pan or barbecue) over high heat. Coat steaks evenly in seed mixture, spray lightly with oil; cook steaks for 5 minutes each side for medium or until cooked to your liking. Cover loosely with foil; rest for 5 minutes.

**4** Meanwhile, boil, steam or microwave broccolini until just tender; drain.

**5** Slice steaks into thick slices across the grain. Serve steak, broccolini and hummus sprinkled with reserved seed mixture.

**WHITE BEAN HUMMUS** Process ingredients until smooth; season with pepper to taste.

**TIP** White bean hummus can be made up to 3 days ahead and stored in an airtight container in the fridge.

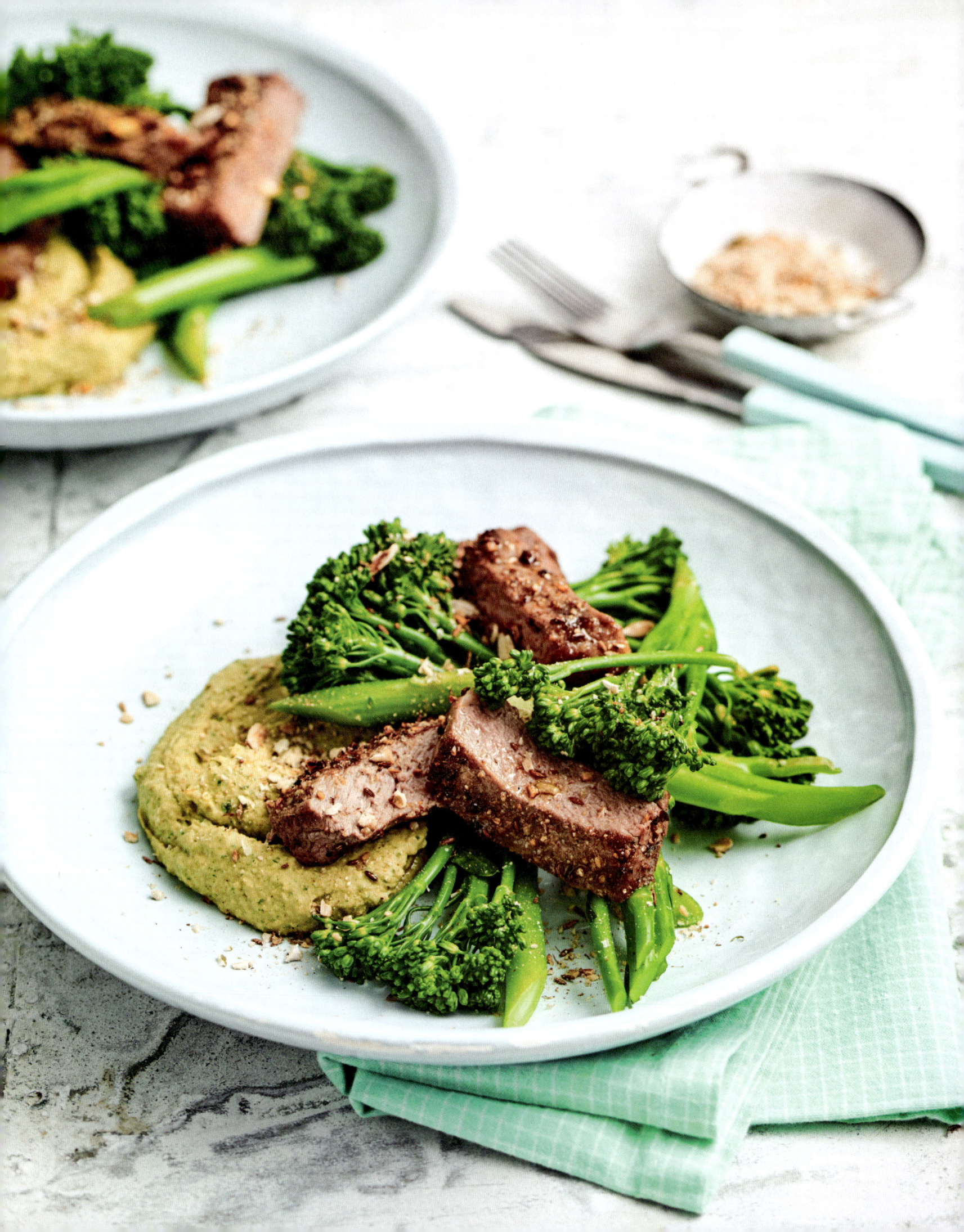

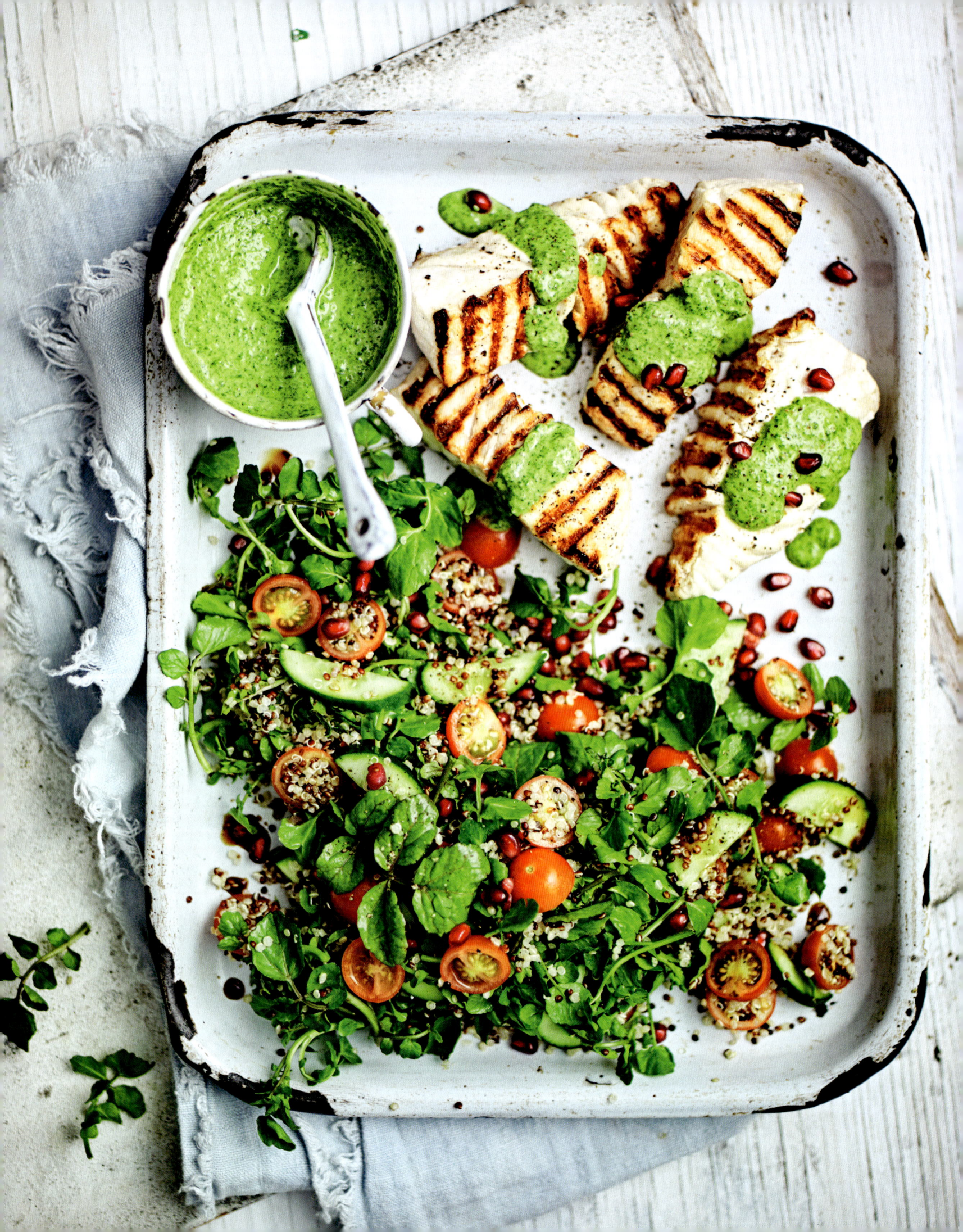

| 12.1g total fat (2.1g saturated fat) | 1731kJ (413 cal) | 36.5g carbohydrate | 34.5g protein | 9.8g fibre | 323mg sodium |

# FISH & QUINOA SALAD
## with green hummus

**PREP + COOK TIME** 35 MINUTES **SERVES** 4

$2/3$ cup (135g) tri-coloured quinoa, rinsed well (see tips)

$1\frac{1}{4}$ cups (310ml) water

500g (1lb) skinless boneless blue-eye trevalla fillets (see tips)

2 teaspoons olive oil

1 cup fresh flat-leaf parsley leaves, chopped coarsely

1 cup fresh coriander (cilantro) leaves, chopped coarsely

1 cup fresh mint leaves, chopped coarsely

1 teaspoon ground sumac

2 fresh long green chillies, seeded, chopped finely

$\frac{1}{2}$ cup (130g) hummus

$1\frac{1}{2}$ tablespoons water

$\frac{1}{4}$ cup (60ml) lemon juice

200g ($6\frac{1}{2}$oz) trimmed watercress

200g ($6\frac{1}{2}$oz) cherry tomatoes, halved

1 small lebanese cucumber (100g), halved lengthways, sliced thinly

$1/3$ cup (50g) pomegranate seeds

1 tablespoon pomegranate molasses

**1** Place quinoa and the water in a medium saucepan over high heat, cover; bring to the boil. Reduce heat to low; cook, covered, for 10 minutes. Stand, covered, for 10 minutes.

**2** Meanwhile, preheat a grill plate (or grill pan or barbecue) on high. Brush fish with oil; cook for 3 minutes each side or until just cooked through. (The cooking time will depend on the thickness of the fish.) Transfer fish to a plate; cover loosely with foil.

**3** To make green hummus, process parsley, coriander, mint, sumac, chilli, hummus, the water and half the lemon juice until smooth.

**4** Place quinoa, watercress, tomato, cucumber, pomegranate seeds and remaining lemon juice in a large bowl; toss to combine.

**5** Serve fish with quinoa salad; drizzle with green hummus and pomegranate molasses.

**DR JO SAYS**

To keep your carbohydrate intake down at a meal, ensure no more than a quarter of your plate comes from starchy foods. As a rule of thumb, aim to have no more than ¾–1 cup of a cooked starchy food in one meal.

**TIPS** Use red or white quinoa instead of tri-coloured, if preferred. Any firm white fish fillet, such as blue-eye trevalla, ling, kingfish or snapper would work well here. You can find hummus in the refrigerated section of most supermarkets.

| | | | | | |
|---|---|---|---|---|---|
| ● 17g total fat (3.4g saturated fat) | ● 1873kJ (447 cal) | ● 46.9g carbohydrate | ● 26.8g protein | ● 7.8g fibre | ● 439mg sodium |

# SICHUAN BEEF NOODLES
## with creamy sesame dressing

**PREP + COOK TIME** 25 MINUTES **SERVES** 4

2 teaspoons sichuan peppercorns

400g (12½oz) beef eye-fillet, sliced thinly across the grain

2 teaspoons reduced-salt soy sauce

2 teaspoons sesame oil

200g (6½oz) buckwheat soba noodles

2 teaspoons vegetable oil

250g (8oz) baby cucumbers, cut into matchsticks

1 bunch red radishes (500g), trimmed, sliced thinly

4 green onions (scallions), cut into matchsticks

**CREAMY SESAME DRESSING**

2 tablespoons rice wine vinegar

2 tablespoons water

1 tablespoon reduced-salt soy sauce

1 tablespoon natural crunchy peanut butter (see tip)

1 tablespoon pure maple syrup

2 teaspoons tahini

2 teaspoons sesame oil

2 teaspoons sriracha

**1** Crush peppercorns coarsely with a mortar and pestle; transfer to a medium bowl. Add beef, soy sauce and 1 teaspoon of sesame oil; toss to combine.

**2** Make creamy sesame dressing.

**3** Cook soba noodles in a large saucepan of boiling water according to packet directions. Rinse under cold water; drain.

**4** Heat a large wok over high heat. Add vegetable oil and remaining sesame oil; stir-fry beef, in batches, for 2 minutes or until browned all over. Transfer to a large bowl.

**5** Combine noodles, cucumber, radish and green onion in a large bowl. Add 2 tablespoons creamy sesame dressing; toss to coat.

**6** Divide noodle mixture and beef among four bowls. Drizzle with remaining dressing.

**CREAMY SESAME DRESSING** Place ingredients in a small bowl; whisk until smooth. (Makes ⅔ cup)

**TIP** Use a salt-reduced brand of natural peanut butter.

**SRIRACHA** (see-rah-jah), also known as 'rooster sauce' because of the picture on the bottle, is named after the city in Thailand where it was produced, Si Racha. This hot, tangy, chilli sauce adds a spicy kick to recipes.

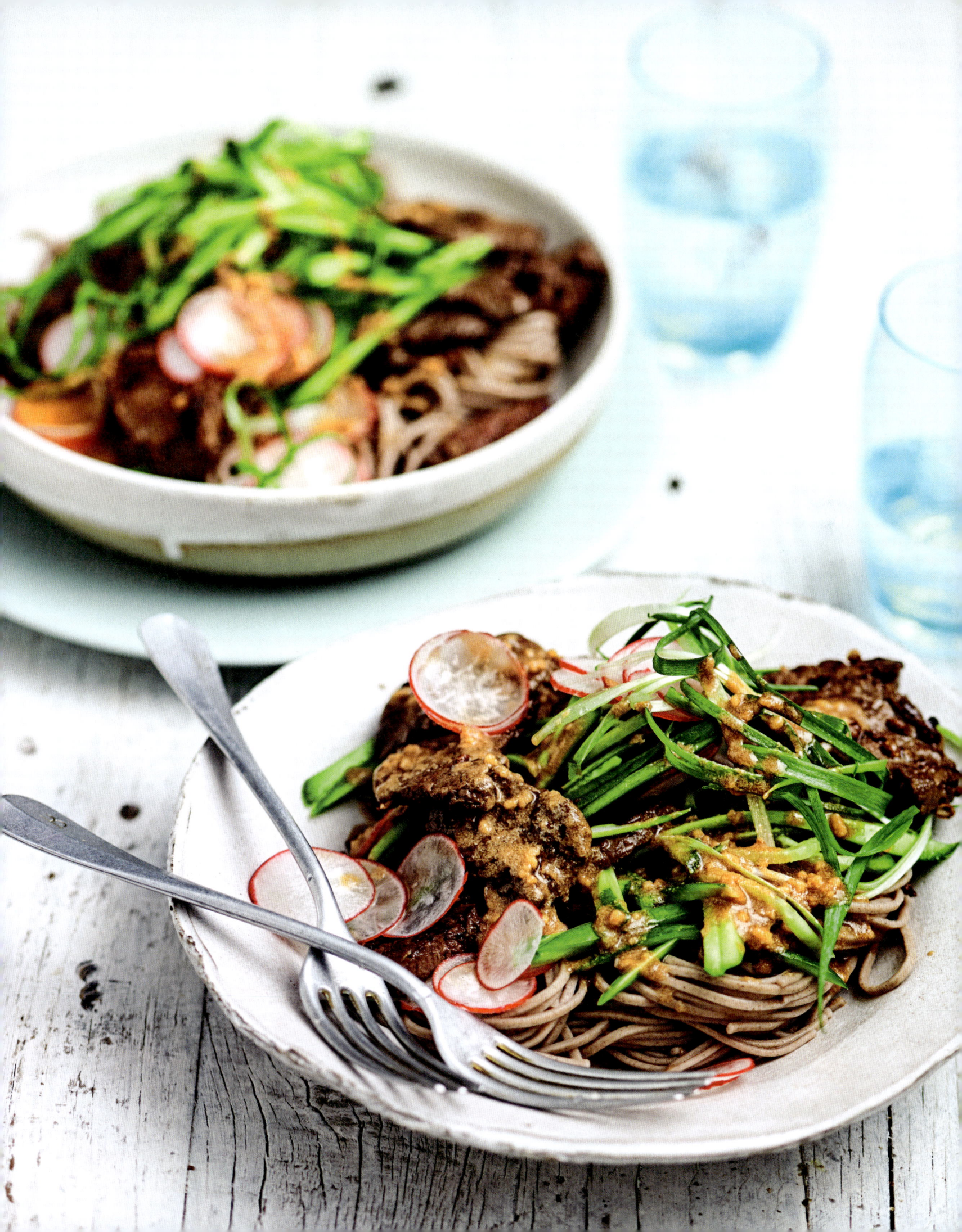

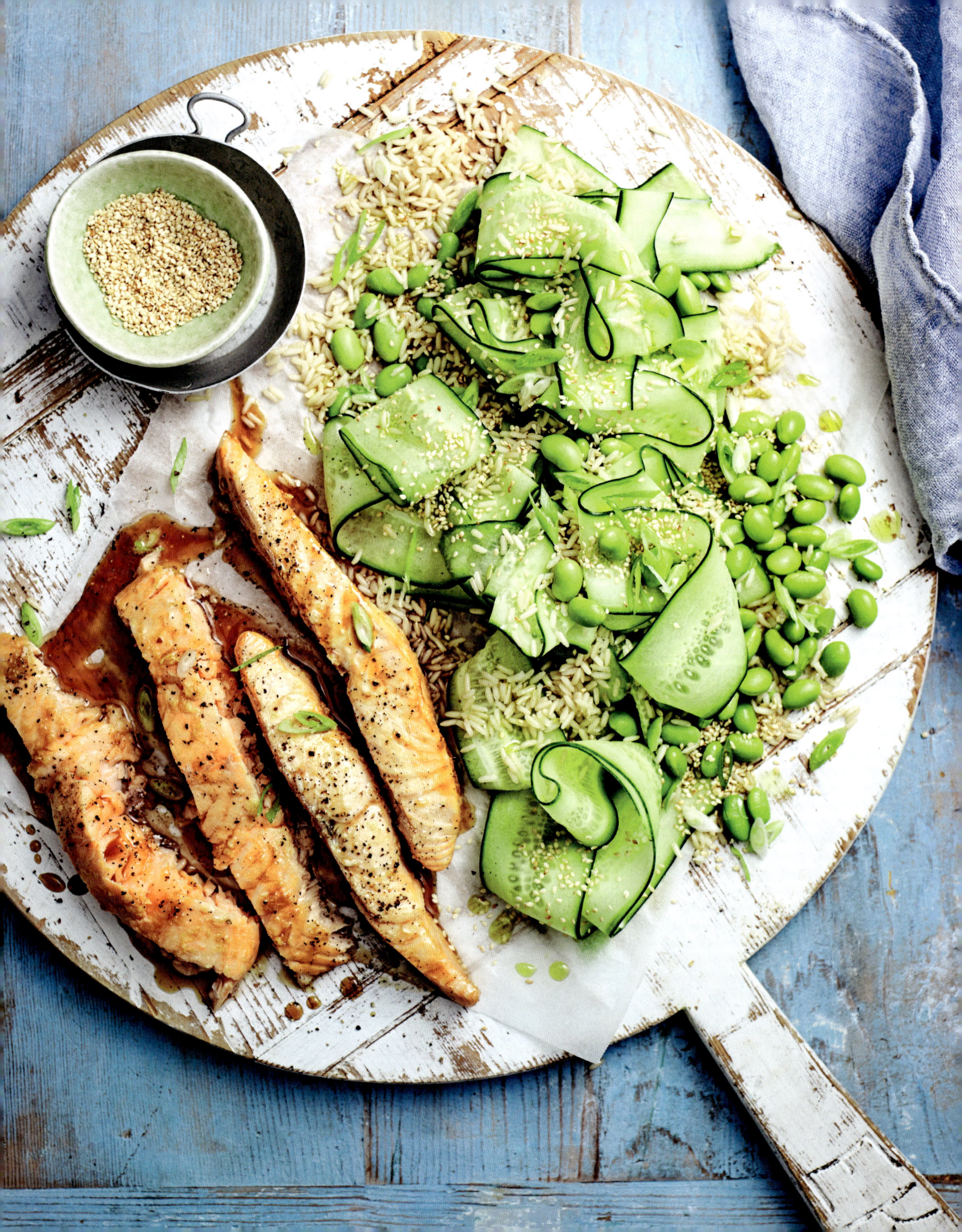

| 23g total fat (4.2g saturated fat) | 1986kJ (474 cal) | 33.8g carbohydrate | 34.1g protein | 3.6g fibre | 589mg sodium |

# TERIYAKI SALMON WITH
## edamame & cucumber rice salad

**PREP + COOK TIME** 35 MINUTES (+ REFRIGERATION) **SERVES** 4

¼ cup (60ml) reduced-salt soy sauce

¼ cup (90g) honey

1 tablespoon grated fresh ginger

1 tablespoon lime juice

1 x 500g (1lb) piece skinless salmon fillet

⅓ cup (65g) doongara low-GI brown rice (see tips)

200g (6½oz) frozen shelled edamame (soya beans)

2 telegraph (hothouse) cucumbers (800g),
  sliced thinly lengthways into ribbons (see tips)

2 tablespoons lemon juice

2 teaspoons sesame oil

1 green onion (scallion), sliced thinly

2 teaspoons sesame seeds, toasted

**1** To make the teriyaki marinade, combine soy sauce, honey, ginger and lime juice in a small bowl. Place salmon in a shallow ovenproof dish; pour over marinade. Turn salmon to coat; refrigerate for at least 30 minutes.

**2** Meanwhile, cook rice according to packet directions.

**3** Boil, steam or microwave edamame until warmed though; cool slightly.

**4** Remove salmon from fridge; stand for 10 minutes to bring to room temperature.

**5** Preheat oven to 200°C/400°F. Line an oven tray with baking paper.

**6** Place salmon on tray; roast for 10 minutes or until cooked to your liking. Transfer salmon to a plate, cover loosely with foil; rest for 5 minutes.

**7** Meanwhile, strain roasting juices into a small saucepan; bring to the boil over medium-high heat. Boil for 5 minutes or until sauce is reduced and thickened slightly.

**8** Combine rice, cucumber, edamame, lemon juice and sesame oil in a large bowl.

**9** Serve salmon with rice salad, drizzled with teriyaki sauce and sprinkled with green onion and sesame seeds.

**DR JO SAYS**

Pure floral honeys are a healthier sugar, particularly for people with diabetes, as they have lower GI values. They also provide a few short-chain carbohydrates that boost the growth of beneficial bacteria in the gut.

**TIPS** Grown exclusively in Australia, doongara is a naturally low GI rice variety, with the added benefit of being hard to overcook, as the grains remain separate. It is available from major supermarkets.

Use a vegetable peeler to thinly slice the cucumber lengthways.

# Remarkably HEALTHY GRAINS

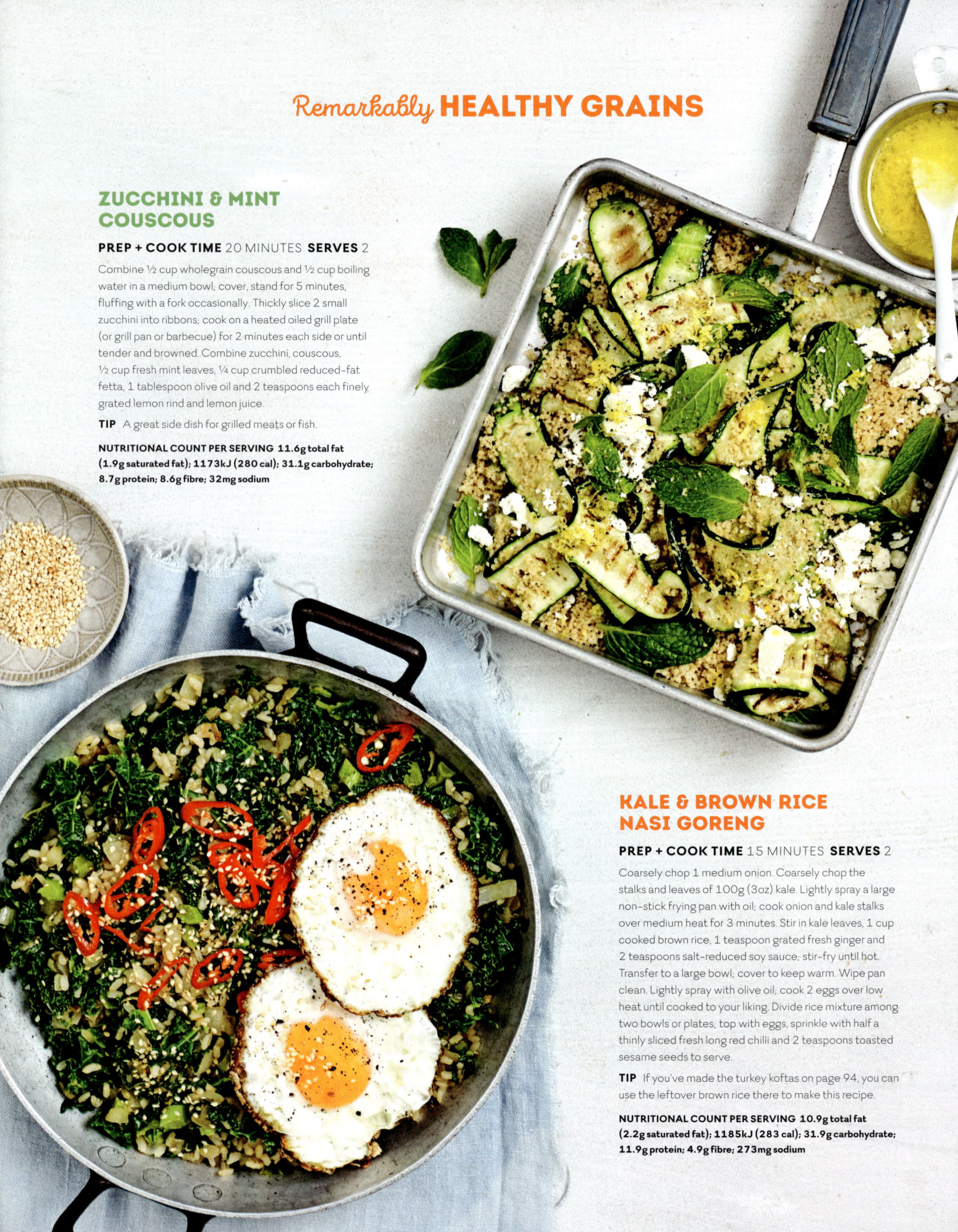

## ZUCCHINI & MINT COUSCOUS

**PREP + COOK TIME** 20 MINUTES **SERVES** 2

Combine ½ cup wholegrain couscous and ½ cup boiling water in a medium bowl; cover, stand for 5 minutes, fluffing with a fork occasionally. Thickly slice 2 small zucchini into ribbons; cook on a heated oiled grill plate (or grill pan or barbecue) for 2 minutes each side or until tender and browned. Combine zucchini, couscous, ½ cup fresh mint leaves, ¼ cup crumbled reduced-fat fetta, 1 tablespoon olive oil and 2 teaspoons each finely grated lemon rind and lemon juice.

**TIP** A great side dish for grilled meats or fish.

**NUTRITIONAL COUNT PER SERVING 11.6g total fat (1.9g saturated fat); 1173kJ (280 cal); 31.1g carbohydrate; 8.7g protein; 8.6g fibre; 32mg sodium**

## KALE & BROWN RICE NASI GORENG

**PREP + COOK TIME** 15 MINUTES **SERVES** 2

Coarsely chop 1 medium onion. Coarsely chop the stalks and leaves of 100g (3oz) kale. Lightly spray a large non-stick frying pan with oil; cook onion and kale stalks over medium heat for 3 minutes. Stir in kale leaves, 1 cup cooked brown rice, 1 teaspoon grated fresh ginger and 2 teaspoons salt-reduced soy sauce; stir-fry until hot. Transfer to a large bowl; cover to keep warm. Wipe pan clean. Lightly spray with olive oil; cook 2 eggs over low heat until cooked to your liking. Divide rice mixture among two bowls or plates; top with eggs, sprinkle with half a thinly sliced fresh long red chilli and 2 teaspoons toasted sesame seeds to serve.

**TIP** If you've made the turkey koftas on page 94, you can use the leftover brown rice there to make this recipe.

**NUTRITIONAL COUNT PER SERVING 10.9g total fat (2.2g saturated fat); 1185kJ (283 cal); 31.9g carbohydrate; 11.9g protein; 4.9g fibre; 273mg sodium**

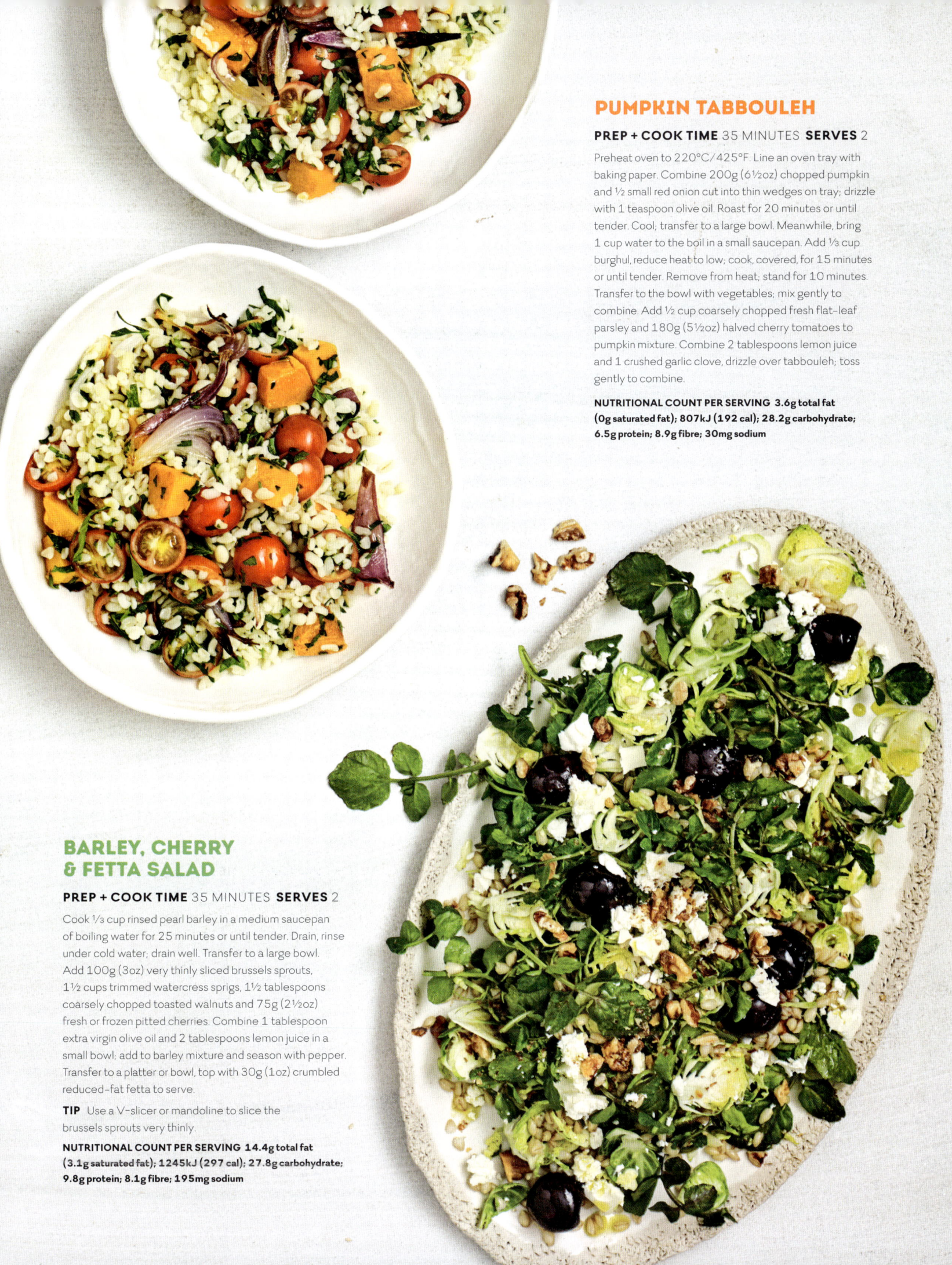

## PUMPKIN TABBOULEH

**PREP + COOK TIME** 35 MINUTES **SERVES** 2

Preheat oven to 220°C/425°F. Line an oven tray with baking paper. Combine 200g (6½oz) chopped pumpkin and ½ small red onion cut into thin wedges on tray; drizzle with 1 teaspoon olive oil. Roast for 20 minutes or until tender. Cool; transfer to a large bowl. Meanwhile, bring 1 cup water to the boil in a small saucepan. Add ⅓ cup burghul, reduce heat to low; cook, covered, for 15 minutes or until tender. Remove from heat; stand for 10 minutes. Transfer to the bowl with vegetables; mix gently to combine. Add ½ cup coarsely chopped fresh flat-leaf parsley and 180g (5½oz) halved cherry tomatoes to pumpkin mixture. Combine 2 tablespoons lemon juice and 1 crushed garlic clove, drizzle over tabbouleh; toss gently to combine.

**NUTRITIONAL COUNT PER SERVING** 3.6g total fat (0g saturated fat); 807kJ (192 cal); 28.2g carbohydrate; 6.5g protein; 8.9g fibre; 30mg sodium

## BARLEY, CHERRY & FETTA SALAD

**PREP + COOK TIME** 35 MINUTES **SERVES** 2

Cook ⅓ cup rinsed pearl barley in a medium saucepan of boiling water for 25 minutes or until tender. Drain, rinse under cold water; drain well. Transfer to a large bowl. Add 100g (3oz) very thinly sliced brussels sprouts, 1½ cups trimmed watercress sprigs, 1½ tablespoons coarsely chopped toasted walnuts and 75g (2½oz) fresh or frozen pitted cherries. Combine 1 tablespoon extra virgin olive oil and 2 tablespoons lemon juice in a small bowl; add to barley mixture and season with pepper. Transfer to a platter or bowl, top with 30g (1oz) crumbled reduced-fat fetta to serve.

**TIP** Use a V-slicer or mandoline to slice the brussels sprouts very thinly.

**NUTRITIONAL COUNT PER SERVING** 14.4g total fat (3.1g saturated fat); 1245kJ (297 cal); 27.8g carbohydrate; 9.8g protein; 8.1g fibre; 195mg sodium

| | | | | | |
|---|---|---|---|---|---|
| ● 18.3g total fat (5g saturated fat) | ● 1937kJ (462 cal) | ● 39.3g carbohydrate | ● 29g protein | ● 10.5g fibre | ● 146mg sodium |

# PASTA WITH SALMON
## & minty pea pesto

**PREP + COOK TIME** 25 MINUTES **SERVES** 4

220g (7oz) wholemeal penne pasta (see tip)
2 cups (240g) frozen peas, thawed
300g (9½oz) skinless boneless salmon fillets
1 cup fresh mint leaves
1 teaspoon finely grated lemon rind
2 tablespoons lemon juice
1 clove garlic, crushed
⅓ cup (25g) finely grated parmesan
1 tablespoon extra virgin olive oil
1 small lemon (65g), cut into wedges
small mint leaves, to garnish

**1** Cook pasta in a large saucepan of boiling water following packet directions until just tender. Remove pasta with a slotted spoon; reserve ⅓ cup of cooking water. Place peas into a colander in the sink; tip remaining cooking water over peas to blanch. Rinse under cold water.

**2** Heat a heavy-based non-stick frying pan over medium-high heat. Cook salmon for 3 minutes each side or until just cooked through. Transfer to a plate; flake with a fork.

**3** To make pesto, process drained peas, mint, lemon rind and juice, garlic, parmesan, oil and reserved cooking water in a food processor, pulsing until well combined but still chunky.

**4** Toss pesto through hot pasta; fold through salmon flakes. Divide pasta and salmon mixture among four bowls or plates, season with pepper. Serve with lemon wedges and mint.

**TIP** Use the same weight of your favourite wholemeal pasta shape instead of penne, if you like.

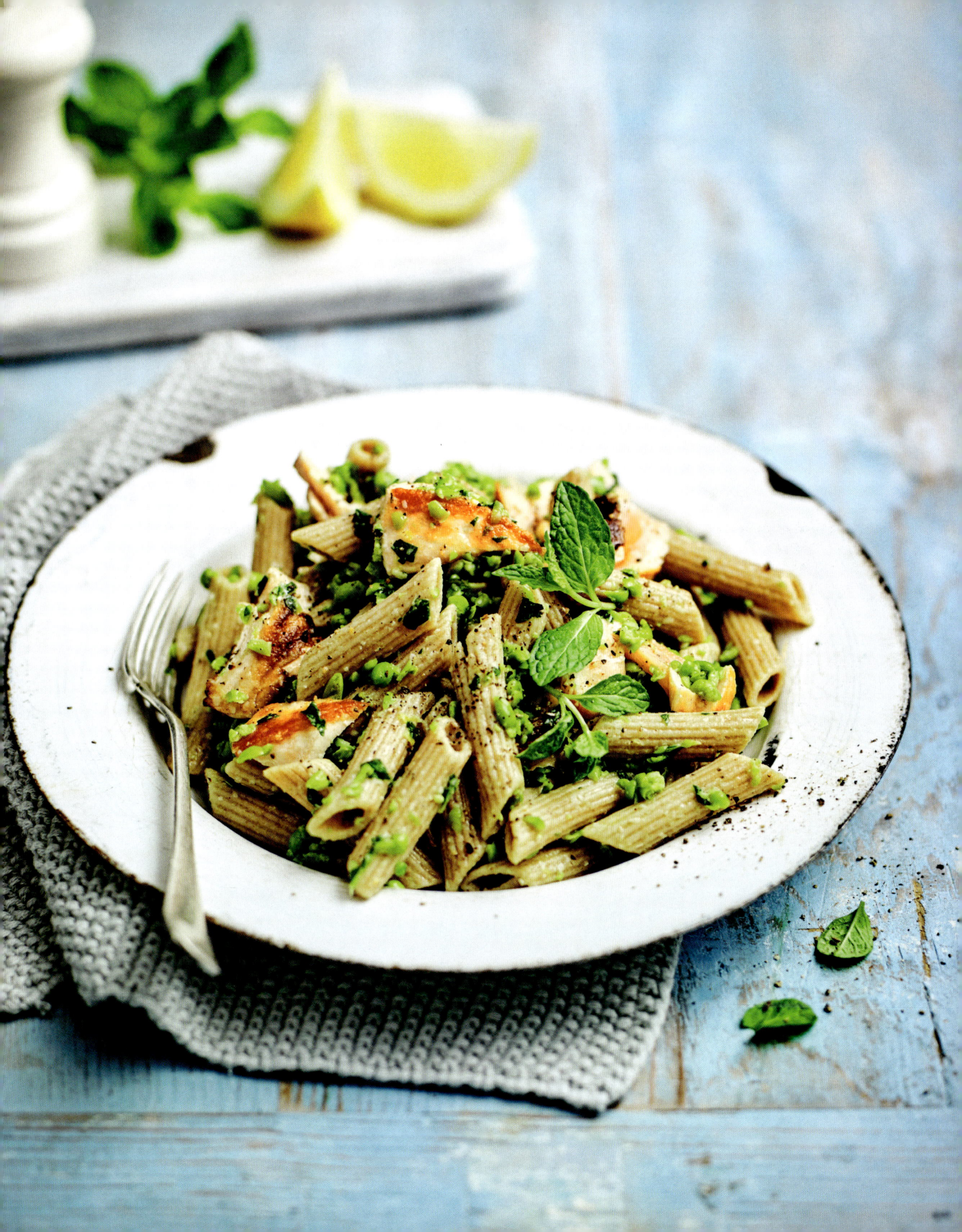

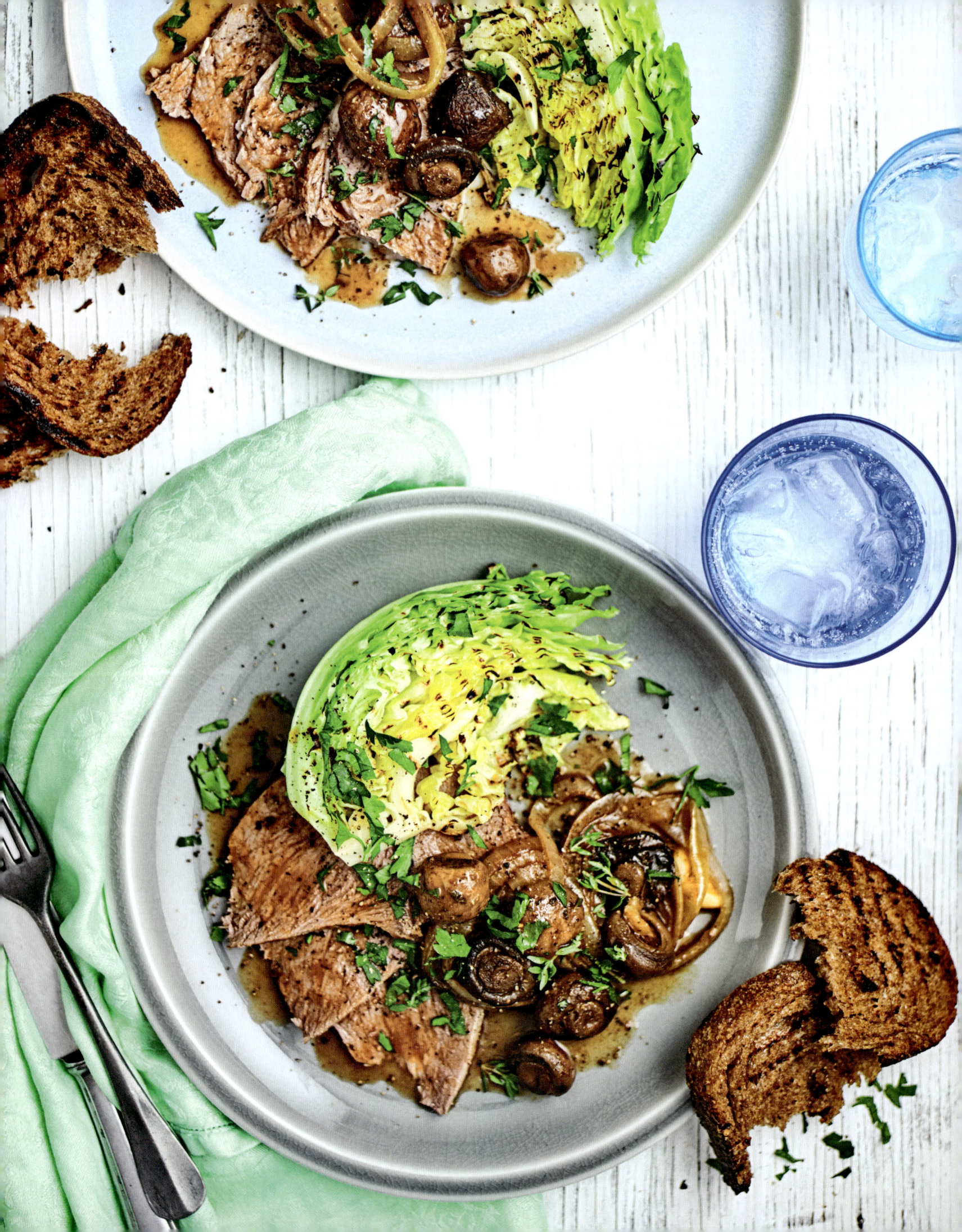

**NUTRITIONAL COUNT PER SERVING**

| • 14.5g total fat (3.9g saturated fat) | • 1749kJ (418 cal) | • 18.4g carbohydrate | • 49.3g protein | • 6.8g fibre | • 305mg sodium |
|---|---|---|---|---|---|

# POT-ROASTED BEEF
## with mushrooms & thyme

**PREP + COOK TIME** 1 HOUR 25 MINUTES **SERVES** 4

1 tablespoon extra virgin olive oil

1kg (2lb) piece beef bolar blade roast, fat trimmed

1 medium onion (150g), sliced thickly

6 cloves garlic, peeled

400g (12½oz) swiss brown mushrooms

2 tablespoons tomato paste

½ cup (125ml) water

4 fresh thyme sprigs

½ small savoy cabbage (600g), cut into 4 wedges

olive-oil spray

4 slices wholemeal sourdough bread (100g)

¼ cup coarsely chopped fresh flat-leaf parsley

**1** Preheat oven to 160°C/325°F.

**2** Heat oil in a flameproof cast iron casserole dish with a tight-fitting lid over medium heat. Add beef; cook, turning occasionally, for 8 minutes or until browned all over. Transfer to a plate.

**3** Add onion, garlic and mushrooms to the dish; cook, stirring, for 5 minutes. Stir in tomato paste; cook for 1 minute. Add the water and thyme; bring sauce to the boil. Return beef to dish. Cover, transfer to oven; cook for 1 hour. Remove from oven; rest for 10 minutes.

**4** Meanwhile, heat a grill pan (or grill plate) over medium-high heat. Spray cabbage wedges with oil; cook for 4 minutes each side or until just cooked through and light grill marks appear. Spray bread lightly with oil; grill for 1 minute each side or until light grill marks appear.

**5** Remove beef; thinly slice 100g (3oz) per serve. Serve beef with mushrooms, sauce, cabbage and grilled bread. Sprinkle with parsley.

**DR JO SAYS**

What you drink also affects your blood glucose. Soft drinks are the obvious no-no, but excess added sugar is found in flavoured coffees, iced tea and fruit juice-based smoothies. Unsweetened coffee and tea are best, and make water your regular drink.

**TIPS** This recipe makes more roast beef than you will need (100g per person). You can freeze the rest (sliced into 100g portions, if you like), or store in an airtight container in the fridge for up to 2 days and use for sandwiches or salads.

**BEEF BOLAR BLADE** is an economical and versatile cut. It is tender and flavoursome, and whole pieces can be slow cooked or pot roasted, or cubed for casseroles and stews. It can also be sliced into thin strips and stir-fried.

| 21.2g total fat (3.9g saturated fat) | 1812kJ (433 cal) | 25g carbohydrate | 31.8g protein | 5.9g fibre | 106mg sodium |
|---|---|---|---|---|---|

# LAMB LEG STEAKS
## with quinoa tabbouleh

**PREP + COOK TIME** 25 MINUTES (+ COOLING) **SERVES** 4

600g (1¼lb) lamb leg steaks, fat trimmed
1½ tablespoons cumin seeds
olive-oil spray
1 medium lemon (140g), cut into wedges

**QUINOA TABBOULEH**
¾ cup (150g) white quinoa, rinsed well (see tip)
1½ cups (375ml) water
1½ cups fresh flat-leaf parsley, chopped finely
200g (6½oz) cherry tomatoes, quartered
4 green onions (scallions), white part chopped finely, green tops shredded
2½ tablespoons extra virgin olive oil
¼ cup (60ml) lemon juice
1 clove garlic, crushed

**1** Make quinoa tabbouleh.

**2** Heat a large non-stick frying pan over high heat. Coat lamb with cumin seeds; spray lightly with oil. Cook lamb for 2 minutes each side for medium or until cooked to your liking. Cover loosely with foil; rest for 5 minutes.

**3** Thickly slice lamb on the diagonal. Serve lamb with tabbouleh and lemon wedges, sprinkle with shredded green onion tops.

**QUINOA TABBOULEH** Place quinoa and the water in a medium saucepan; bring to the boil. Reduce heat to low; cook for 10 minutes. Stand, covered, for 5 minutes. Fluff with a fork; transfer to a large bowl to cool. Add parsley, tomato, white part of onion, and combined oil, lemon juice and garlic to cooled quinoa; toss to combine.

**TIP** Use red or tri-colour quinoa instead of white quinoa, if you like.

**DR JO SAYS**
Portion size is key to keeping your weight and blood glucose under control. Filling half your plate at most meals with non-starchy vegies is the best means of maximising your intake of nutrients while lowering the kilojoules and the carbohydrates.

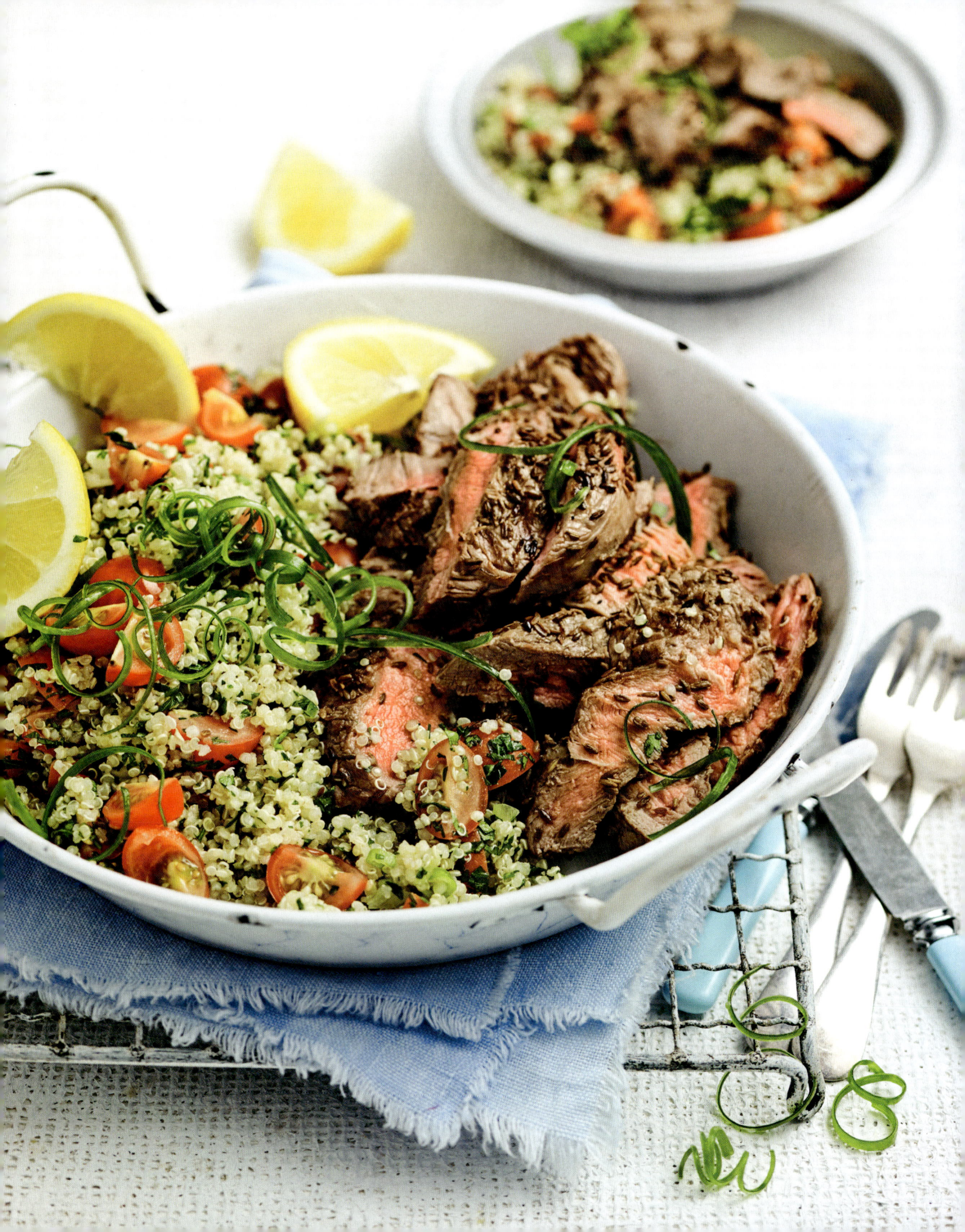

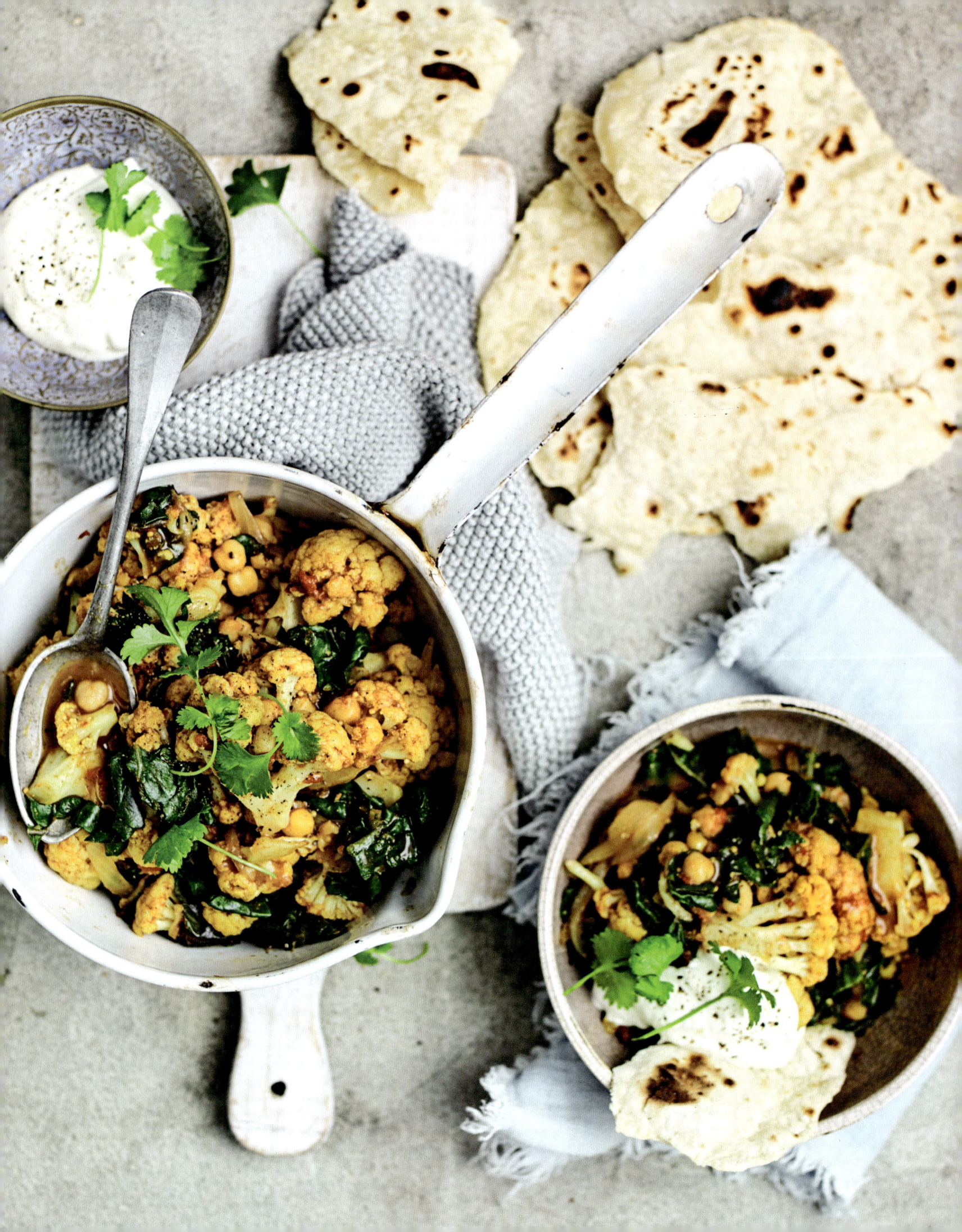

| | | | | | |
|---|---|---|---|---|---|
| ● 15.7g total fat (5g saturated fat) | ● 1863kJ (445 cal) | ● 49.5g carbohydrate | ● 17.9g protein | ● 16.6g fibre | ● 407mg sodium |

# LOADED CHICKPEA MASALA
## with spelt chapatis

**PREP + COOK TIME** 40 MINUTES (+ STANDING) **SERVES** 4

1 tablespoon olive oil

1 large onion (200g), sliced thinly

1 clove garlic, crushed

1 tablespoon finely chopped fresh ginger

2 teaspoons yellow mustard seeds

2 teaspoons garam masala

1 teaspoon ground coriander

$\frac{1}{2}$ teaspoon ground turmeric

$\frac{1}{4}$ teaspoon cayenne pepper

400g (12$\frac{1}{2}$oz) can diced tomatoes

$\frac{2}{3}$ cup (160ml) canned light coconut milk

$\frac{1}{3}$ cup (80ml) water

1 small cauliflower (1kg), cut into florets

400g (12$\frac{1}{2}$oz) can no-added-salt chickpeas
   (garbanzo beans), drained, rinsed

1 bunch silver beet (swiss chard) (750g),
   stems removed, leaves chopped coarsely

$\frac{1}{3}$ cup (95g) low-fat natural Greek-style yoghurt

$\frac{1}{4}$ cup fresh coriander (cilantro) sprigs

**SPELT CHAPATIS**

1 cup (150g) white spelt flour, plus extra for dusting

$\frac{1}{4}$ teaspoon fine sea salt

$\frac{1}{4}$ cup (60ml) warm water, plus extra if needed

1 tablespoon olive oil

1 Prepare spelt chapati dough; set aside to rest.

2 Heat olive oil in a large saucepan over medium–high heat. Add onion; cook, stirring, for 5 minutes or until soft. Add garlic and ginger; stir for 1 minute or until fragrant. Add mustard seeds; once they start popping, add remaining spices and stir for 1 minute or until fragrant.

3 Add tomatoes, coconut milk and the water to pan; bring to the boil. Add cauliflower and chickpeas; bring back to the boil. Reduce heat to low–medium; cook, covered, for 15 minutes or until cauliflower is tender.

4 Meanwhile, continue to make spelt chapatis.

5 Stir silver beet through chickpea mixture; simmer for 3 minutes or until wilted.

6 Serve chickpea masala topped with yoghurt and coriander sprigs; accompany with chapatis.

**SPELT CHAPATIS** Combine flour and salt in a medium bowl. Slowly add the warm water and oil, combining the mixture with your hands until a soft dough forms. Stand dough for 15 minutes. (Meanwhile, start step 2.) Divide dough into four balls. Dust balls with extra flour; flatten each one into a circle. Using a floured rolling pin, roll dough out on a lightly floured surface into four round chapatis approximately 3mm ($\frac{1}{8}$in) thick. Heat a medium heavy-based frying pan over high heat until hot. Cook one piece of dough at a time for 1 minute or until bubbles start to form on the surface. Turn; cook for a further 1 minute or until golden. Repeat with remaining dough to make a total of four chapatis. Wrap in a clean tea towel to keep warm.

**TIP** The chapatis are best served straight after cooking. This recipe is not suitable to freeze.

| 9.2g total fat (3g saturated fat) | 1260kJ (301 cal) | 27.3g carbohydrate | 23.2g protein | 8g fibre | 172mg sodium |
|---|---|---|---|---|---|

# LAMB CUTLETS
## with roasted panzanella salad

PREP + COOK TIME 40 MINUTES SERVES 4

1 medium orange sweet potato (400g), cut into
   large pieces
2 medium red onions (340g), cut into thin wedges
4 cloves garlic, crushed
¼ cup (60ml) extra virgin olive oil
250g (8oz) mixed cherry tomatoes
1 medium red capsicum (bell pepper) (200g), seeded,
   sliced thickly
80g (2½oz) wholegrain sourdough bread, torn coarsely
1 tablespoon finely chopped fresh rosemary leaves
olive-oil spray
12 french-trimmed lamb cutlets (600g)
60g (2oz) baby spinach leaves
½ cup fresh basil leaves
½ cup fresh flat-leaf parsley leaves
1 medium lebanese cucumber (170g),
   halved lengthways, sliced thickly
1½ tablespoons red wine vinegar

1 Preheat oven to 200°C/400°F.

2 Place sweet potato, onion, half the garlic and 1 tablespoon of the oil in a roasting pan; toss well to coat vegetables. Roast for 20 minutes; add tomato, capsicum and bread to pan; toss to coat. Roast for a further 15 minutes or until sweet potato is tender and bread is crisp.

3 Meanwhile, place rosemary, remaining garlic and another tablespoon of the oil in a small bowl; stir to combine. Spray a large frying pan with oil; heat over high heat. Cook lamb, in batches, for 1 minute each side. Press rosemary mixture evenly onto lamb. Place lamb on vegetables in roasting pan, and roast for the final 5 minutes of cooking time.

4 Place spinach, basil, parsley and cucumber in a large bowl. Combine remaining 1 tablespoon olive oil and the red wine vinegar in a small bowl. Add warm vegetables and dressing to spinach mixture; toss gently to combine.

5 Transfer panzanella salad to a platter or divide among four plates, top with lamb; season with pepper.

**DR JO SAYS**
Sourdough bread is generally a good bread choice, as the acidity lowers the GI. Look for a wholegrain variety for more fibre and maximum nutrition.

TIP Swap mint leaves for parsley leaves, if you prefer.

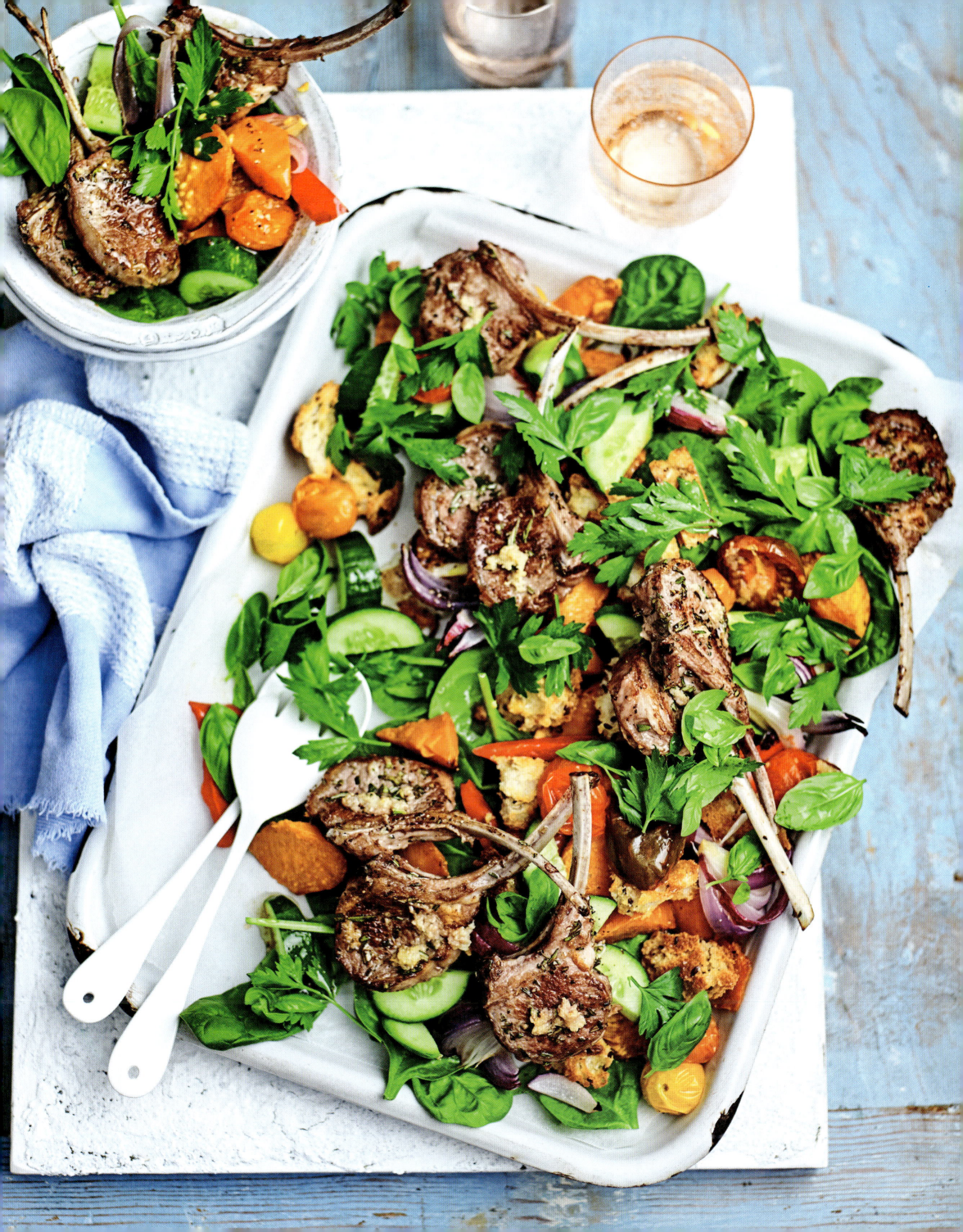

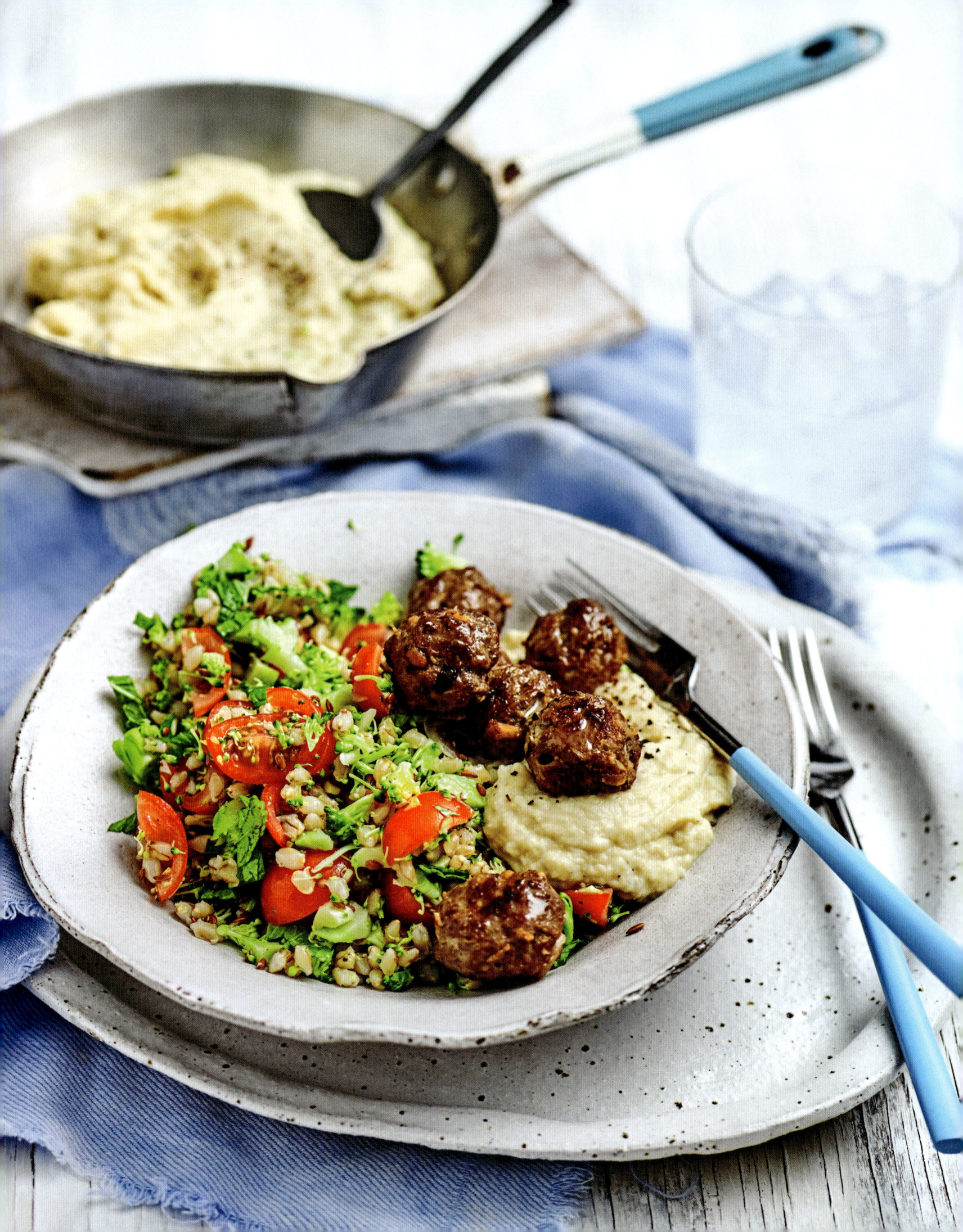

NUTRITIONAL COUNT PER SERVING

| ● 20.7g total fat (4.6g saturated fat) | ● 1814kJ (433 cal) | ● 24.3g carbohydrate | ● 30.6g protein | ● 12.8g fibre | ● 112mg sodium |

# LAMB KOFTA
## with broccoli barley salad

**PREP + COOK TIME** 1 HOUR 10 MINUTES (+ REFRIGERATION & STANDING) **SERVES** 4

400g (12½oz) lean minced (ground) lamb

2 tablespoons pine nuts, toasted

2 cloves garlic, crushed

1 medium onion (150g), grated

1½ teaspoons ground cumin

½ teaspoon dried oregano

**BABA GHANOUSH**

1 large eggplant (500g)

1 clove garlic, crushed

1 tablespoon unhulled tahini

2 tablespoons lemon juice

2 tablespoons natural Greek-style yoghurt

**BROCCOLI BARLEY SALAD**

½ cup (100g) pearl barley

300g (9½oz) broccoli, chopped finely

½ cup fresh mint leaves, chopped coarsely

1 tablespoon flaxseeds (linseeds)

2 tablespoons lemon juice

1 clove garlic, crushed

2 teaspoons extra virgin olive oil

250g (8oz) cherry tomatoes, quartered

**1** Combine lamb, pine nuts, garlic, onion, cumin and oregano in a large bowl; season with pepper, mix well. Cover; refrigerate for 1 hour.

**2** Meanwhile, make baba ghanoush and broccoli barley salad.

**3** Roll level tablespoons of the lamb mixture into balls (to make a total of 28 meatballs). Preheat a large non-stick frying pan over high heat. Cook koftas for 10 minutes or until browned and cooked through.

**4** Serve kofta with broccoli barley salad and baba ghanoush. Accompany with lemon wedges, if you like.

**BABA GHANOUSH** Prick eggplant all over with a sharp knife. Set a wire rack over the largest gas burner on your stove (see tip) over medium-high heat. Cook eggplant on rack over flame, turning occasionally, for 12 minutes or until charred and soft. Transfer to a heatproof bowl, cover with plastic wrap; stand for 20 minutes. Gently rub and discard skin. Blend or process eggplant flesh with remaining ingredients to form a smooth puree.

**BROCCOLI BARLEY SALAD** Cook barley in a saucepan of boiling water for 25 minutes or until tender; drain. Transfer to a bowl; cool for 5 minutes. Just before serving, add remaining ingredients to barley; stir gently to combine, season with pepper.

**DR JO SAYS**

Daily consumption of flaxseed (linseed) can improve glycaemic control in those with diabetes and improve cardiovascular risk factors. This is likely due to the presence of plant omega-3 fat, specific types of fibre and lignans.

**TIPS** If you don't have a gas burner you can use a barbecue, oven grill (broiler) or grill pan to cook the eggplant; adjust the cooking time accordingly.

**DID YOU KNOW?** Lignans are phytonutrients, which are compounds produced by plants. Plants use phytonutrients to stay healthy, and now scientists are finding that some of these are beneficial to humans.

**NUTRITIONAL COUNT PER SERVING**

| | | | | | |
|---|---|---|---|---|---|
| 14.5g total fat (3.9g saturated fat) | 1991kJ (475 cal) | 36.1g carbohydrate | 47.1g protein | 7.3g fibre | 442mg sodium |

# ROSEMARY LAMB ROAST
## with yoghurt flatbread & tzatziki

**PREP + COOK TIME** 1 HOUR 15 MINUTES (+ STANDING) **SERVES** 6

2 x 450g (14½oz) lamb mini roasts

2 cloves garlic, quartered

8 fresh rosemary sprigs

100g (3oz) baby spinach leaves

250g (8oz) cherry tomatoes, halved

1 small red onion (100g), halved, sliced thinly

1 tablespoon olive oil

1 tablespoon lemon juice

1 teaspoon dried oregano

1 small lemon (65g), cut into wedges

**YOGHURT FLATBREAD**

2 cups (320g) wholemeal self-raising flour

1 cup (280g) low-fat natural Greek-style yoghurt

1 teaspoon finely grated lemon rind

olive-oil spray

**TZATZIKI**

1 cup (280g) low-fat natural Greek-style yoghurt

1 lebanese cucumber (130g), grated, squeezed
   of excess moisture

½ cup fresh mint leaves, chopped finely

¼ teaspoon sea salt flakes

**1** Preheat oven to 200°C/400°F.

**2** Using a sharp knife, make four 1cm (½in) deep cuts at intervals across each lamb roast; insert garlic and rosemary into each cut. Place lamb on a greased wire rack over a roasting pan; pour in hot water to a depth of 1cm (½in). Transfer to oven; roast for 30 minutes for medium–rare, or until cooked to your liking. Cover lamb loosely with foil; rest for 15 minutes, then cut into thin slices.

**3** Meanwhile, make yoghurt flatbread and tzatziki.

**4** Combine spinach, tomato, onion, oil and lemon juice in a medium bowl; sprinkle with oregano.

**5** Divide flatbreads, lamb, salad and tzatziki among six plates; serve with lemon wedges.

**YOGHURT FLATBREAD** Place flour, yoghurt and lemon rind in a medium bowl; combine with a wooden spoon until a dough forms. Tip dough onto a lightly floured surface; knead gently until smooth. Place in a cleaned bowl, cover with a tea towel; stand for at least 20 minutes. Divide dough into six portions; using a floured rolling pin, roll each on a lightly floured surface into a 3mm (⅛in) thick oval approximately 15cm x 20cm (6in x 8in) in size. Lightly spray a grill pan (or grill plate) with a little oil; heat over medium–high heat. Cook one flatbread at a time for 1 minute on each side or until puffed and golden.

**TZATZIKI** Combine ingredients in a medium bowl; season with pepper. Cover; refrigerate until needed.

**TIP** Using yoghurt in the flatbread replaces the yeast, making this a great way to cook your own flatbread in a flash.

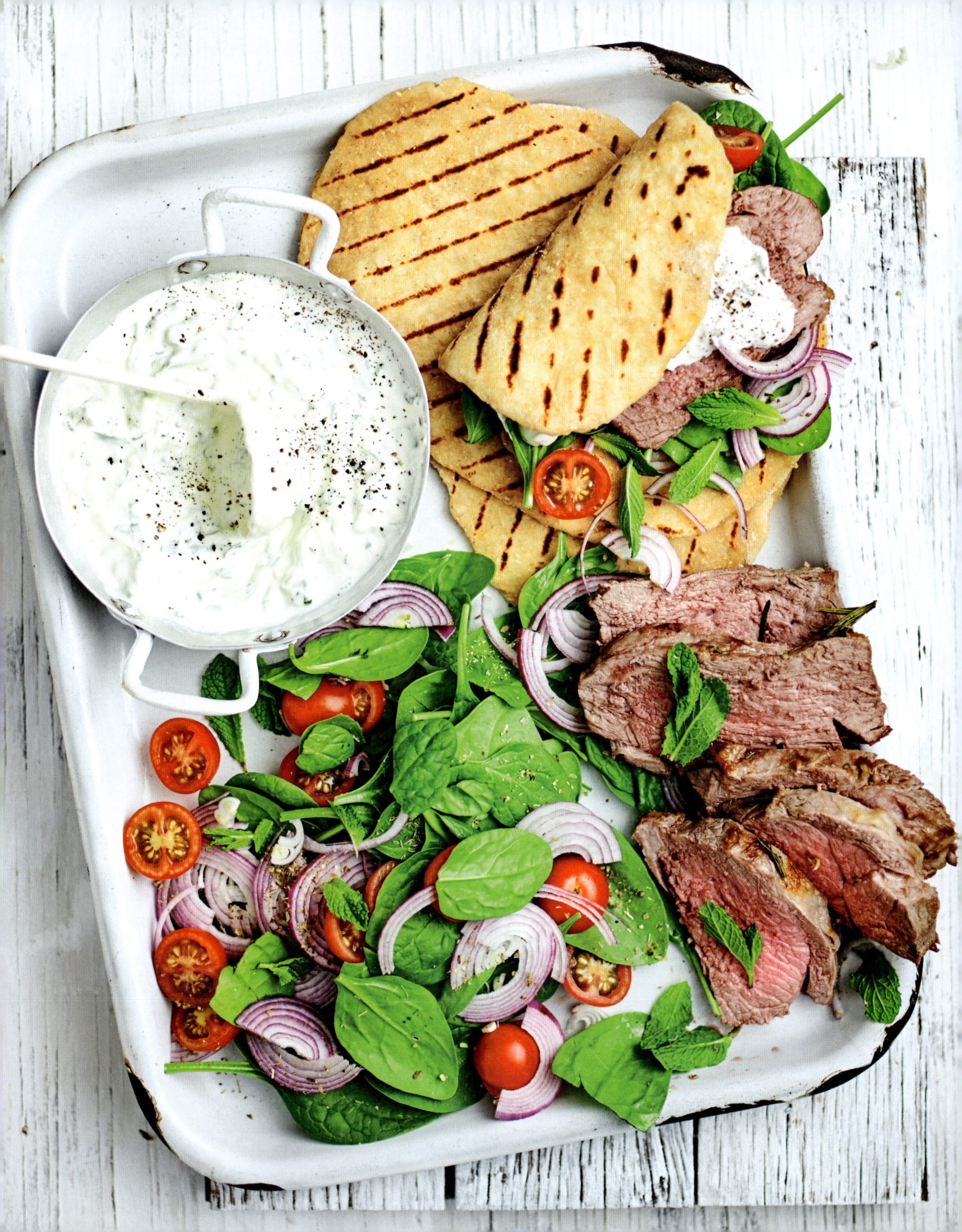

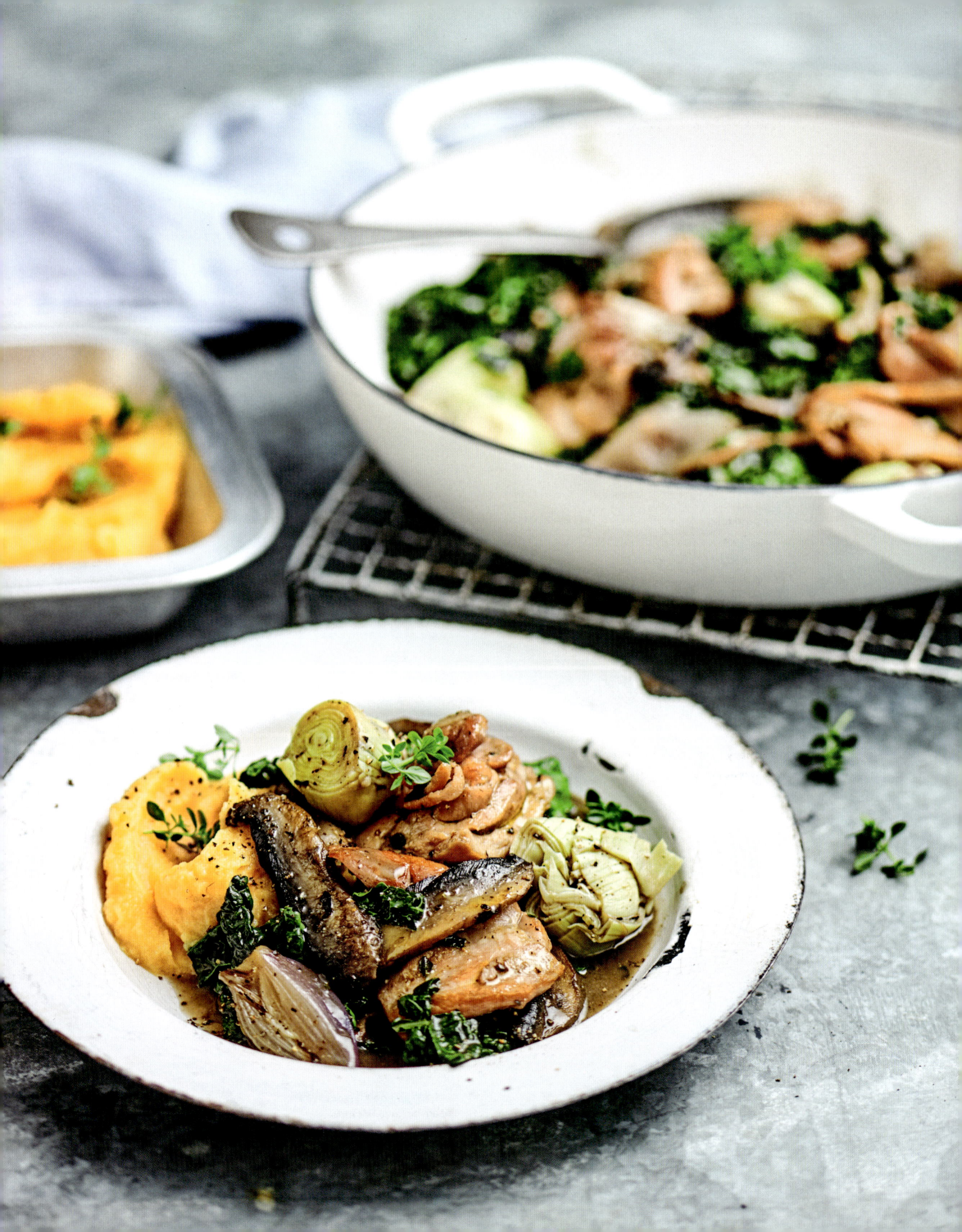

**NUTRITIONAL COUNT PER SERVING**

| 12.6g total fat (3.4g saturated fat) | 1482kJ (354 cal) | 17.3g carbohydrate | 30.3g protein | 10.8g fibre | 745mg sodium |

# BRAISED CHICKEN
## with mushrooms & artichokes

**PREP + COOK TIME** 1 HOUR **SERVES** 4

1 tablespoon olive oil

2 shortcut bacon rashers (75g), sliced thinly

400g (12½oz) chicken thigh fillets, fat trimmed, halved

6 shallots (150g), peeled, halved lengthways

400g (12½oz) portobello mushrooms, sliced thickly

4 small cloves garlic, sliced very thinly

4 sprigs lemon thyme, plus extra to serve

½ cup (125ml) dry white wine

2 tablespoons plain (all-purpose) flour

1 cup (250ml) salt-reduced chicken stock

1 cup (250ml) water

280g (9oz) marinated artichoke hearts, drained

1 bunch cavolo nero (tuscan cabbage) (200g), stalks removed, leaves chopped coarsely

**GOLDEN MASH**

500g (1lb) celeriac (celery root), chopped coarsely

150g (4½oz) orange sweet potatoes, chopped coarsely

½ cup (125ml) milk

**1** Heat oil in large heavy-based saucepan over high heat. Add bacon; cook, stirring constantly, for 3 minutes or until crisp. Transfer to a large bowl. Add chicken to pan; cook, turning once, for 4 minutes or until browned lightly. Add to bowl with bacon.

**2** Reduce heat to medium, add shallots to pan; cook, stirring frequently, for 5 minutes or until golden brown. Add mushroom, garlic, thyme and wine; bring to a simmer. Simmer for 4 minutes or until mushroom softens and liquid is almost evaporated.

**3** Sprinkle flour over mushroom mixture; cook, stirring, for 1 minute. Add stock and the water, stirring to combine with flour until smooth. Return chicken and bacon to pan; bring to a simmer over low-medium heat; cook, covered, for 15 minutes or until shallots are tender and chicken is cooked through.

**4** Meanwhile, make golden mash.

**5** Add artichokes and cavolo nero to chicken in pan; cook for 5 minutes or until cavolo nero wilts. Top with extra lemon thyme sprigs; serve with mash.

**GOLDEN MASH** Cook celeriac and sweet potato in a medium saucepan of boiling water for 20 minutes or until very tender; drain well. Blend or process vegetables and milk until smooth. Season to taste with pepper.

**TIP** The recipe can be prepared up to the end of step 3 a day ahead; store, covered, in the fridge. Reheat while making golden mash.

| ● 16g total fat (3.9g saturated fat) | ● 1587kJ (379 cal) | ● 15.9g carbohydrate | ● 34.9g protein | ● 11.2g fibre | ● 189mg sodium |
|---|---|---|---|---|---|

# STEAK & CANNELLINI BEAN
## bubble-n-squeak with salsa verde

**PREP + COOK TIME** 35 MINUTES **SERVES** 4

1 large lemon (200g)

1½ cups fresh flat-leaf parsley, chopped coarsely

2 teaspoons dijon mustard

1 teaspoon baby capers in vinegar, drained, rinsed

2 tablespoons extra virgin olive oil

1 clove garlic, crushed

¼ cup (60ml) water

200g (6½oz) brussels sprouts, trimmed, sliced thinly

4 spring onions, chopped coarsely

2 x 400g (12½oz) cans no-added-salt cannellini beans, drained, rinsed

olive-oil spray

600g (1¼lb) beef rump steaks, fat trimmed

**1** For the salsa verde, finely grate lemon rind; juice lemon. Process 1 cup of the parsley, 1 teaspoon of the mustard, capers, lemon rind and juice, oil and garlic until finely chopped and well combined.

**2** To make the bubble-n-squeak, place the water in a medium saucepan; bring to the boil over high heat. Add sprouts and onion; cook for 2 minutes or until just tender. Add cannellini beans and remaining parsley and mustard; cook for 2 minutes or until warmed through. Using a vegetable masher, crush mixture to form a coarse puree. Cover to keep warm.

**3** Meanwhile, heat a heavy-based frying pan over high heat. Spray pan with oil; cook steaks for 2 minutes each side for medium-rare or until cooked to your liking. Transfer to a plate, cover loosely with foil; rest for 5 minutes. Return all resting juices to pan and cook over low heat for 1 minute or until reduced by half; season to taste with pepper. Slice steaks across the grain.

**4** Divide bubble-n-squeak and steak among four plates. Spoon salsa verde and pan juices over steak, season with pepper to serve.

**TIP** Use half mint and half flat-leaf parsley in the salsa verde, if you like.

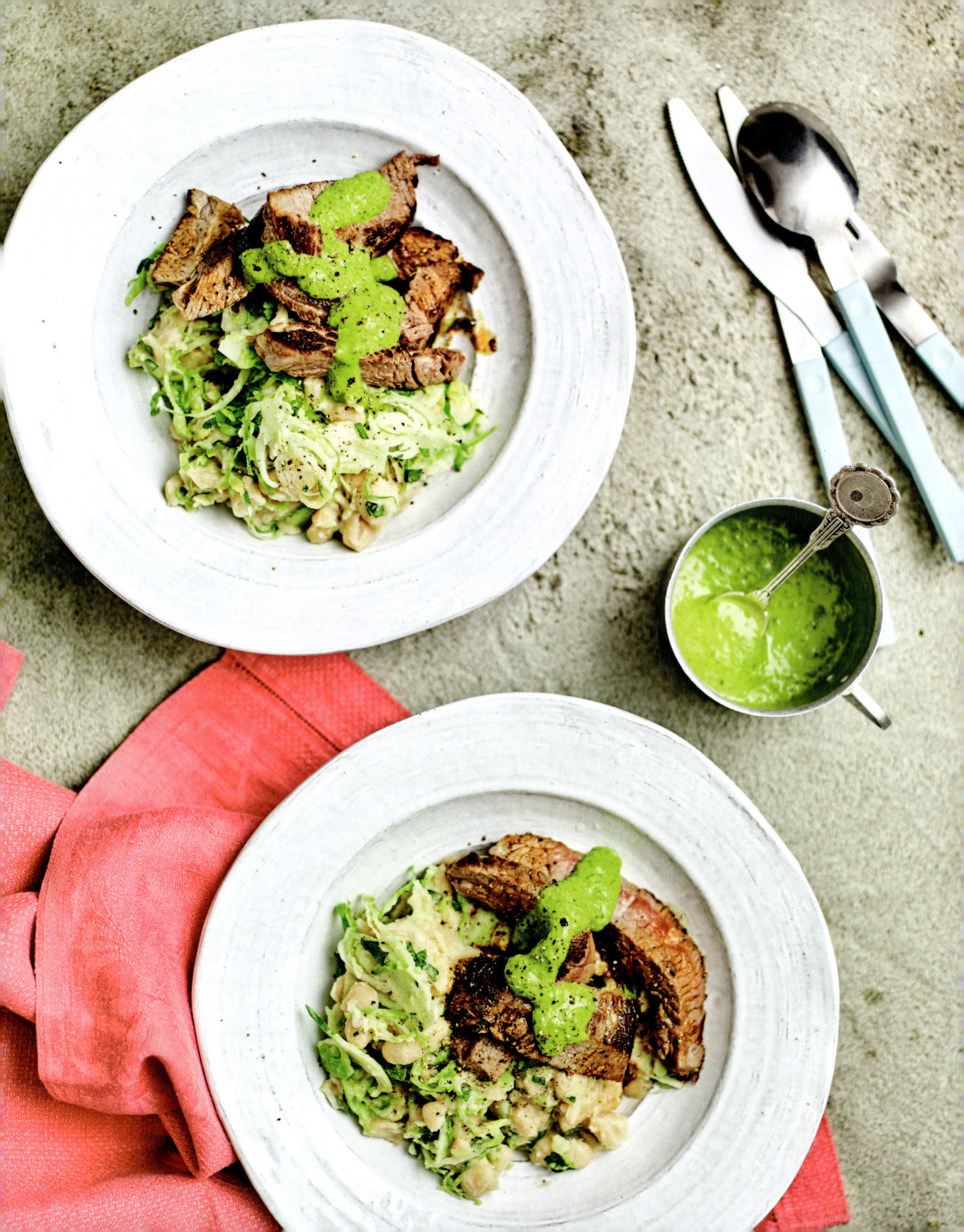

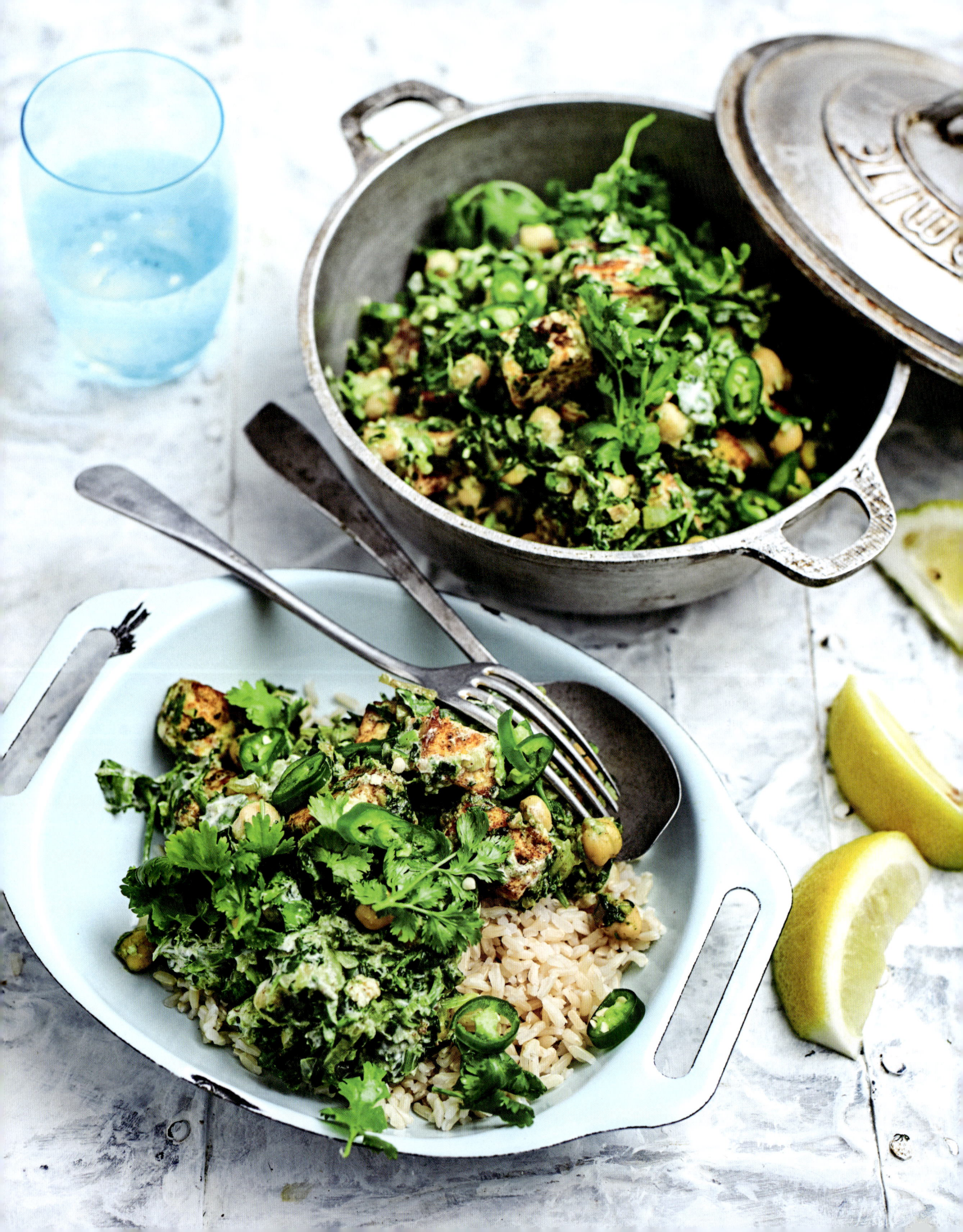

| ● 16g total fat (6.7g saturated fat) | ● 1735kJ (414 cal) | ● 43.2g carbohydrate | ● 19.8g protein | ● 8.7g fibre | ● 119mg sodium |

# Spinach & paneer CURRY

**PREP + COOK TIME** 35 MINUTES **SERVES** 4

¾ cup (150g) doongara low-GI brown rice
1 tablespoon olive oil
1 medium onion (150g), sliced thinly
1 tablespoon finely chopped fresh ginger
2 cloves garlic, crushed
1 bunch fresh coriander (cilantro), leaves separated,
 roots and stems washed, chopped coarsely
1 fresh long green chilli, sliced thinly
120g (4oz) baby spinach leaves
200g (6½oz) paneer cheese, cut into
 2cm (¾in) cubes
1 tablespoon garam masala
2 teaspoons ground cumin
400g (12½oz) can salt-reduced chickpeas
 (garbanzo beans), drained, rinsed
⅓ cup (95g) natural yoghurt
1 small lemon (65g), cut into wedges

**1** Cook rice according to packet directions. Drain; cover to keep warm.

**2** Meanwhile, heat 2 teaspoons of the oil in a medium heavy-based frying pan over medium–high heat. Add onion; cook, stirring, for 5 minutes or until soft. Add ginger, garlic, coriander stems and roots, and half the green chilli; cook for 1 minute or until fragrant. Add spinach; cook for 1 minute or until just wilted.

**3** Transfer spinach mixture to a food processor with coriander leaves; pulse until chopped coarsely.

**4** Heat remaining oil in same pan over medium–high heat. Add paneer; cook, turning, for 2 minutes. Add spices; cook, stirring, for 1 minute or until fragrant.

**5** Return spinach mixture to pan, add chickpeas and yoghurt; remove from heat, stir until well combined.

**6** Divide rice and paneer mixture among four bowls. Sprinkle with remaining chilli; serve with lemon wedges.

**DOONGARA RICE** is grown exclusively in Australia; it is a naturally low GI rice variety, with the added benefit of being hard to overcook, as the grains remain separate. Doongara rice is available from major supermarkets.

**PANEER** (or panir) is a fresh unripened cows'-milk cheese similar to pressed ricotta. It originates from the region that encompasses Iran, Afghanistan, India and Pakistan. It has a crumbly texture and mild flavour, and is usually available, near the fetta and haloumi, in major supermarkets, and some health food shops and Indian grocery stores.

**DR JO SAYS**
Aim to have at least one vegetarian meal a week. A Finnish study in men found that replacing 1% of energy from animal protein with plant protein reduced the risk of type 2 diabetes by 18%.

| ● 16.8g total fat (3.8g saturated fat) | ● 1912kJ (456 cal) | ● 37.7g carbohydrate | ● 29.4g protein | ● 7.4g fibre | ● 555mg sodium |
| --- | --- | --- | --- | --- | --- |

# COQ AU VIN
## with endive salad

**PREP + COOK TIME** 1 HOUR 5 MINUTES **SERVES** 4

1 tablespoon olive oil

4 chicken lovely legs (520g) (see tip)

8 red shallots (200g), peeled, trimmed, halved if large

50g (1½oz) shortcut bacon rashers, chopped coarsely

400g (12½oz) swiss brown mushrooms

2 cloves garlic, sliced thinly

1 tablespoon fresh thyme leaves

2 fresh bay leaves

⅓ cup (80ml) water

1 tablespoon plain (all-purpose) flour

½ cup (125ml) red wine

½ cup (125ml) salt-reduced chicken stock

300g (9½oz) mixed heirloom baby carrots, trimmed, peeled

¾ cup (150g) pearl couscous

1 cup (250ml) boiling water

### ENDIVE SALAD

1 shortcut bacon rasher (35g), cut into matchsticks

1 bunch curly endive (300g), leaves picked

1 tablespoon extra virgin olive oil

2 teaspoons red or white wine vinegar

**1** Preheat oven to 180°C/350°F.

**2** Heat oil in a medium flameproof roasting pan or cast iron casserole dish over medium heat. Add chicken; cook, turning occasionally, for 8 minutes or until browned all over. Transfer chicken to a plate; cover to keep warm.

**3** Add shallot, bacon, mushrooms, garlic, herbs and the water to pan. Reduce heat to low; cook, covered, stirring occasionally, for 5 minutes.

**4** Sprinkle flour over mixture in pan; cook, stirring, for 2 minutes. Add wine and stock; stir until well combined. Return chicken to pan. Cover with foil or a lid, transfer to oven; roast for 15 minutes. Remove lid, add carrots; return, uncovered, to oven and roast for a further 12 minutes or until carrots and chicken are tender.

**5** Place couscous and the boiling water in a medium heavy-based saucepan; bring to the boil. Reduce heat to low; cook, covered, for 8 minutes or until couscous is tender. Drain.

**6** Meanwhile, make endive salad.

**7** Serve coq au vin with couscous and salad.

**ENDIVE SALAD** Cook bacon in a small frying pan over medium heat until crisp; drain on paper towel. Combine endive and bacon in a medium bowl. Combine oil and vinegar in a small bowl. Drizzle salad with dressing; toss gently to coat.

**DR JO SAYS**

Alcohol can cause hypo-glycaemia while drinking and for 24 hours afterwards. Stick to the recommended only two drinks a day, eat while drinking and test your blood glucose regularly for the next 24 hours, particularly before going to bed.

**TIP** Chicken lovely legs are trimmed, skinless chicken drumsticks. You can find them at chicken speciality shops and major supermarkets.

This diabetes-friendly version of coq au vin, served with pearl couscous instead of crusty bread or potato puree, still boasts the rich flavour of the traditional version.

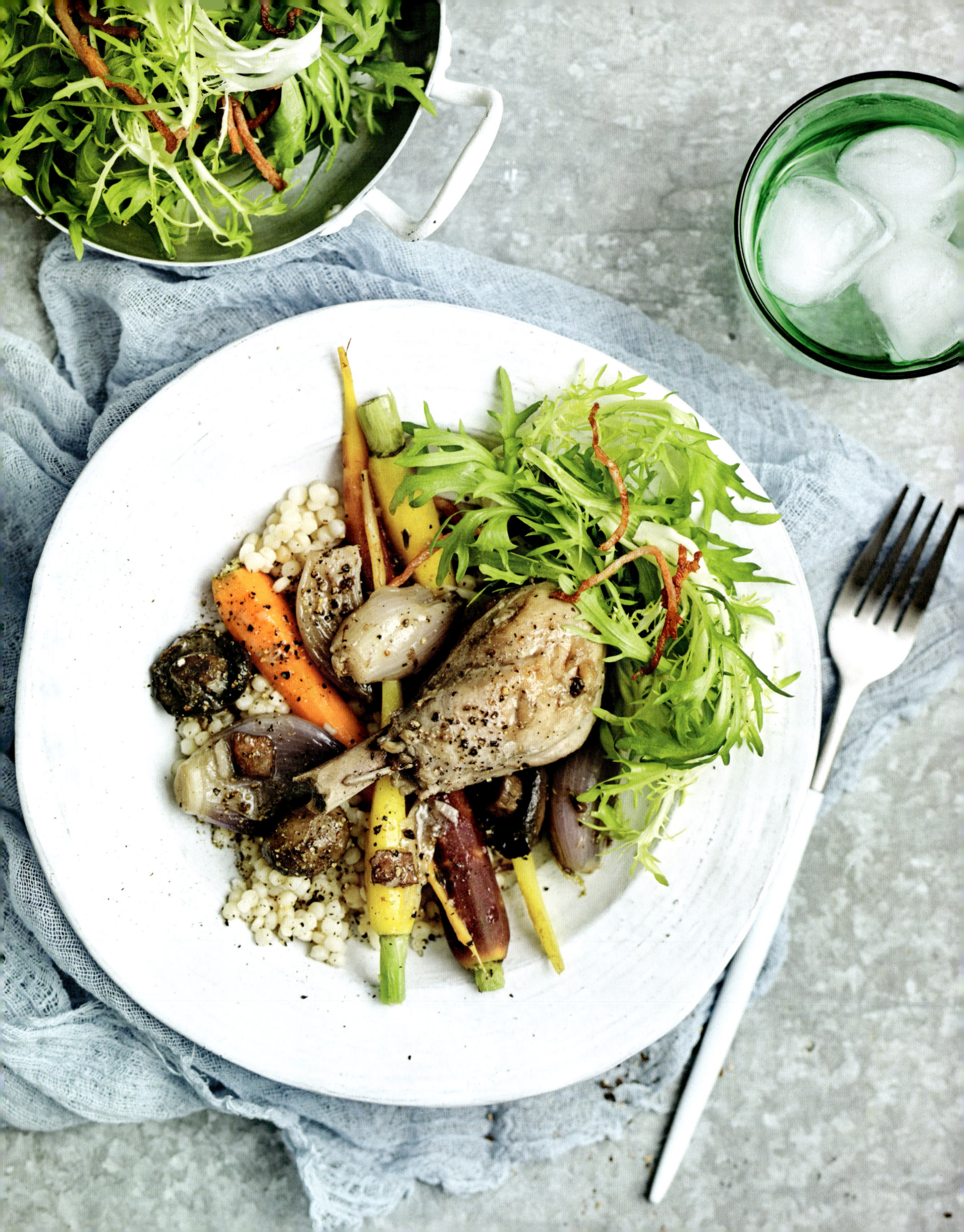

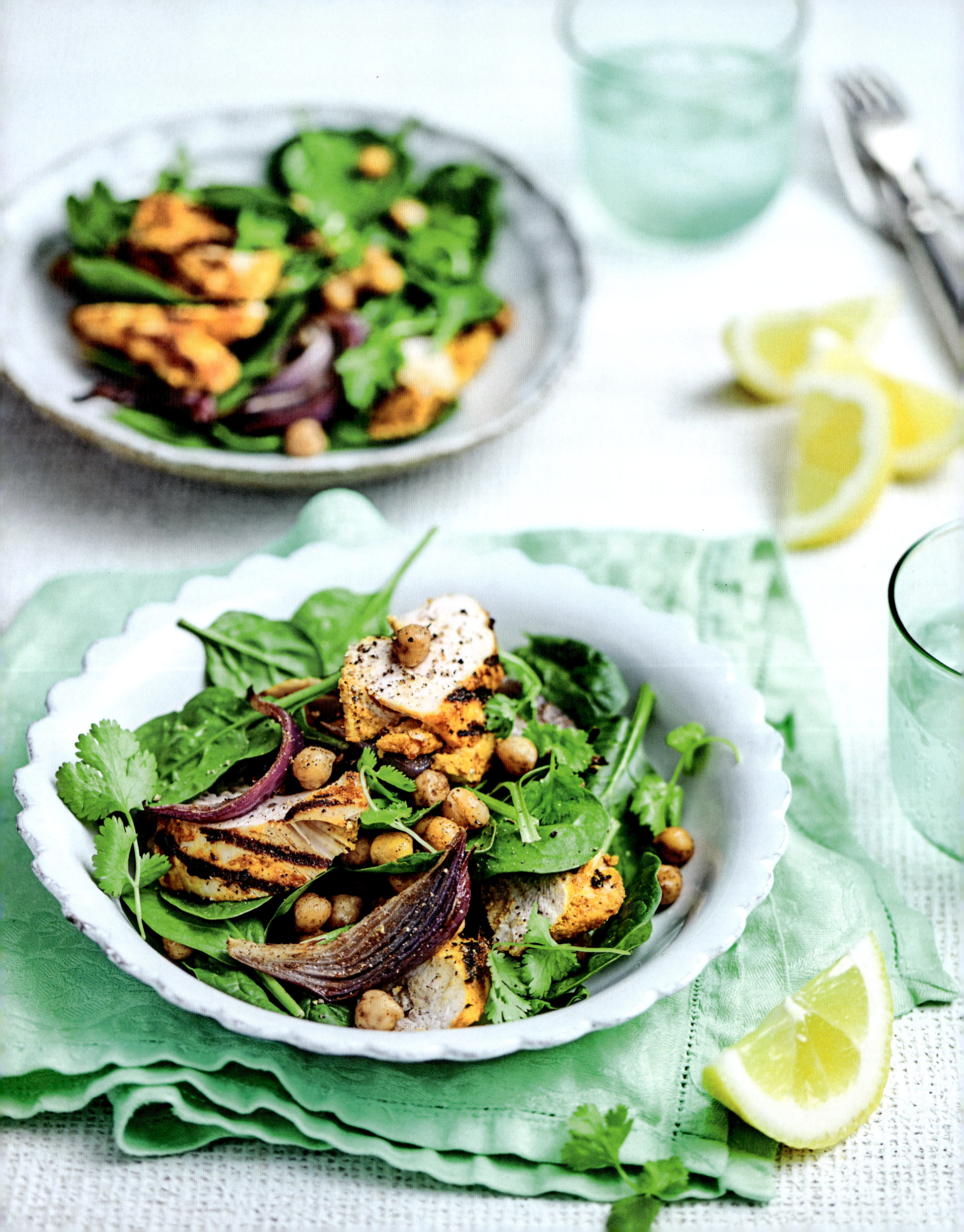

| • 16.1g total fat (4.3g saturated fat) | • 1624kJ (387 cal) | • 18.8g carbohydrate | • 37.2g protein | • 9g fibre | • 420mg sodium |
|---|---|---|---|---|---|

# TANDOORI CHICKEN
## with roast chickpea salad

**PREP + COOK TIME** 40 MINUTES (+ REFRIGERATION) **SERVES** 4

¾ cup (230g) low-fat natural Greek-style yoghurt

1 tablespoon finely grated fresh ginger

6 cloves garlic, crushed

1 tablespoon tandoori paste

1 teaspoon garam masala

2 teaspoons ground cumin

1 teaspoon ground coriander

1 fresh long red chilli, chopped coarsely

2 teaspoons grated fresh turmeric (see tips)

600g (1¼lb) chicken thigh fillets (see tips)

1 medium lemon (140g), cut into wedges

**ROAST CHICKPEA SALAD**

400g (12½oz) can salt-reduced chickpeas (garbanzo beans), drained, rinsed

1 medium red onion (170g), cut into wedges

1 tablespoon extra virgin olive oil

2 teaspoons garam masala

160g (5oz) baby spinach leaves

½ cup fresh coriander (cilantro) leaves

2 tablespoons lemon juice

**1** Blend or process yoghurt, ginger, garlic, tandoori paste, spices, chilli and turmeric until smooth.

**2** Place chicken in a large ziptop bag; pour over yoghurt marinade, massaging into chicken to cover all over. Refrigerate for at least 1 hour.

**3** Meanwhile, make roast chickpea salad.

**4** Heat a grill plate (or grill pan) on high heat; line with baking paper. Cook chicken on grill plate, covered with a roasting pan, for 5 minutes each side, or until grill marks appear and chicken is cooked through (see tips). Cover loosely with foil; rest for 5 minutes.

**5** Slice chicken, add to chickpea salad; toss to combine. Season with pepper to taste; serve with lemon wedges.

**ROAST CHICKPEA SALAD** Preheat oven to 200°C/400°F. Grease and line a large oven tray. Combine chickpeas, onion, oil and garam masala in a medium bowl. Spread on lined tray; roast for 20 minutes or until chickpeas are golden and onion is tender. Leave to cool. Transfer chickpeas and onion to a large bowl; add spinach, coriander and lemon juice. Season to taste with pepper.

**DR JO SAYS**
Having diabetes increases the risk of heart disease, so it's important to eat for both good blood glucose and a healthy heart. Excess salt can lead to high blood pressure – a key risk factor for heart attack and stroke. Using spices helps cut the salt while adding flavour.

**TIPS** Use 1 teaspoon ground turmeric if fresh turmeric is unavailable. Be careful when using fresh turmeric, as it can stain your skin, clothes, bench top and plastic cooking equipment and utensils.

You can also marinate the chicken in a large glass or stainless steel bowl, covered, in the fridge. Cook the chicken on a barbecue grill plate with the lid closed, if you prefer.

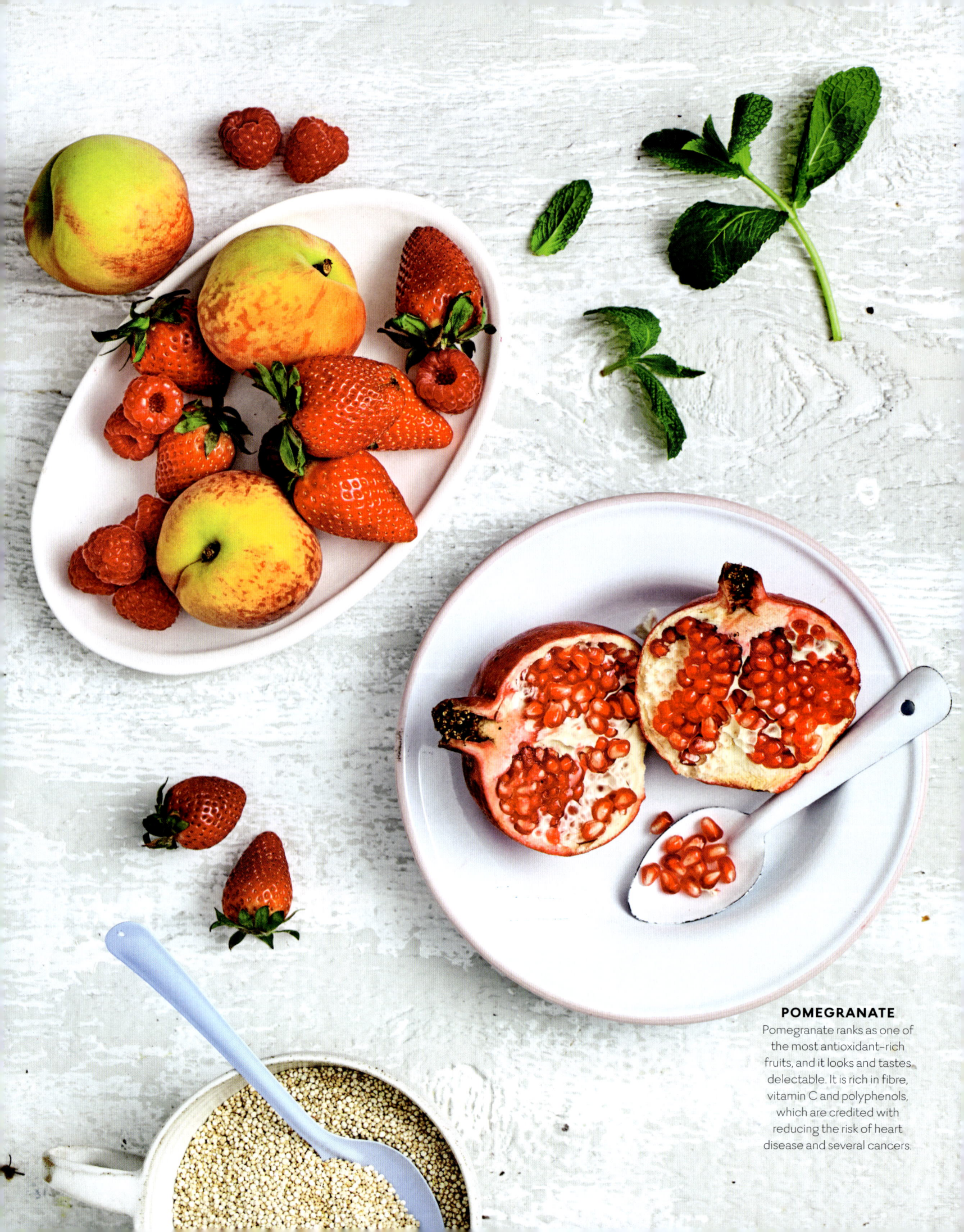

**POMEGRANATE**
Pomegranate ranks as one of the most antioxidant-rich fruits, and it looks and tastes delectable. It is rich in fibre, vitamin C and polyphenols, which are credited with reducing the risk of heart disease and several cancers.

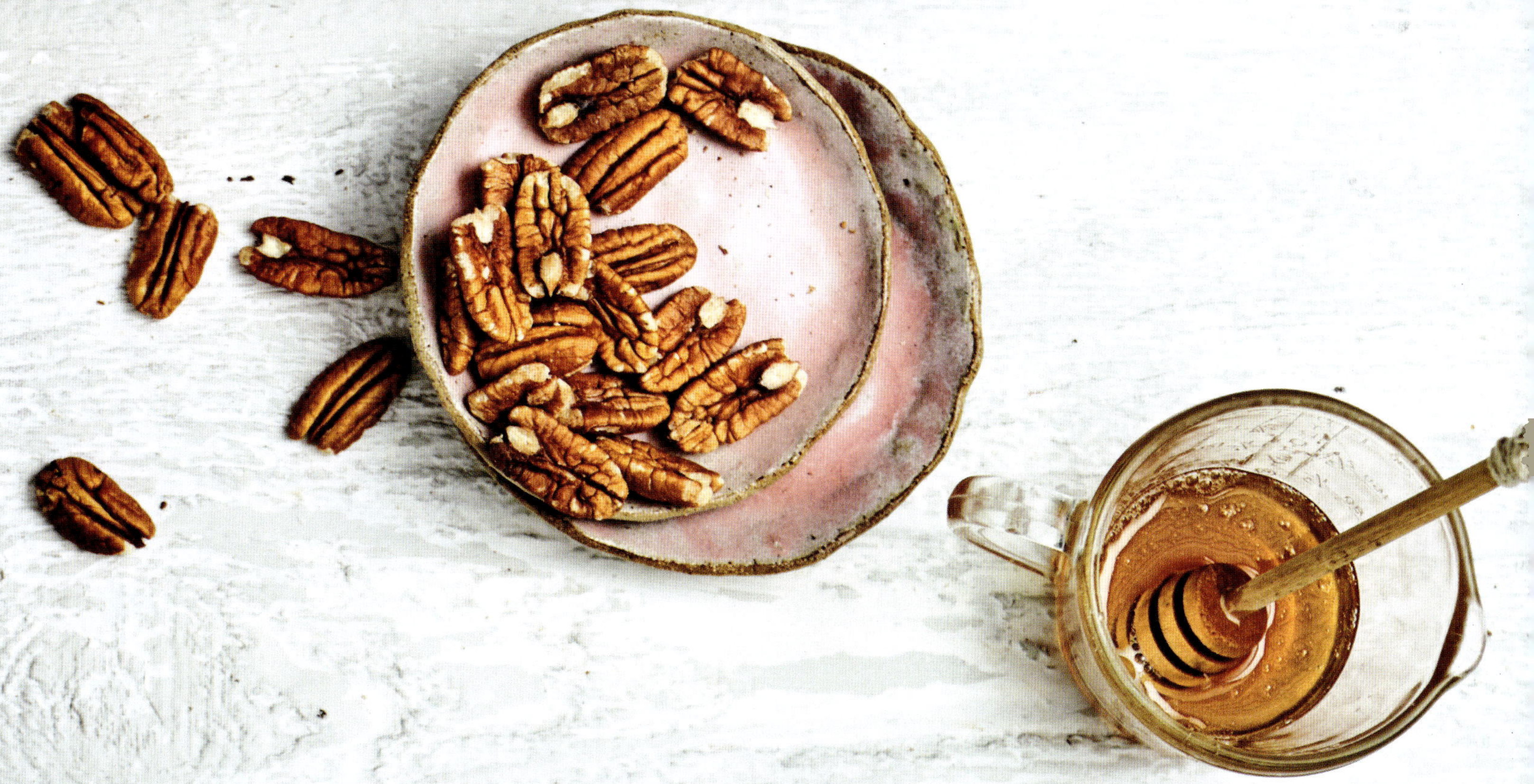

# DESSERT

Most of us love a sweet treat at least now and again. The good news is, it is entirely possible to enjoy a dessert without it leading to high blood glucose spikes and negative impacts on health. It all comes down to using quality ingredients, limiting added sugars and using healthy fat sources. Portion size is, of course, also key. Make dessert an occasional indulgence that you savour and truly enjoy.

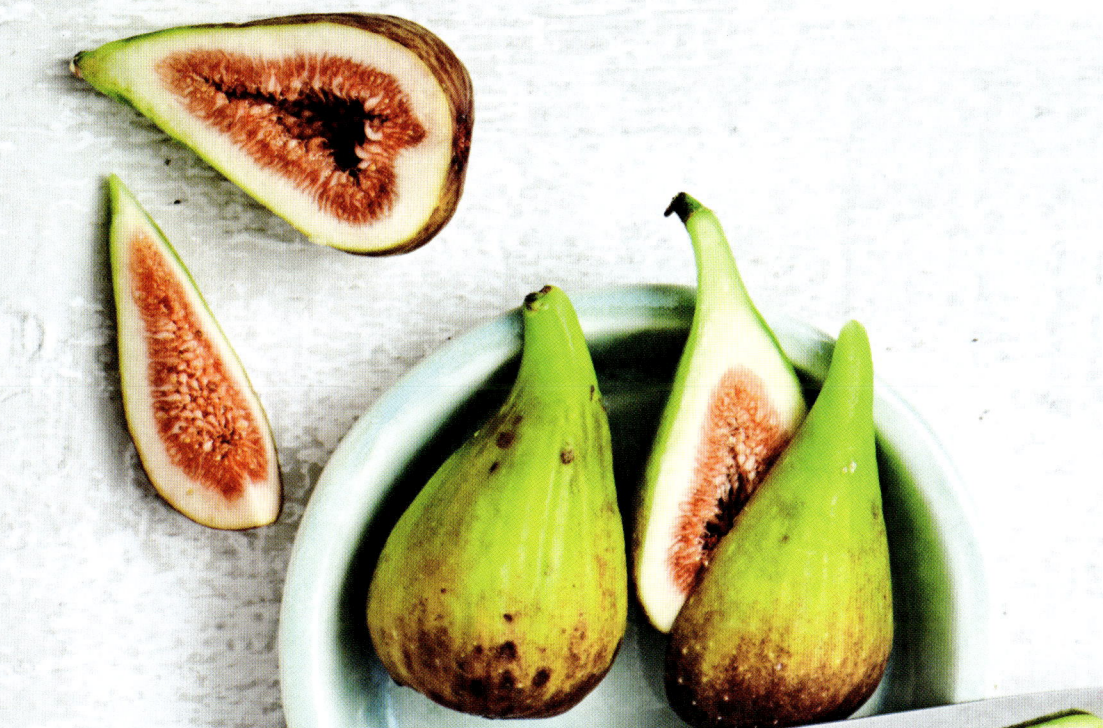

## FIGS

The Ancient Greeks believed so fervently that figs were health promoting, they fed them to their athletes competing in the original Olympic games. They are a great source of fibre and delicious served with cheese, or grilled and served with a dollop of greek yoghurt.

**NUTRITIONAL COUNT PER PIECE**

| | | | | | |
|---|---|---|---|---|---|
| ● 1.9g total fat (1.6g saturated fat) | ● 210kJ (50 cal) | ● 5.9g carbohydrate | ● 2.1g protein | ● 1.2g fibre | ● 11mg sodium |

# SKIM MILK MARSHMALLOWS
## with berries

**PREP + COOK TIME** 25 MINUTES (+ STANDING) **MAKES** 16 (2 PIECES PER SERVING)

⅔ cup (160ml) skim milk
¼ cup (90g) honey
½ cup (75g) frozen raspberries, thawed
2 tablespoons powdered gelatine
½ cup (40g) desiccated coconut
125g (4oz) fresh raspberries

**1** Grease and line a 20cm (8in) square cake pan with freezer film or plastic wrap.

**2** Blend ⅓ cup milk with the honey and thawed raspberries until mixture is smooth. Press through a sieve into the bowl of an electric mixer; discard solids in strainer. Fit whisk attachment to mixer; whisk milk mixture on medium speed.

**3** Meanwhile, sprinkle gelatine over remaining cold milk in a heatproof jug. Stir with a fork; stand jug in a small saucepan of boiling water until gelatine dissolves.

**4** With the electric mixer operating on high, slowly add the gelatine mixture to raspberry mixture; whisk on high speed for 4 minutes. Working quickly, spoon marshmallow into pan. Smooth top with an offset palette knife or the back of a spoon. Stand for 2 hours or until set.

**5** Place coconut on a tray. Remove marshmallow from the pan; use a hot knife to cut the marshmallow evenly into 16 squares. Roll each square in coconut. Serve two marshmallows per person with a quarter of the raspberries.

**TIP** Marshmallows are best made on the day of serving.
As this makes 16 squares, and the portion size is only 2 pieces per person, it's a good reason to get friends and family around to cut down on the temptation to sneak a few more!

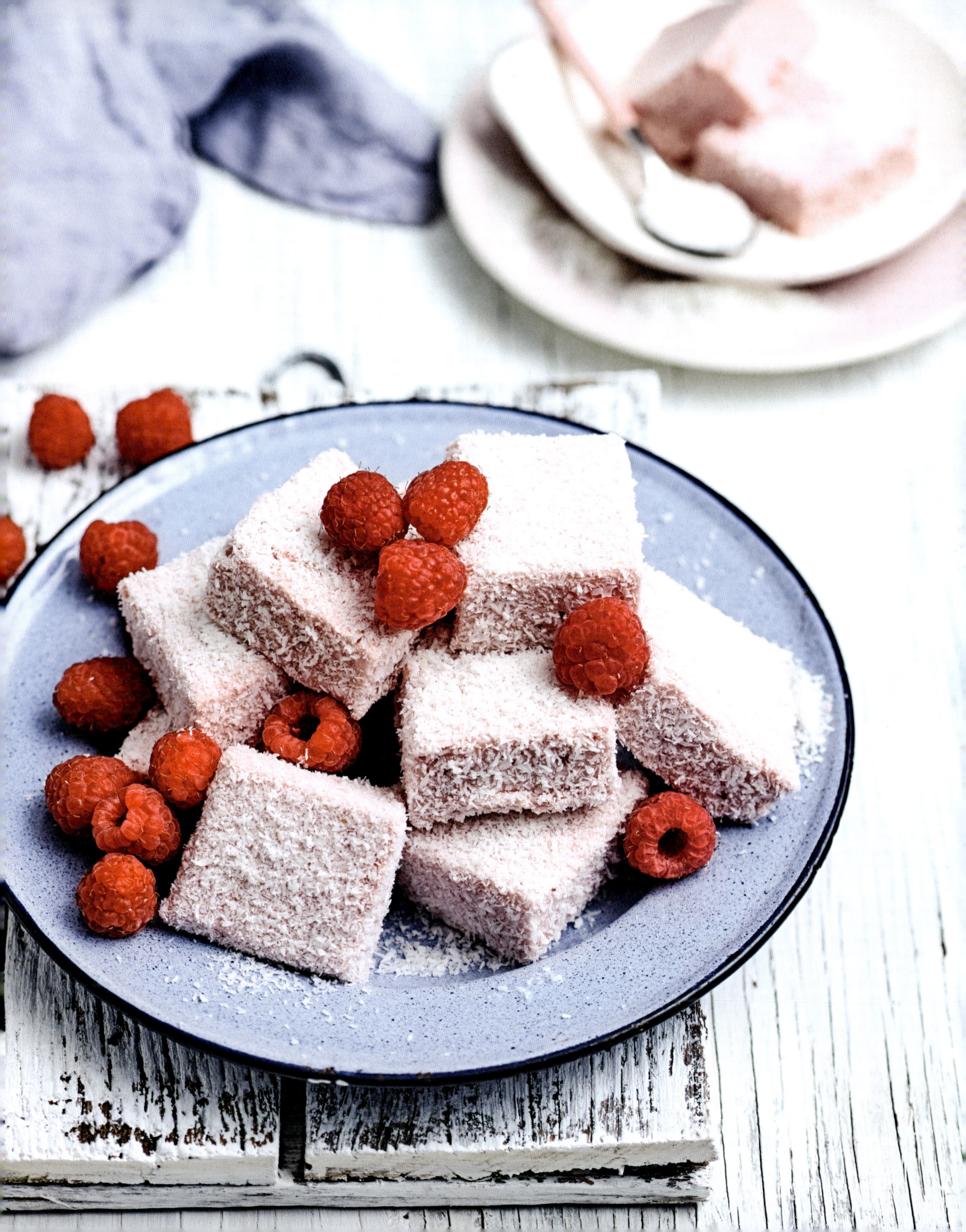

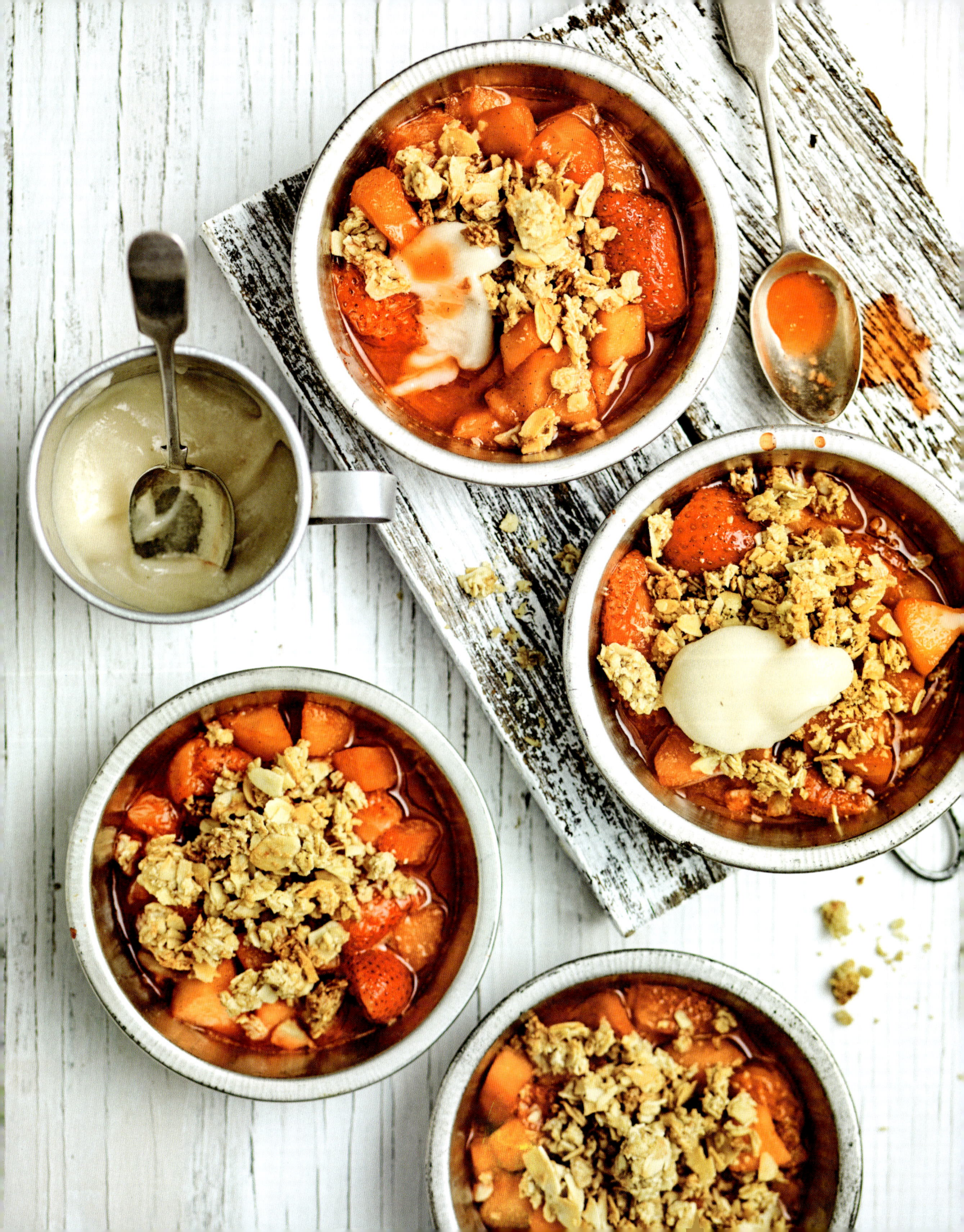

| ● 6.7g total fat (1.8g saturated fat) | ● 797kJ (190 cal) | ● 26.4g carbohydrate | ● 4.1g protein | ● 5.2g fibre | ● 5mg sodium |

# BERRY & APPLE CRUMBLE
## with custard apple 'custard'

**PREP + COOK TIME** 30 MINUTES **SERVES** 4

$1/3$ **cup (30g) rolled oats**

$1/4$ **cup (20g) flaked almonds**

**10g ($1/2$oz) unsalted butter**

**$1½$ tablespoons brown sugar**

**1 teaspoon water**

**2 medium granny smith apples (300g)**

**$1/4$ cup (60ml) water, extra**

**$1½$ teaspoons vanilla bean paste**

**250g (8oz) strawberries, washed, halved**

**CUSTARD APPLE 'CUSTARD'**

**1 medium custard apple (150g)**

**1** Preheat oven to 170°C/340°F. Line a small oven tray with baking paper.

**2** Beat oats, almonds, butter, 1 tablespoon of the sugar and the 1 teaspoon of water with an electric mixer until combined. Tip into tray, spread roughly to form clumps; bake for 10 minutes or until light golden and crunchy.

**3** Meanwhile, make custard apple 'custard'.

**4** Peel, core and dice apple coarsely. Place remaining sugar, the extra water, apple and vanilla in a medium saucepan over high heat; cook, stirring, for 2 minutes or until water comes to the boil. Add strawberries, stir to combine; cook for a further 8 minutes or until apple is soft and liquid is reduced by a third.

**5** Divide apple mixture among four heatproof ¾ cup (180ml) ramekins or serving bowls; top each with a quarter of the crumble mixture. Serve each with a quarter of the custard apple 'custard'.

**CUSTARD APPLE 'CUSTARD'** Halve custard apple; discard all seeds, being careful not to discard any flesh. Process flesh in a small food processor until smooth. Cover, placing plastic wrap directly on the surface of the puree.

**DR JO SAYS**

Nuts, including almonds, have been shown to reduce the risk of heart disease, stroke and type 2 diabetes, while improving cardiovascular health in those with diabetes.

**TIP** Here the pureed custard apple replaces regular custard to great effect, without all the kilojoules.

**CUSTARD APPLES** are a sub-tropical fruit with a pale green knobbly skin, a sweet creamy white flesh and brown seeds. Remove the seeds and eat the flesh when soft.

| ● 7g total fat (2.7g saturated fat) | ● 569kJ (135 cal) | ● 12g carbohydrate | ● 4.9g protein | ● 1.6g fibre | ● 96mg sodium |
|---|---|---|---|---|---|

# Ginger-poached rhubarb
# ALMOND FILLO TARTS

**PREP + COOK TIME** 30 MINUTES (+ COOLING) **SERVES** 4

olive-oil spray
2 sheets fillo pastry (30g)
¾ cup (210g) natural Greek-style yoghurt
2 tablespoons light sour cream
1 tablespoon small fresh mint leaves
1 tablespoon natural flaked almonds, toasted lightly
GINGER-POACHED RHUBARB
300g (9½oz) rhubarb, cut into 3cm (1¼in) pieces
1cm (½in) piece fresh ginger, sliced thinly
1 cup (250ml) low-joule dry ginger ale
1 teaspoon stevia granules

**1** Preheat oven to 200°C/400°F. Lightly spray four holes of a 6-hole (¾ cup/180ml) texas muffin pan with oil.

**2** Spray one pastry sheet with oil, top with remaining sheet; press lightly to seal. Cut in half; cut each half into quarters. Overlap 2 pieces to form a rough square; carefully line muffin holes with pastry.

**3** Bake pastry for 5 minutes or until browned lightly and crisp. Stand in pans for 5 minutes. Using a small metal spatula, carefully transfer pastry cases from pans to wire racks; leave to cool.

**4** Meanwhile, make ginger-poached rhubarb.

**5** Combine yoghurt and sour cream in a small bowl.

**6** Just before serving, divide yoghurt mixture among pastry cases. Top each with a quarter of the cooled rhubarb; drizzle evenly with any syrup. Top with torn mint leaves and flaked almonds to serve.

**GINGER-POACHED RHUBARB** Place rhubarb in a single layer in a medium frying pan, add ginger, ginger ale and stevia; bring to the boil. Reduce heat to medium–high; cook for 3 minutes (depending on thickness of rhubarb) or until just tender, without stirring so as not to break up the rhubarb. Carefully remove rhubarb with a slotted spoon; transfer to a large plate to cool. Bring syrup to the boil over high heat; boil for 3 minutes or until reduced and syrupy. Pour over rhubarb; leave to cool, then discard ginger slices from rhubarb.

**TIPS** Use 1 tablespoon of coarsely chopped pistachios instead of the almond flakes, if you like.

The rhubarb can be cooked the day before; store in an airtight container, large enough so the rhubarb holds its shape, in the fridge.

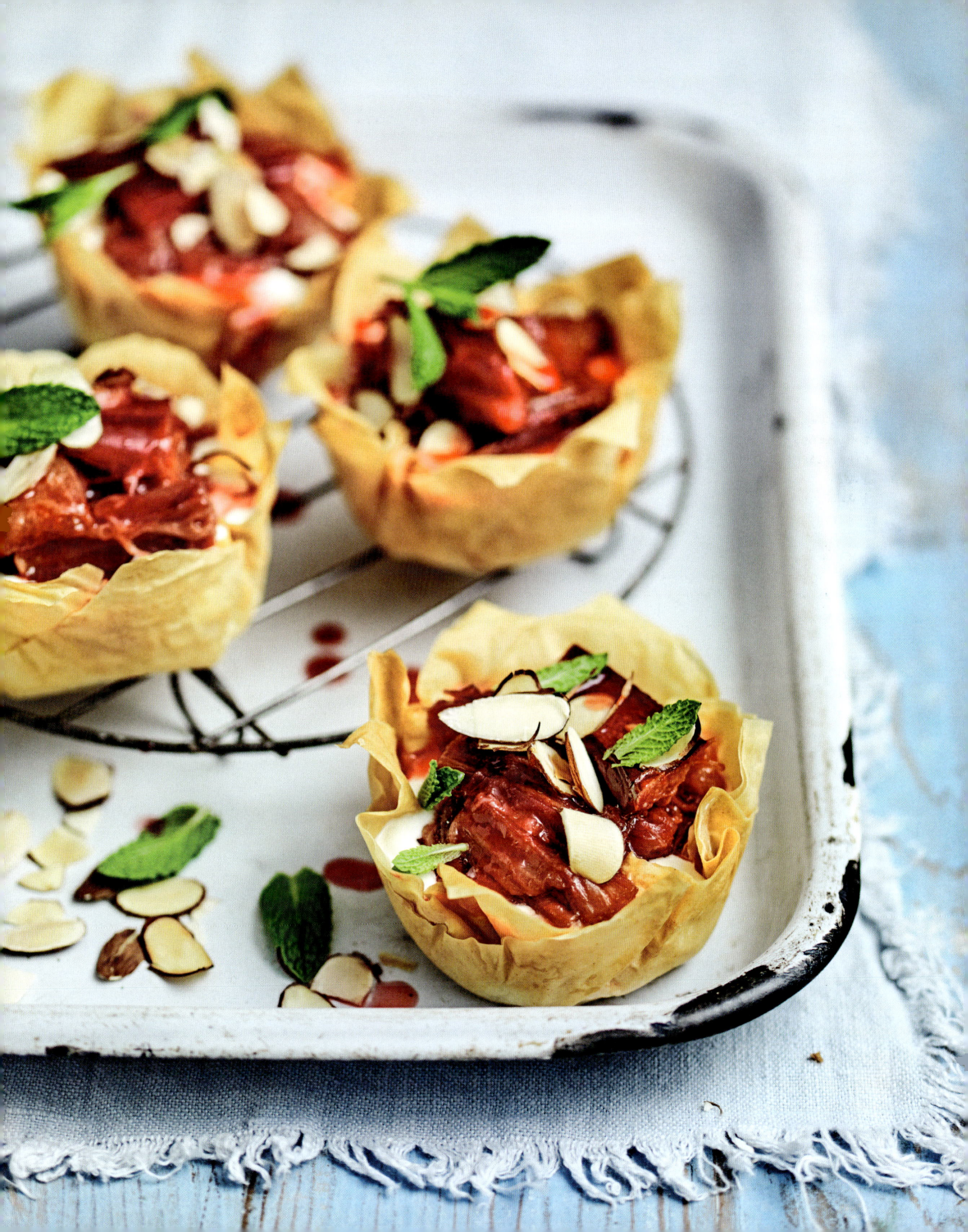

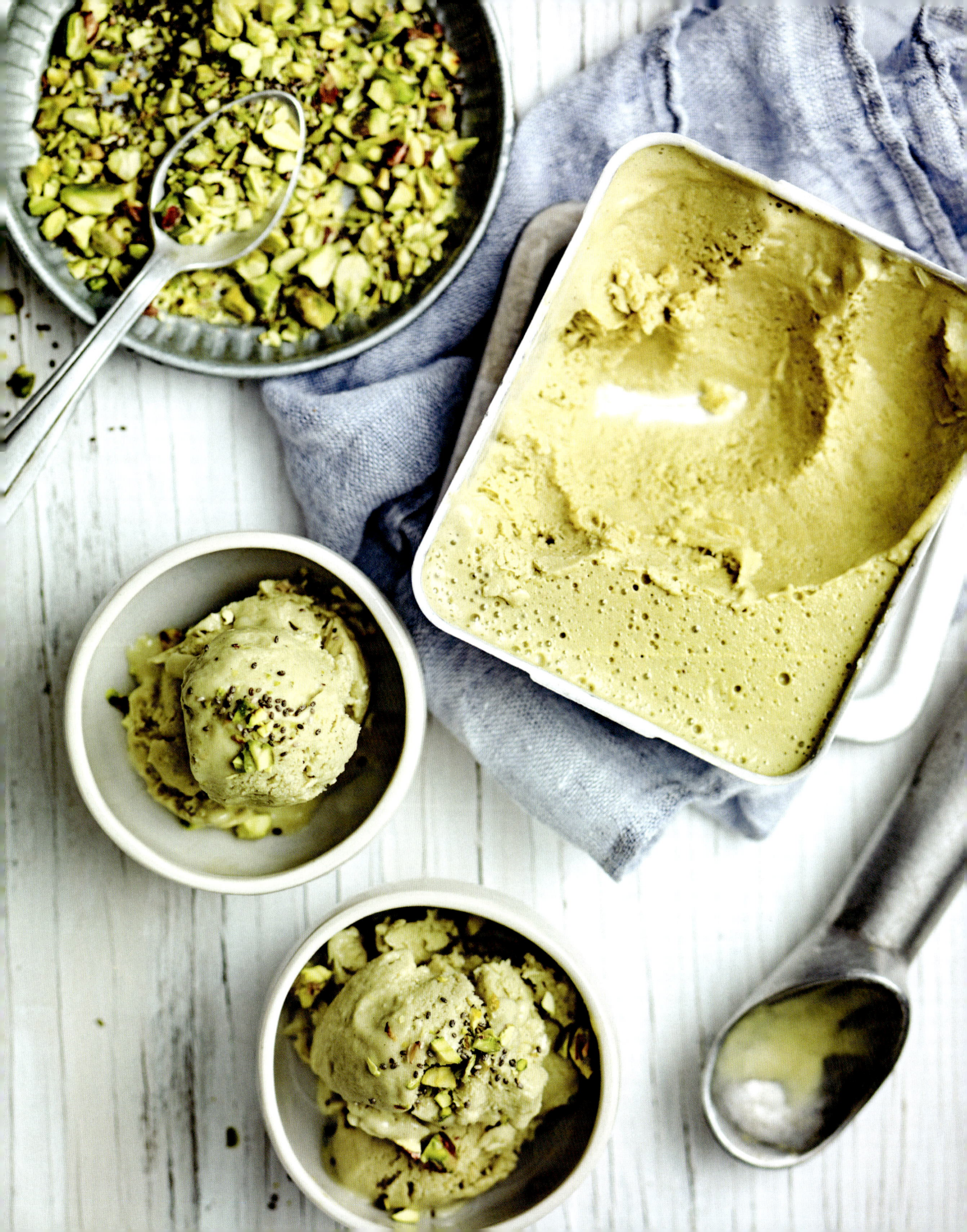

| ● 2.6g total fat (1g saturated fat) | ● 528kJ (126 cal) | ● 20.7g carbohydrate | ● 3.7g protein | ● 3.4g fibre | ● 22mg sodium |
|---|---|---|---|---|---|

# Banana matcha
# FRO-YO

**PREP + COOK TIME** 10 MINUTES (+ FREEZING) **SERVES** 4

2 medium very ripe bananas (400g), sliced
½ cup (140g) natural Greek-style yoghurt
1 teaspoon matcha powder
1 teaspoon vanilla bean paste
2 teaspoons honey
2 teaspoons black chia seeds
2 tablespoons pistachios, chopped finely

**1** Place bananas in a small airtight freezer-proof container. Freeze for at least 4 hours or until frozen.

**2** Process frozen bananas, yoghurt, matcha powder, vanilla and honey until a smooth soft-serve fro-yo consistency forms. Freeze for a further 1 hour or until mixture is firm enough to scoop.

**3** Combine chia and pistachios in a small bowl. Divide fro-yo among four small bowls, sprinkle evenly with chia mixture to serve.

**TIP** The fro-yo can be served as soon as it is processed, but it will be the consistency of soft-serve frozen yoghurt rather than firm.

**DR JO SAYS**
Nuts and seeds are terrific snacks that deliver heart-healthy nutrients, while having almost no carbohydrates, so they won't raise your blood glucose levels.

| 5.3g total fat (1.8g saturated fat) | 578kJ (138 cal) | 17.3g carbohydrate | 4.9g protein | 0.9g fibre | 47mg sodium |

# BUTTERMILK PANNA COTTA
## with strawberry salad

**PREP + COOK TIME** 25 MINUTES (+ COOLING & REFRIGERATION) **SERVES** 6

5 small gelatine leaves (25g) (see tips)
¾ cup (180ml) milk
2 teaspoons fresh thyme leaves,
   chopped finely (see tips)
1¼ cups (310ml) buttermilk
⅓ cup (80ml) pure maple syrup
1 teaspoon pure vanilla extract
**STRAWBERRY SALAD**
250g (8oz) strawberries, diced
1 tablespoon extra virgin olive oil
1 tablespoon fresh thyme leaves

**1** Soak gelatine sheets in a bowl of cold water for 5 minutes or until softened.

**2** Place milk and thyme leaves in a small saucepan; bring to a simmer, taking care not to boil. Squeeze excess water from gelatine, add to hot milk; whisk well to dissolve. Remove milk mixture from heat; cool completely. Blend or process until smooth; strain into a large jug.

**3** Stir buttermilk, maple syrup and vanilla into gelatine mixture. Divide mixture evenly among 6 x 100ml (3oz) dariole moulds. Refrigerate for 4 hours or overnight to set.

**4** Just before serving, make strawberry salad.

**5** Carefully turn out panna cotta onto small plates; serve with strawberry salad.

**STRAWBERRY SALAD** Combine ingredients in a small bowl.

**TIPS** We used McKenzie's brand gelatine leaves here.
If you have one, use a stick blender to blend the gelatine mixture as it works well with the smaller amount of liquid.
Swap mint for the thyme, if you like.

**DARIOLE MOULDS** are small cylindrical moulds. They were originally used in France to bake darioles (hence the name), small puff pastry cases filled with an almond-based pastry cream. Use any small serving dishes you have of a similar capacity.

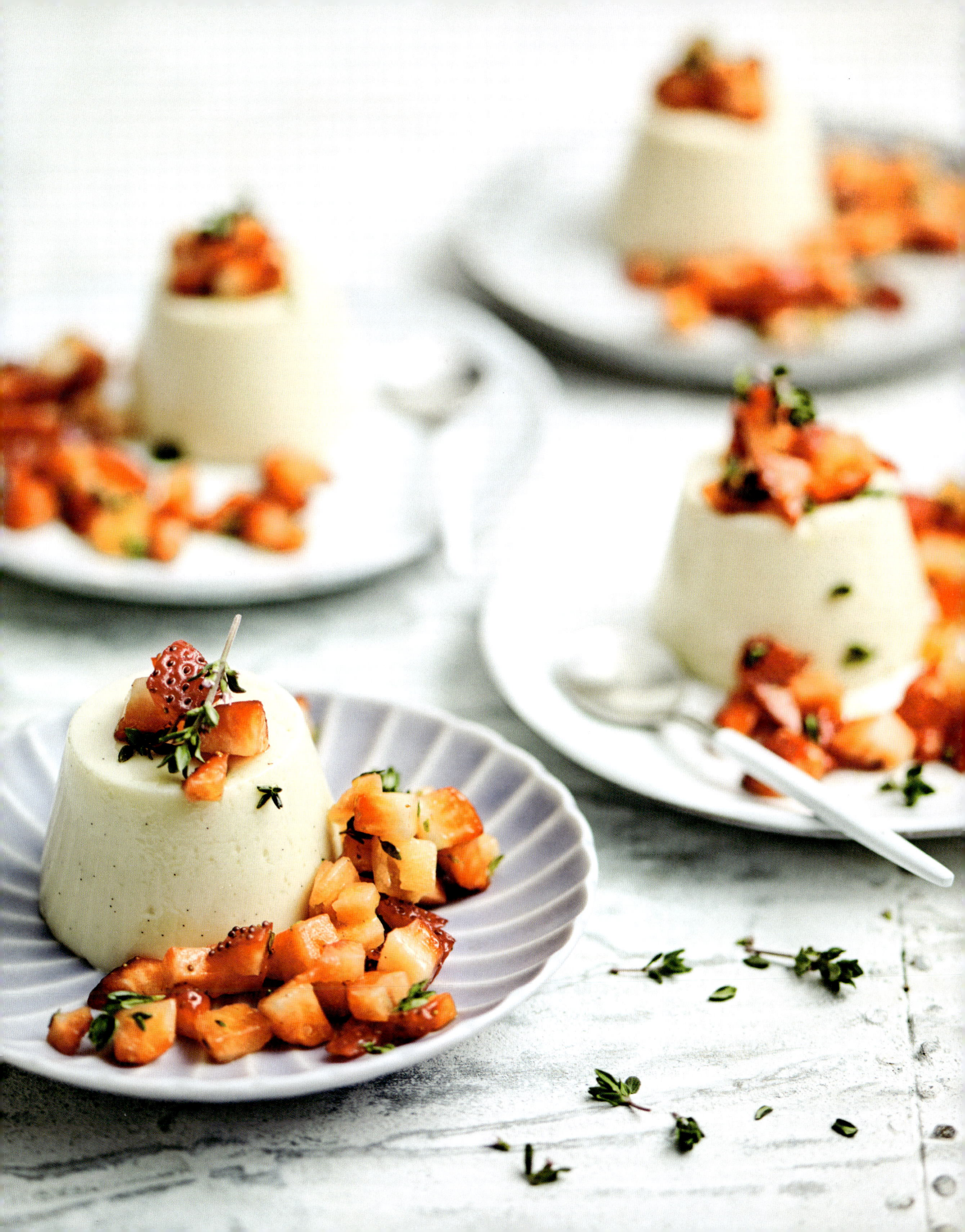

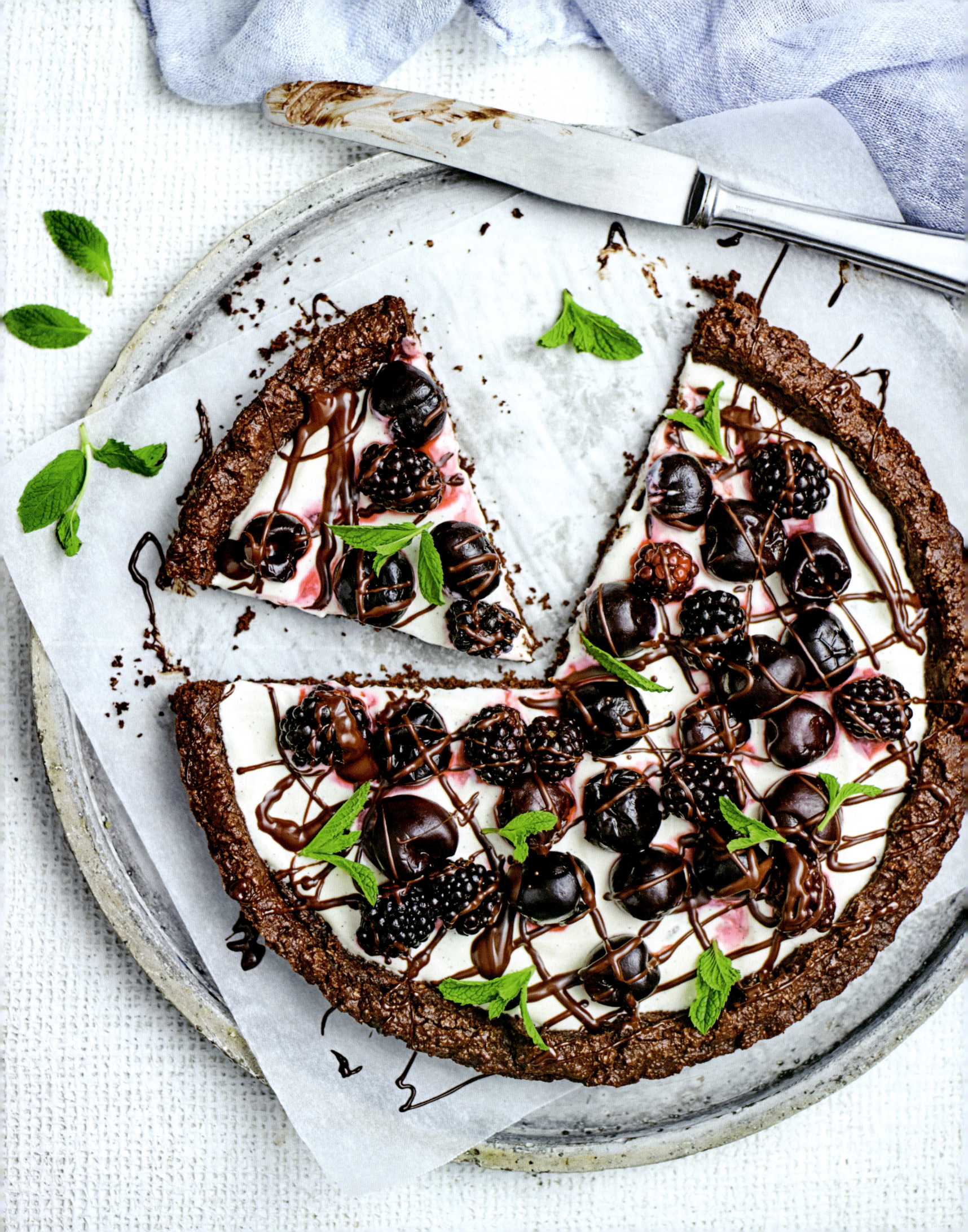

| | | | | | |
|---|---|---|---|---|---|
| ● 9.1g total fat (4.1g saturated fat) | ● 726kJ (173 cal) | ● 16.4g carbohydrate | ● 5.2g protein | ● 3.2g fibre | ● 56mg sodium |

# Fruits of the forest
# COOKIE 'PIZZA'

**PREP + COOK TIME** 35 MINUTES (+ COOLING) **SERVES** 8

¾ cup (70g) rolled oats
¼ cup (30g) almond meal
¼ cup (30g) dutch-processed cocoa
½ teaspoon baking powder
30g (1oz) unsalted butter, melted
¼ cup (60ml) pure maple syrup
1½ tablespoons light sour cream
1 egg
1 egg white
½ cup (140g) natural yoghurt
2 teaspoons vanilla bean paste
20g (¾oz) dark (semi-sweet) chocolate (70% cocoa)
1 cup (150g) fresh cherries, pitted
½ cup (75g) blueberries
½ cup (75g) fresh or frozen blackberries
small fresh mint leaves, to serve

**1** Preheat oven to 180°C/350°F. Grease and line a 22cm (9in) loose-based tart tin.

**2** Pulse oats in a food processor until they resemble flour. Transfer to a large bowl; sift in almond meal, cocoa and baking powder.

**3** Place butter, maple syrup, sour cream, egg and egg white in a medium bowl; whisk until combined. Fold egg mixture into oat mixture until combined; transfer mixture to tin.

**4** Spread oat mixture over base of tin, creating a 2cm (¾in) rim up side of tin to form a 'crust' around the edge. Bake for 15 minutes or until firm and dry; cool completely in tin.

**5** Meanwhile, mix yoghurt and vanilla bean paste in a small bowl until combined; refrigerate until required.

**6** Melt chocolate. Remove cookie base from tin; spread with yoghurt mixture. Arrange cherries and berries on top. Drizzle with chocolate and sprinkle with mint to serve.

### DR JO SAYS

Oats are rich in soluble fibre, which helps to slow the absorption of glucose. Steer clear, however, of instant oats, as these have a higher GI. Instead, opt for traditional or steel-cut oats.

**TIP** To melt chocolate, place broken pieces in a microwave-safe bowl, then microwave it using short bursts of low power (50%). Check every 10-20 seconds by pressing with a spatula — it could be melted even though it's retained its shape.

To melt using the stove top, stir broken chocolate in a small heatproof bowl over a small saucepan of simmering water (don't let water touch base of bowl) until just melted.

# Exceptionally Good ICE-CREAM SANDWICHES

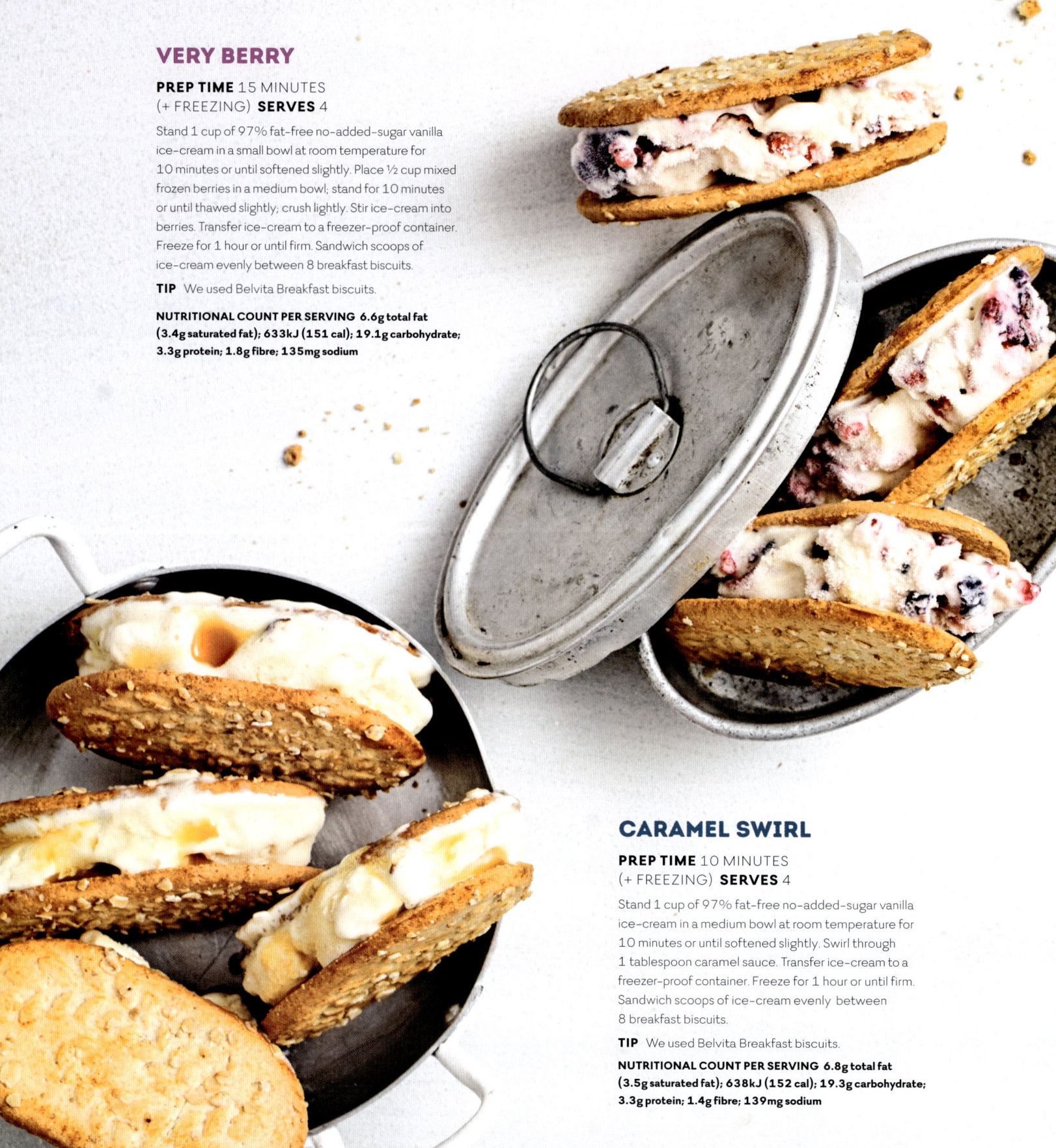

## VERY BERRY

**PREP TIME** 15 MINUTES
(+ FREEZING) **SERVES** 4

Stand 1 cup of 97% fat-free no-added-sugar vanilla ice-cream in a small bowl at room temperature for 10 minutes or until softened slightly. Place ½ cup mixed frozen berries in a medium bowl; stand for 10 minutes or until thawed slightly; crush lightly. Stir ice-cream into berries. Transfer ice-cream to a freezer-proof container. Freeze for 1 hour or until firm. Sandwich scoops of ice-cream evenly between 8 breakfast biscuits.

**TIP** We used Belvita Breakfast biscuits.

**NUTRITIONAL COUNT PER SERVING** 6.6g total fat (3.4g saturated fat); 633kJ (151 cal); 19.1g carbohydrate; 3.3g protein; 1.8g fibre; 135mg sodium

## CARAMEL SWIRL

**PREP TIME** 10 MINUTES
(+ FREEZING) **SERVES** 4

Stand 1 cup of 97% fat-free no-added-sugar vanilla ice-cream in a medium bowl at room temperature for 10 minutes or until softened slightly. Swirl through 1 tablespoon caramel sauce. Transfer ice-cream to a freezer-proof container. Freeze for 1 hour or until firm. Sandwich scoops of ice-cream evenly between 8 breakfast biscuits.

**TIP** We used Belvita Breakfast biscuits.

**NUTRITIONAL COUNT PER SERVING** 6.8g total fat (3.5g saturated fat); 638kJ (152 cal); 19.3g carbohydrate; 3.3g protein; 1.4g fibre; 139mg sodium

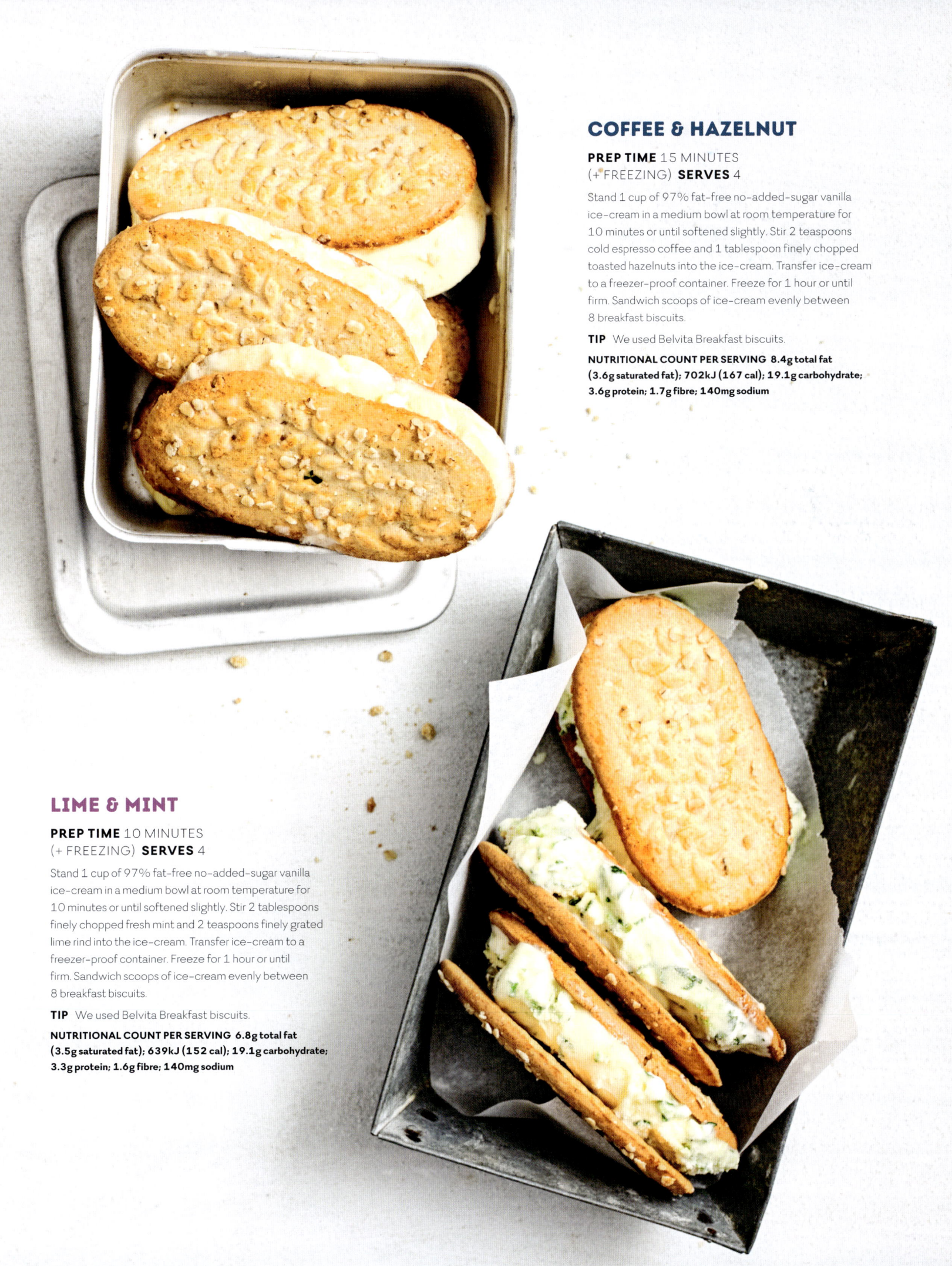

## COFFEE & HAZELNUT

**PREP TIME** 15 MINUTES
(+ FREEZING) **SERVES** 4

Stand 1 cup of 97% fat-free no-added-sugar vanilla ice-cream in a medium bowl at room temperature for 10 minutes or until softened slightly. Stir 2 teaspoons cold espresso coffee and 1 tablespoon finely chopped toasted hazelnuts into the ice-cream. Transfer ice-cream to a freezer-proof container. Freeze for 1 hour or until firm. Sandwich scoops of ice-cream evenly between 8 breakfast biscuits.

**TIP** We used Belvita Breakfast biscuits.

**NUTRITIONAL COUNT PER SERVING** 8.4g total fat (3.6g saturated fat); 702kJ (167 cal); 19.1g carbohydrate; 3.6g protein; 1.7g fibre; 140mg sodium

## LIME & MINT

**PREP TIME** 10 MINUTES
(+ FREEZING) **SERVES** 4

Stand 1 cup of 97% fat-free no-added-sugar vanilla ice-cream in a medium bowl at room temperature for 10 minutes or until softened slightly. Stir 2 tablespoons finely chopped fresh mint and 2 teaspoons finely grated lime rind into the ice-cream. Transfer ice-cream to a freezer-proof container. Freeze for 1 hour or until firm. Sandwich scoops of ice-cream evenly between 8 breakfast biscuits.

**TIP** We used Belvita Breakfast biscuits.

**NUTRITIONAL COUNT PER SERVING** 6.8g total fat (3.5g saturated fat); 639kJ (152 cal); 19.1g carbohydrate; 3.3g protein; 1.6g fibre; 140mg sodium

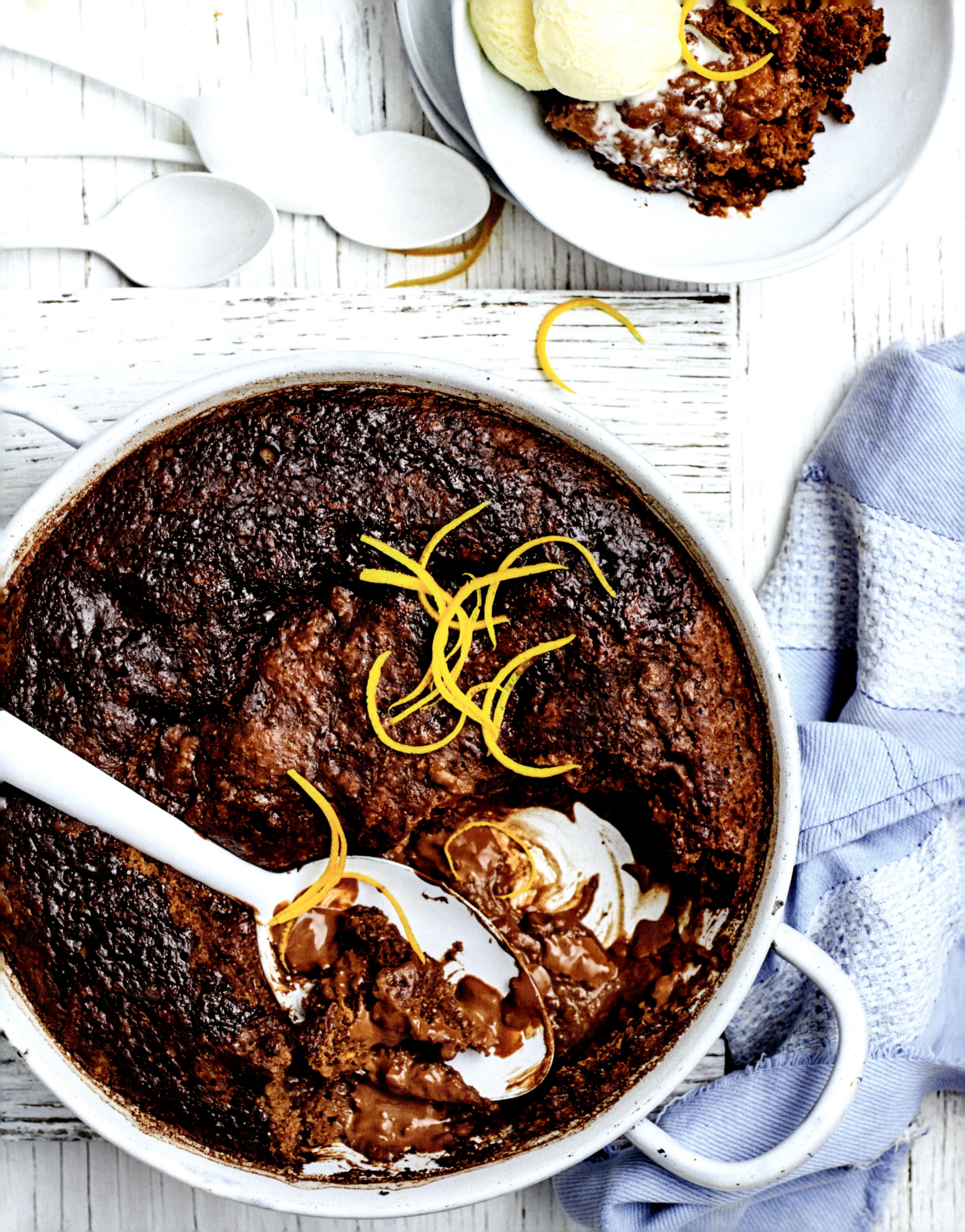

| ● 5.3g total fat (2.6g saturated fat) | ● 677kJ (161 cal) | ● 22g carbohydrate | ● 5.8g protein | ● 2.3g fibre | ● 178mg sodium |
|---|---|---|---|---|---|

# Jaffa self-saucing PUDDING

**PREP + COOK TIME** 45 MINUTES **SERVES** 6

1 large orange (300g) (see tips)
1/3 cup (50g) self-raising flour
1/3 cup (55g) wholemeal self-raising flour (see tips)
1/4 cup (30g) dutch-processed cocoa
1/4 cup (55g) brown sugar
1/3 cup (80ml) skim milk
1 egg
1 cup (250ml) boiling water
300g (9½oz) no-added-sugar, low-fat
  vanilla ice-cream

**1** Preheat oven to 150°C/300°F. Lightly grease a 1 litre (4 cup) ovenproof dish.

**2** Finely grate orange as needed to get 1 tablespoon rind; shred remaining rind into long strips. Juice orange (you need 1 tablespoon juice).

**3** Sift flours and 1½ tablespoons of the cocoa into a large bowl. Add 1½ tablespoons of the sugar; stir to combine.

**4** Whisk milk, egg, orange juice and finely grated rind in a medium bowl. Add to flour mixture; fold until just combined.

**5** Spoon pudding mixture into dish. Place dish on an oven tray. Combine remaining cocoa and sugar in a small bowl; sprinkle over pudding. Carefully pour over the boiling water; bake for 25 minutes or until set.

**6** Sprinkle pudding with shredded orange rind and serve with ice cream.

**TIPS** You will need one large orange for this recipe – the larger the better to get the amount of rind needed.
If you don't have wholemeal self-raising flour, you can use all regular self-raising flour instead.

| 1.2g total fat (0.7g saturated fat) | 382kJ (91 cal) | 16.3g carbohydrate | 2g protein | 3.1g fibre | 139mg sodium |

# *Fruit salad*
# RICE PAPER ROLLS

**PREP + COOK TIME** 35 MINUTES **SERVES** 6

1 small mango (300g)
¼ cup (60ml) lime juice
¼ cup (60ml) canned light coconut milk
2 teaspoons vanilla bean paste
12 small rice paper rounds (60g) (see tips)
2 medium kiwifruit (170g), peeled, sliced
125g (4oz) strawberries, sliced
1 lebanese cucumber (130g), peeled, seeded,
  cut into matchsticks
½ cup fresh mint leaves, plus extra, to garnish

**1** Coarsely chop a third of the mango flesh. Slice remaining mango into thin batons.

**2** For mango coconut dipping sauce, blend or process chopped mango, lime juice, coconut milk and vanilla until mixture is smooth.

**3** Cover a chopping board with a damp clean tea towel. Place one sheet of rice paper at a time in a bowl of warm water until softened. Place on tea towel; top rice paper with one-twelfth of the sliced mango, kiwifruit, strawberry, cucumber and mint leaves in a line along the centre of the sheet. Fold bottom half of the rice paper up, then fold in both sides and roll over to enclose the filling.

**4** Repeat with remaining rice paper and filling ingredients to make a total of 12 rolls. Place rolls on a plastic wrap-lined tray; cover with damp paper towel. Refrigerate until ready to serve.

**5** Serve rice paper rolls with mango coconut dipping sauce, sprinkled with extra mint leaves.

**DR JO SAYS**

Include whole fruit in your daily diet but do avoid fruit juices. Juicing concentrates the sugars into an easy-to-consume form and discards the fibre and many of the beneficial phytochemicals.

**TIPS** Be sure to use ripe fruit for this recipe, as they give the best flavour.
We used 15cm (6in) diameter rice paper rounds here. They are available from major supermarkets and Asian food stores.

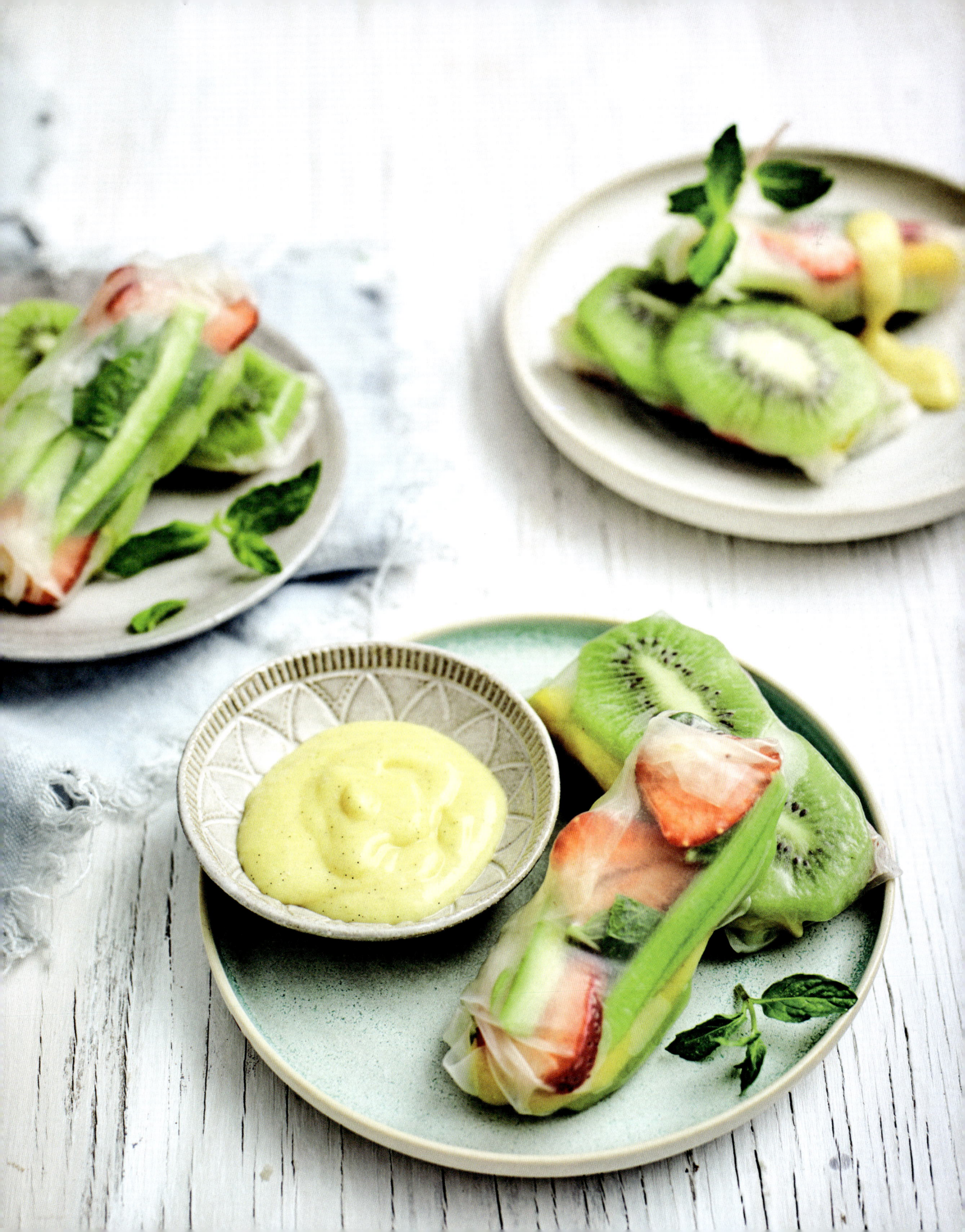

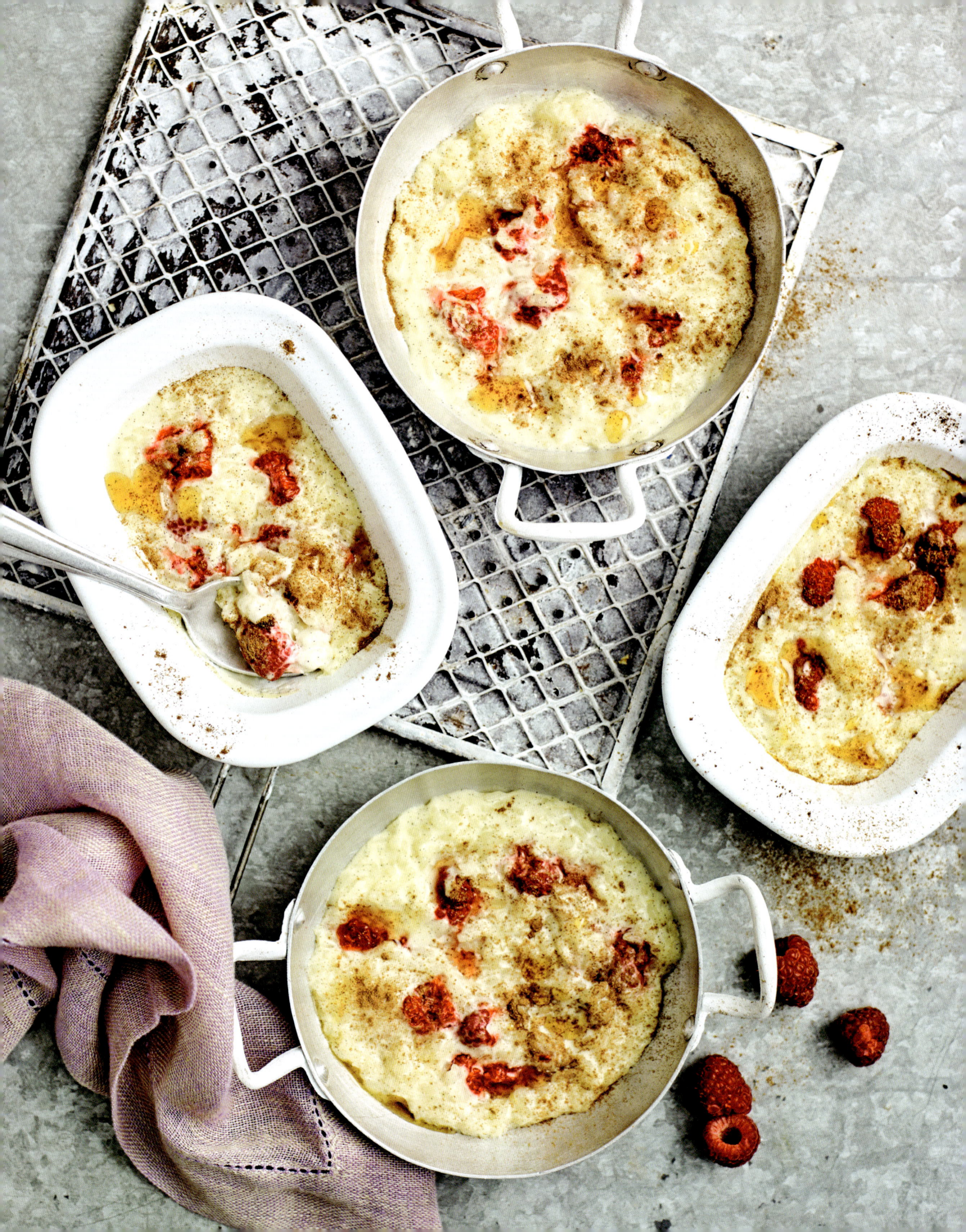

| | | | | | |
|---|---|---|---|---|---|
| 3g total fat (1.8g saturated fat) | 651kJ (155 cal) | 26.2g carbohydrate | 5.5g protein | 1.4g fibre | 51mg sodium |

# BAKED RICE PUDDINGS
## with raspberries

**PREP + COOK TIME** 35 MINUTES **SERVES** 4

$1/3$ cup (65g) white medium-grain rice
2 cups (500ml) milk
$3/4$ cup (180ml) water
$1 1/2$ tablespoons pure maple syrup
$1/2$ teaspoon finely grated lemon rind
1 vanilla bean, split, seeds scraped
$1/4$ cup (35g) fresh raspberries, torn
$1/2$ teaspoon ground cinnamon

**1** Rinse rice under cold running water until water runs clear.
**2** Place milk, the water, 1 tablespoon maple syrup, rind and vanilla bean and seeds in a small saucepan; bring to a simmer. Add rice, stirring to separate grains; bring to the boil. Reduce heat to low; cook, stirring occasionally, for 20 minutes or until rice is tender and liquid reduces and thickens.
**3** Discard vanilla bean; divide rice mixture among four $1/2$ cup (125ml) shallow ovenproof dishes. Top each with a quarter of the raspberries; fold gently to mix, taking care not to break up raspberries further. Drizzle with remaining maple syrup; sprinkle with cinnamon.
**4** Preheat oven grill (broiler) to high; grill for 3 minutes or until tops are golden. Serve warm.

**TIP** Use orange rind instead of lemon rind, and nutmeg instead of cinnamon, if preferred.

| ● 4.5g total fat (1.2g saturated fat) | ● 745kJ (178 cal) | ● 18.8g carbohydrate | ● 14.5g protein | ● 2g fibre | ● 167mg sodium |
|---|---|---|---|---|---|

# Innocent chocolate &
# CHERRY CLAFOUTIS

**PREP + COOK TIME** 35 MINUTES (+ REFRIGERATION) **SERVES** 4

¾ cup (180ml) skim milk
¼ cup (60ml) water
2 eggs
1 egg white
1 teaspoon vanilla bean paste
2 teaspoons liquid stevia with agave
½ cup (75g) white spelt flour
1 teaspoon baking powder
1 tablespoon dutch-processed cocoa,
  plus extra for dusting
¾ cup (135g) frozen pitted cherries
olive-oil spray
⅓ cup (95g) low-fat natural Greek-style yoghurt

**1** Preheat oven to 180°C/350°F.

**2** Place milk, the water, eggs, egg white, vanilla and stevia in a medium bowl. Sift together flour, baking powder and cocoa; whisk into egg mixture until batter is smooth. Strain into a medium jug; cover. Refrigerate batter for 30 minutes.

**3** Arrange four ½ cup (125ml) ceramic ovenproof flan dishes on an oven tray; divide cherries evenly among dishes. Bake for 3 minutes or until cherry juices start to run.

**4** Carefully spray hot dishes with oil; pour ½ cup batter into each dish. Return immediately to oven; bake for a further 12 minutes or until batter is well risen around edges and just set in the centre.

**5** Top each clafoutis with 1 tablespoon yoghurt; dust lightly with extra cocoa to serve.

**TIP** Use pitted fresh cherries instead of frozen cherries, if they are in season.

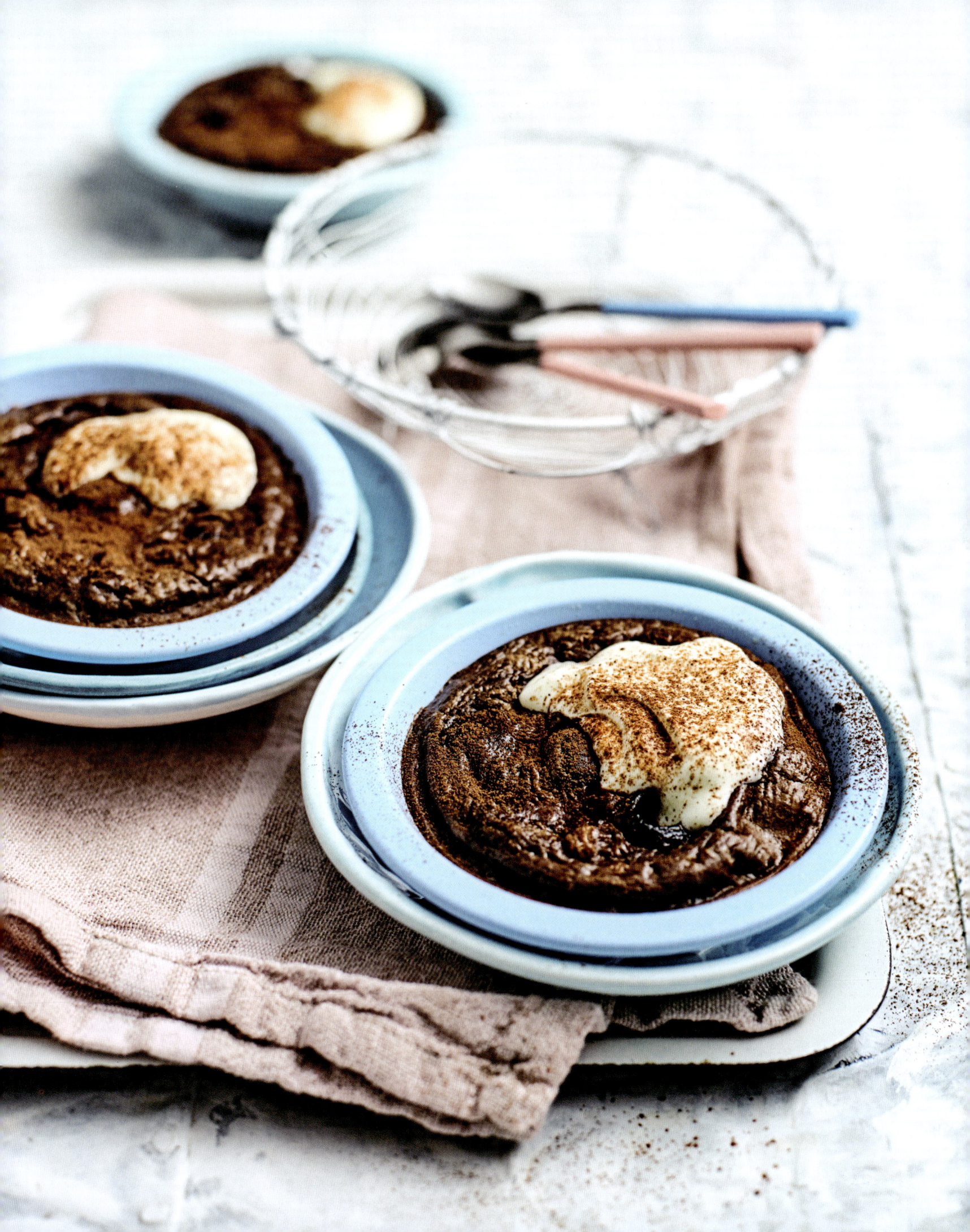

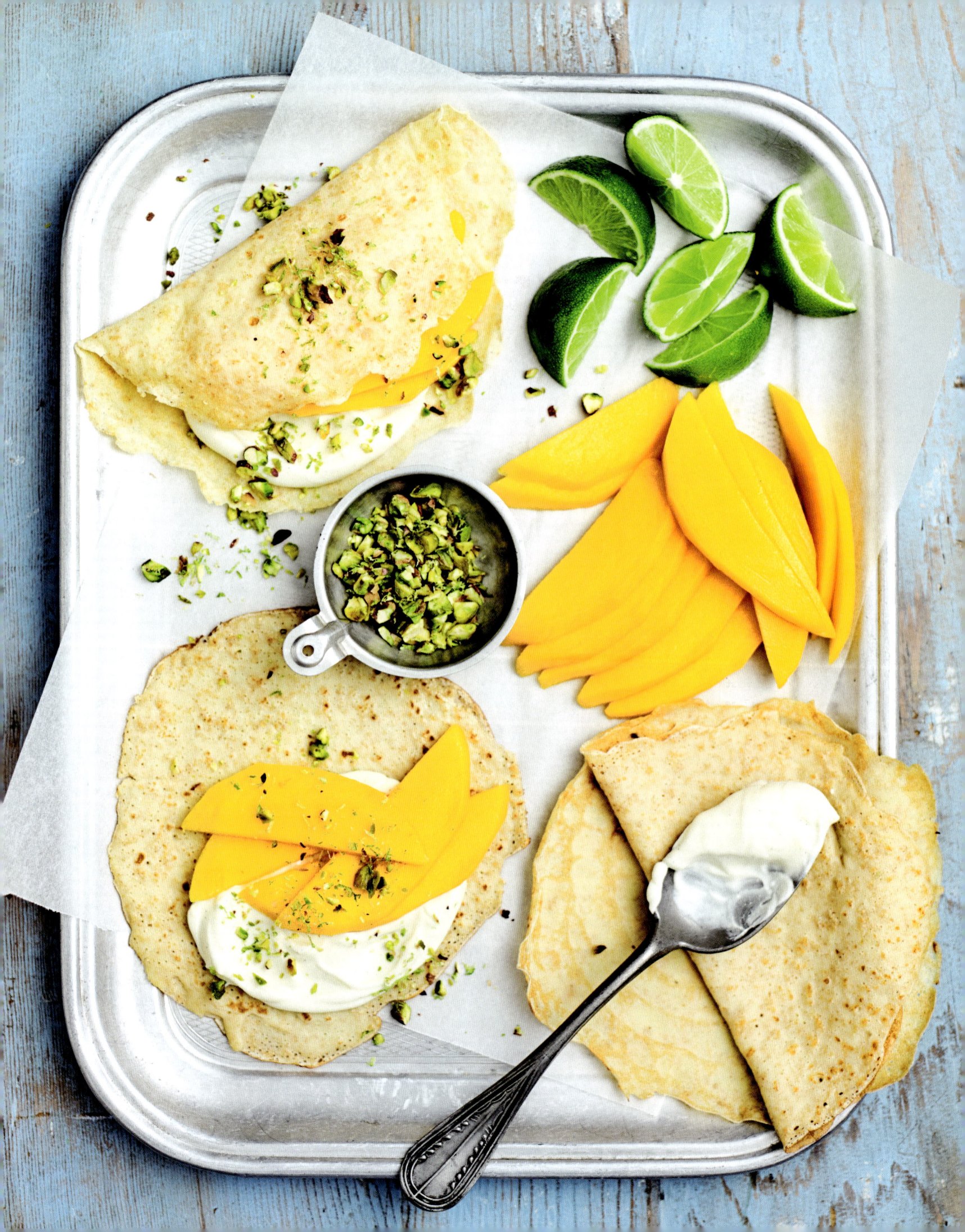

| | | | | | |
|---|---|---|---|---|---|
| ● 7.1g total fat (3.2g saturated fat) | ● 722kJ (172 cal) | ● 16.2g carbohydrate | ● 9g protein | ● 2.8g fibre | ● 101mg sodium |

# CRÊPES WITH
## mango & ricotta cream

**PREP + COOK TIME** 30 MINUTES (+ REFRIGERATION) **SERVES** 4

¼ cup (40g) wholemeal plain (all-purpose) flour
1 egg
⅓ cup (80ml) milk
olive-oil spray
1 small mango (300g), sliced thinly
1 tablespoon coarsely chopped pistachios
pinch ground cardamom
½ teaspoon finely grated lime rind
1 lime (65g), cut into wedges
**RICOTTA CREAM**
150g (4½oz) fresh ricotta
1½ teaspoons powdered stevia
½ teaspoon vanilla bean paste
2 tablespoons milk

**1** Place flour, egg and milk in a medium bowl; whisk until smooth. Cover; refrigerate for 30 minutes.

**2** Meanwhile, make ricotta cream.

**3** Spray a 16cm (6½in) heavy-based non-stick frying pan with oil; heat over medium–high heat. Pour a quarter of the batter (about 2 tablespoons) into pan, swirling pan to make a 16cm diameter crêpe; cook for 1 minute or until golden underneath. Turn crêpe; cook for a further 1 minute or until golden on the other side. Repeat with remaining batter to make three more crêpes.

**4** Spoon a quarter of the ricotta cream onto one side of the crêpe; top with a quarter of the mango slices. Fold crêpe over to enclose filling. Repeat with remaining crêpes, ricotta cream and mango.

**5** Combine pistachios, cardamom and rind in a small bowl; sprinkle over crêpes. Serve with lime wedges.

**RICOTTA CREAM** Blend ingredients with a stick blender until combined and thickened; it should be the consistency of sour cream. Cover; refrigerate until required.

**TIPS** Swap ground cinnamon or nutmeg for cardamom, if preferred. If you don't have a stick blender, use a small food processor to blend the ricotta cream.

| ● 4.4g total fat (2.8g saturated fat) | ● 609kJ (145 cal) | ● 17.4g carbohydrate | ● 7.8g protein | ● 1.3g fibre | ● 82mg sodium |

# yoghurt mango
# JELLIES

**PREP + COOK TIME** 20 MINUTES (+ REFRIGERATION) **SERVES** 4

10g lite mango jelly crystals
¾ cup (180ml) boiling water
1¼ cups (310ml) cold water
2 tablespoons boiling water, extra
2 teaspoons powdered gelatine
500g (1lb) plain yoghurt
1 tablespoon honey
½ small ripe mango (150g), diced
2 tablespoons passionfruit pulp

**1** Place jelly crystals and the boiling water in a medium heatproof bowl; stir to dissolve crystals. Add the cold water; stir to combine.

**2** Place the extra boiling water in a small heatproof bowl, sprinkle gelatine over; stir to dissolve gelatine.

**3** Heat 1 cup yoghurt and the honey in a microwave-safe bowl on HIGH in 30 second bursts until warm. Add gelatine; mix well. Fold through the remaining yoghurt, then whisk in the jelly mixture.

**4** Divide jelly mixture among four 1 cup (250ml) glasses. Refrigerate for 6 hours or overnight until set.

**5** Top jellies evenly with mango and passionfruit to serve.

**TIP** Swap your favourite flavour of lite jelly crystals for the mango flavour used here, if you like.

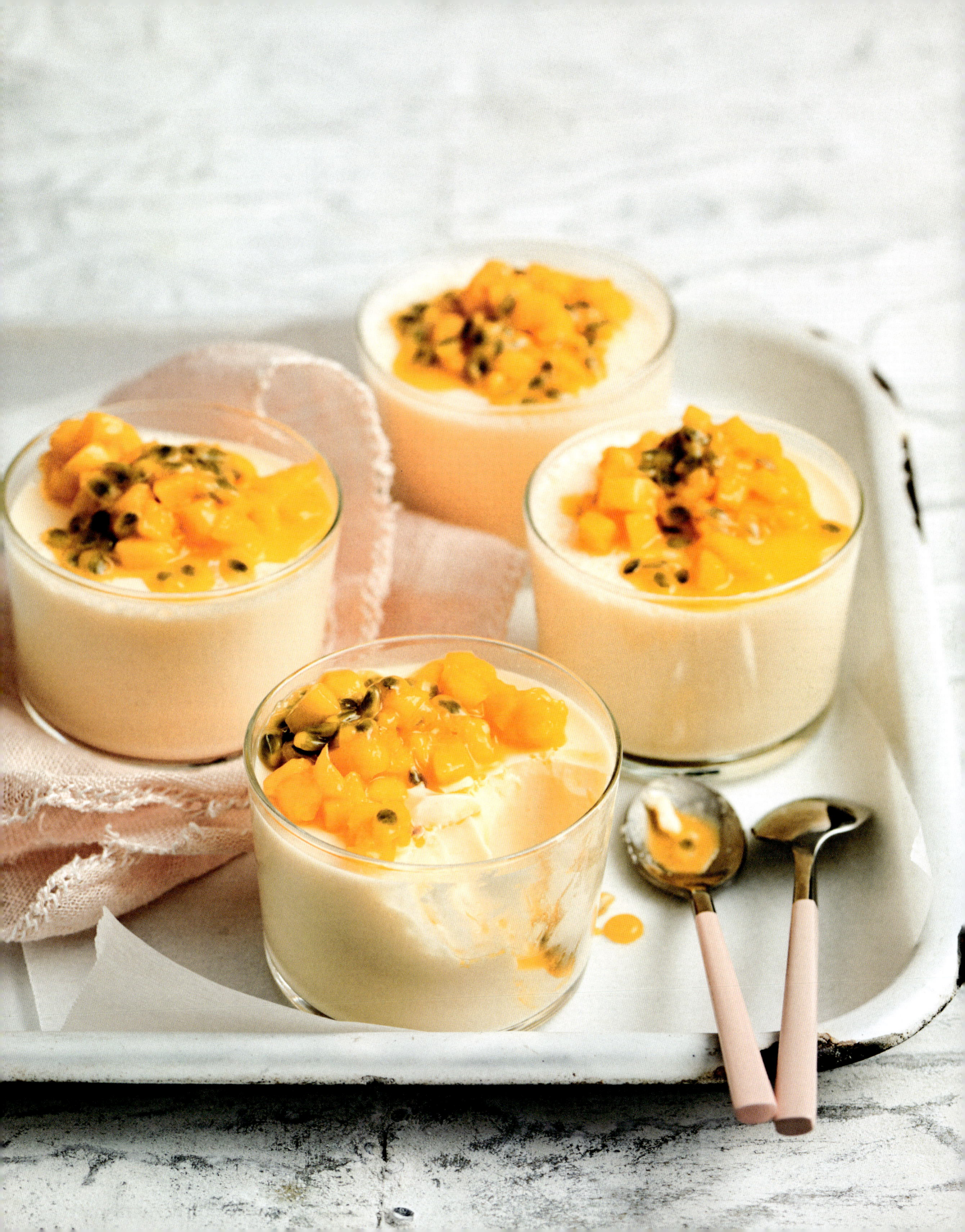

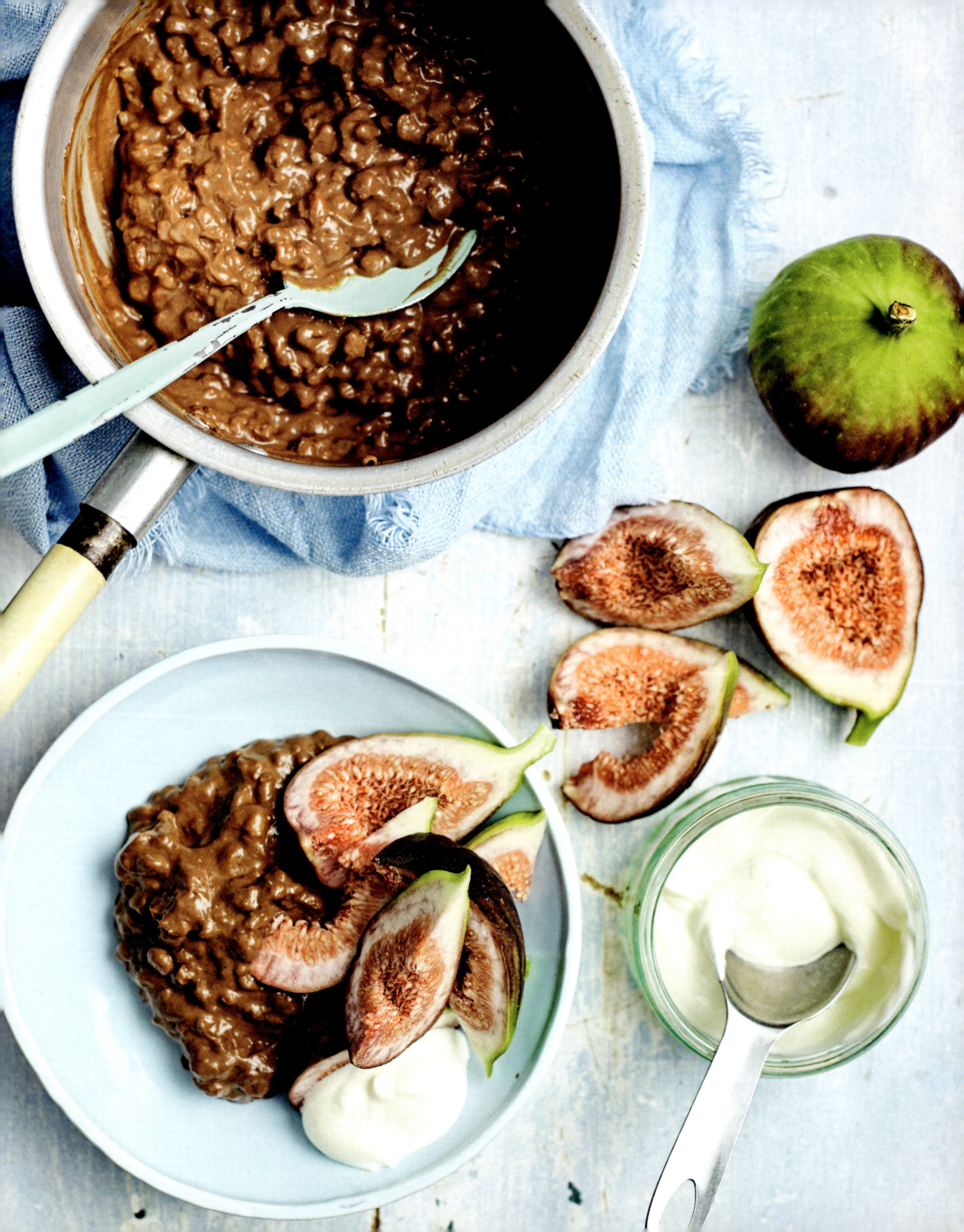

| ● 6.9g total fat (3.5g saturated fat) | ● 746kJ (178 cal) | ● 21.2g carbohydrate | ● 6.2g protein | ● 4.9g fibre | ● 43mg sodium |

# MOCHA FARRO PUDDING
## with figs

**PREP + COOK TIME** 1 HOUR 30 MINUTES (+ COOLING) **SERVES** 4

¼ cup (50g) roasted farro
2½ cups (625ml) water
2 teaspoons coffee granules (see tip)
1 stick cinnamon
1 teaspoon pure vanilla extract
40g (1½oz) dark (semi-sweet) chocolate (70% cocoa), chopped finely
1 teaspoon honey
1 egg yolk
⅓ cup (80ml) low-fat milk
4 small figs (200g), sliced
⅓ cup (95g) low-fat natural Greek-style yoghurt

1 Place farro and 1½ cups of the water in a small heavy-based saucepan; bring to the boil. Reduce heat to low; cook, covered, for 30 minutes. Drain, if necessary.

2 Return farro to the saucepan with the remaining water, coffee, cinnamon and vanilla; bring to the boil. Reduce heat to low; cook, covered, stirring occasionally, for 50 minutes or until the farro is cooked but still slightly firm to the bite. Discard cinnamon stick.

3 Stir chocolate and honey through the farro mixture. Whisk egg yolk and milk in a small bowl; stir through farro. Cook, stirring, over low heat, for 4 minutes or until mixture is thickened. Remove from heat; cool for 15 minutes.

4 Divide farro pudding among four small bowls. Top evenly with figs and yoghurt to serve.

**TIP** Turn this into a delicious chocolate pudding by omitting the coffee and replacing it with the same amount of dutch-processed cocoa powder instead.

**FARRO**, or emmer, is an ancient wheat grain originating in Italy. It is similar to spelt and barley, but retains a firm, chewy texture when cooked.

| 11.1g total fat (6.4g saturated fat) | 715kJ (170 cal) | 12.7g carbohydrate | 4.2g protein | 0.8g fibre | 47mg sodium |

# Blueberry basil
# ICE-CREAM POPS

**PREP + COOK TIME** 50 MINUTES (+ COOLING, REFRIGERATION & FREEZING) **SERVES** 12

250g (8oz) blueberries (see tips)
¼ cup (60ml) water
1½ cups firmly packed fresh basil leaves, shredded
1 cup (250ml) pouring cream
1 cup (250ml) milk
4 egg yolks
½ cup (125ml) pure maple syrup
1½ cups (375g) pot-set natural Greek-style yoghurt

**1** Place blueberries and the water in a small saucepan; cook, covered, over medium heat for 4 minutes or until blueberries release their juices and collapse. Remove lid; cook for a further 4 minutes or until thick and syrupy. Remove from heat; stir through basil. Stand until cooled to room temperature.

**2** Place cream and milk in a small heavy-based saucepan, bring to a simmer over medium-low heat; do not boil.

**3** Process cooled blueberry mixture in a small blender or food processor until a smooth puree forms. Push through a fine mesh strainer over a bowl; discard solids.

**4** Whisk egg yolks and maple syrup until thick and pale. Add warm milk mixture in a thin stream, whisking constantly until combined.

**5** Return mixture to saucepan over medium heat; cook, stirring constantly, for 10 minutes or until mixture thickens and coats the back of a wooden spoon (you may need to move the pan slightly off the heat to ensure the mixture doesn't boil during this time). Remove from heat.

**6** Place yoghurt in a medium heatproof bowl. Press custard mixture through a strainer over yoghurt; whisk until combined. Refrigerate for 30 minutes or until chilled.

**7** Grease and line a 1.5 litre (6 cup) loaf pan with baking paper, extending paper 2cm (¾in) above edge of pan. Pour chilled yoghurt mixture into pan; drizzle over blueberry mixture. Using a spatula, gently swirl blueberry mixture to create a marbled effect. Freeze for 2 hours or until mixture is partially set.

**8** Cover pan firmly with foil. Using the tip of a small sharp knife, make 12 small evenly-spaced cuts into the foil. Insert ice-block sticks (see tips) through cuts and into the ice-cream. Freeze for a further 4 hours or overnight until firm.

**9** To serve, stand ice-cream in pan at room temperature for 5 minutes to soften slightly, then remove from pan; remove paper lining. Use a hot, dry serrated knife to cut ice-cream into 12 even-sized serves. Serve immediately or return to freezer, wrapped individually in freezer wrap.

**TIPS** Use fresh rather than frozen blueberries for this recipe, as they give the best colour and flavour. For a different flavour combination, swap the blueberries and basil with raspberries and mint.

You will need 12 ice-block sticks. Trim a quarter length off the ends of the sticks so they are not too long. Or, if you like, omit the ice-block sticks, and simply set the ice-cream in the loaf pan, then scoop it to serve.

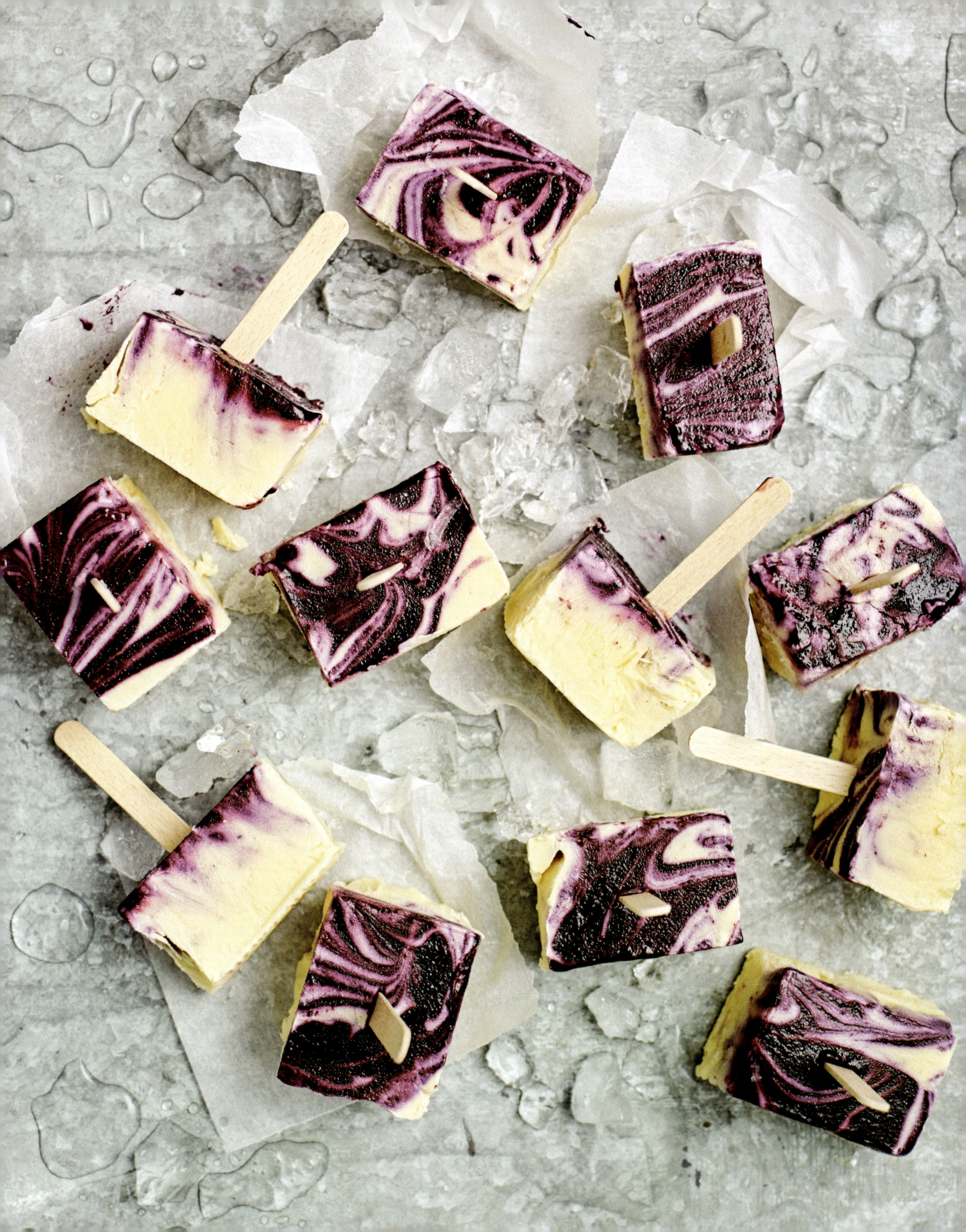

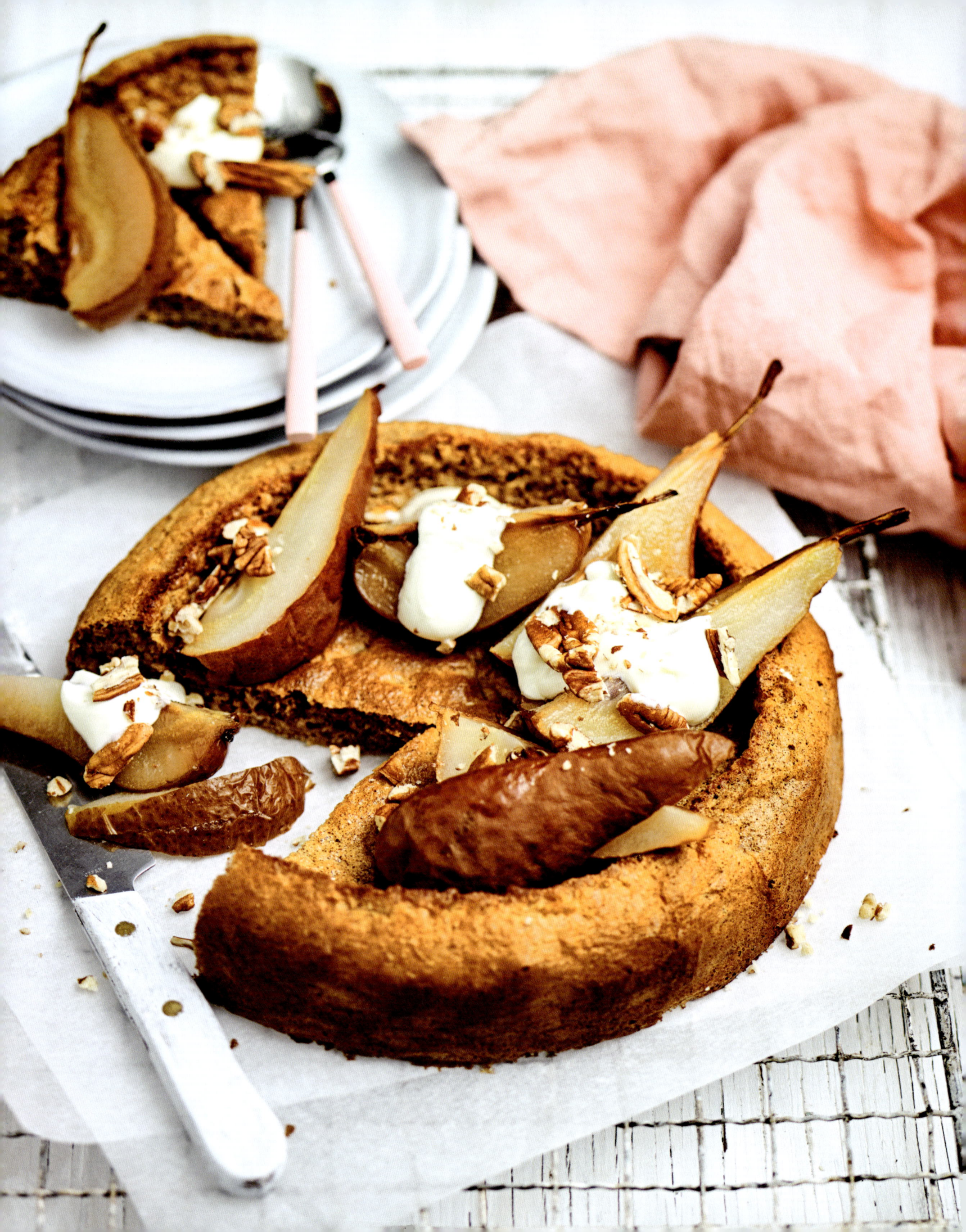

**NUTRITIONAL COUNT PER SERVING**

| 11.1g total fat (3.6g saturated fat) | 750kJ (179 cal) | 15.1g carbohydrate | 4.4g protein | 2.5g fibre | 68mg sodium |
|---|---|---|---|---|---|

# Pecan & pear
# SPICED SOUFFLÉ CAKE

**PREP + COOK TIME** 1 HOUR 20 MINUTES (+ COOLING) **SERVES** 10

2 medium pears (460g), halved lengthways

$2/3$ cup (80g) pecans

4 large eggs

$1/4$ cup (90g) honey

1 teaspoon vanilla bean paste

$3/4$ teaspoon ground nutmeg

$1/2$ teaspoon ground cinnamon

$1/4$ teaspoon ground cloves

2 tablespoons wholemeal plain (all-purpose) flour

1 tablespoon cornflour (cornstarch)

$1/4$ teaspoon sea salt flakes

40g ($1\frac{1}{2}$oz) butter, melted, cooled

$1/3$ cup (95g) natural Greek-style yoghurt

**1** Preheat oven to 180°C/350°F. Line an oven tray with baking paper. Grease and line base and side of a 22cm (9in) springform cake tin.

**2** Place pears, skin-side up, on oven tray. Roast for 40 minutes. Meanwhile, place pecans on another oven tray; roast on another oven shelf for the last 5 minutes of pear roasting time. Cool.

**3** Process $1/2$ cup of the pecans until ground finely. Coarsely chop remaining pecans; reserve. Cut each pear half into 5 wedges (to make 20 wedges in total); core if you like.

**4** Whisk eggs, honey and spices with an electric mixer for 10 minutes or until ribbons form when beaters are lifted. Sift combined flours and salt over egg mixture. Add ground pecans and butter; use a large whisk to gently incorporate ingredients.

**5** Pour batter into tin. Bake cake on lower oven shelf for 20 minutes. Cool in tin for 5 minutes before turning, top-side up, onto a wire rack to cool completely.

**6** Cut cake into 10 equal slices; sprinkle with reserved pecans. Serve one cake slice and two pear wedges per person with a drizzle of yoghurt.

**TIP** The cake is best made on the day of serving. This is a lovely cake for a special occasion, or when having family and friends around for lunch or dinner.

| ● 10.1g total fat (1g saturated fat) | ● 703kJ (168 cal) | ● 13.9g carbohydrate | ● 4.6g protein | ● 2.2g fibre | ● 23mg sodium |
|---|---|---|---|---|---|

# BLUEBERRY DOUGHNUTS
## *with lemon drizzle*

**PREP + COOK TIME** 35 MINUTES (+ COOLING) **MAKES** 8

**3 egg whites**
**¼ cup (60ml) pure maple syrup**
**¾ cup (90g) almond meal**
**½ cup (80g) wholemeal plain (all-purpose) flour**
**2 tablespoons light olive oil**
**80g (2½oz) fresh blueberries**
**¼ cup (40g) 100% sugar-free natural icing mix**
**3 teaspoons lemon juice**
**1 teaspoon finely grated lemon rind**

**1** Preheat oven to 180°C/350°F. Grease eight holes of a ⅓ cup (80ml) doughnut pan.

**2** Beat egg whites with an electric mixer on medium speed for 2 minutes or until foamy. With motor operating, add maple syrup; beat for 3 minutes or until firm peaks form. Sift in combined almond meal and flour; whisk in oil until a smooth batter forms. Transfer batter to a disposable piping bag; snip off the end to make a 1cm (½in) opening.

**3** Place doughnut pan on a large oven tray. Pipe half the almond batter into base of greased holes; divide blueberries evenly over batter. Pipe remaining batter over blueberries. Bake for 12 minutes, turning tray once during baking.

**4** Stand doughnuts in pan for 2 minutes before turning onto a wire rack to cool completely.

**5** Place sifted icing mix and the lemon juice in a small bowl; stir until icing mix dissolves and icing is smooth.

**6** Drizzle cooled doughnuts with icing; sprinkle with rind.

**DR JO SAYS**
Avoid buying commercial biscuits, cakes and pastries. These are loaded with the wrong types of fat, too much added sugar and refined starch, leading to large fluctuations in your blood glucose control and increasing your risk of heart disease.

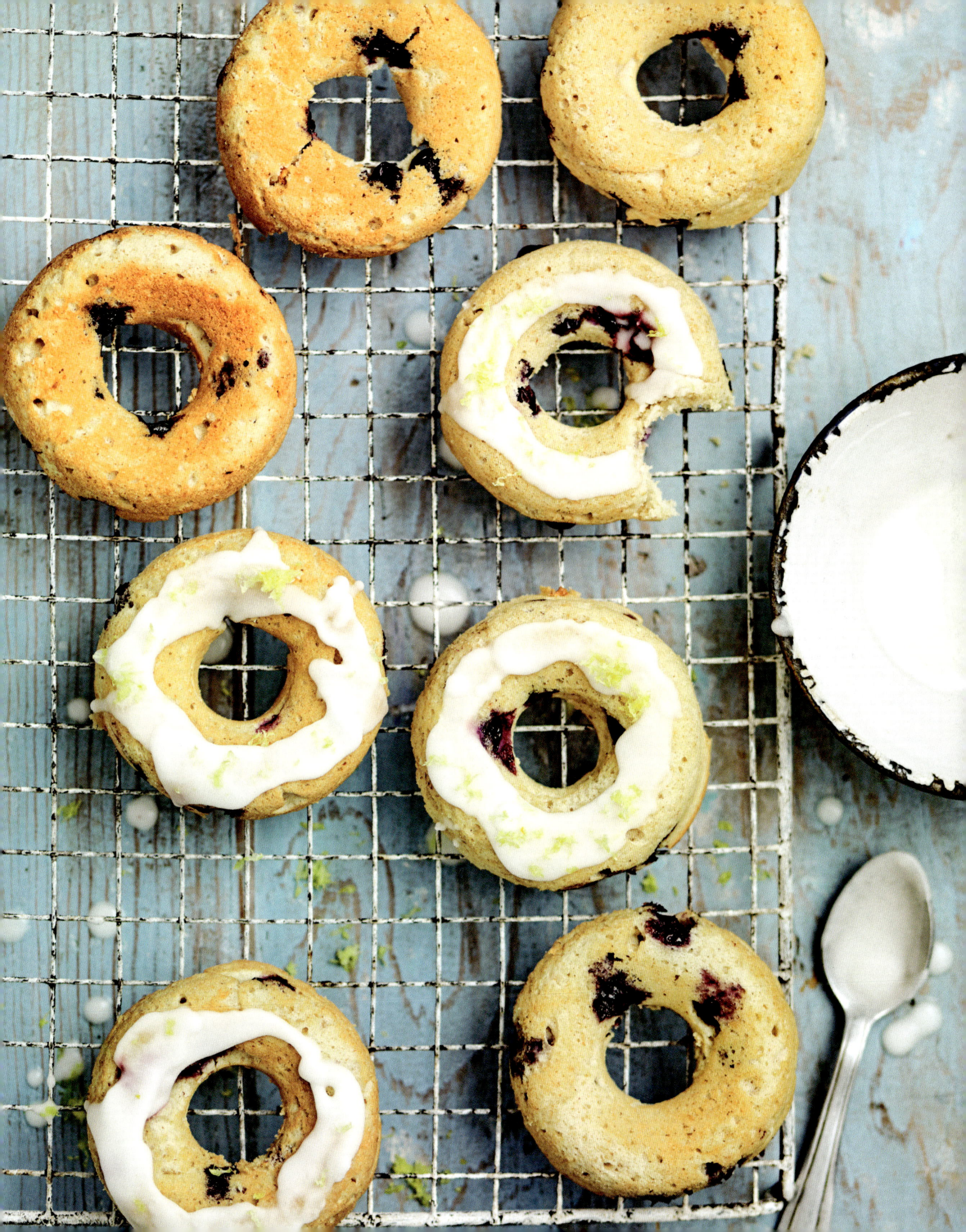

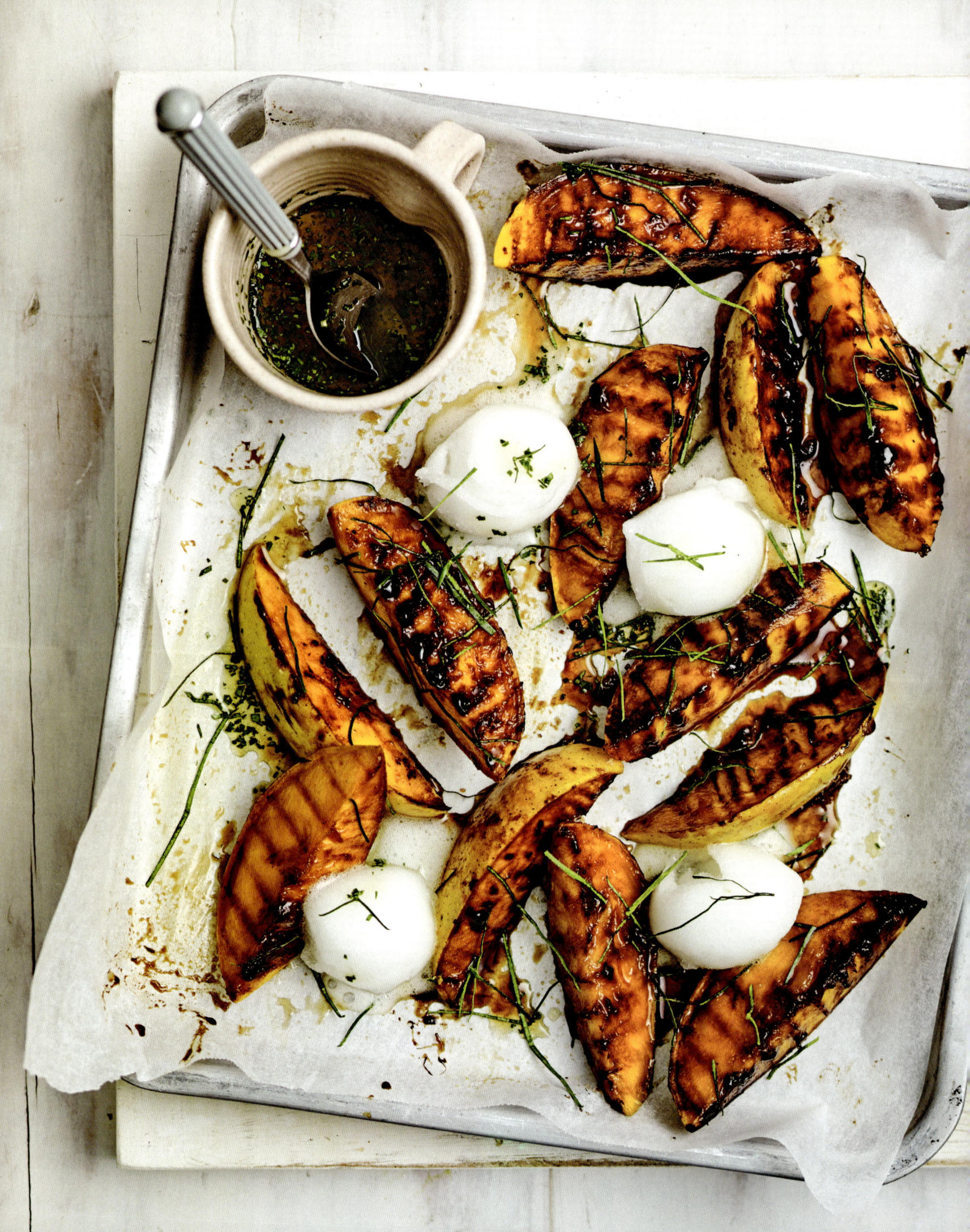

| ● 1.7g total fat (1.4g saturated fat) | ● 518kJ (123 cal) | ● 25.6g carbohydrate | ● 1.4g protein | ● 2.1g fibre | ● 5mg sodium |

# GRILLED MANGO CHEEKS
## with lime drizzle

**PREP + COOK TIME** 10 MINUTES **SERVES** 4

2 small mangoes (600g)
1 tablespoon brown sugar
4 fresh kaffir lime leaves
1 tablespoon pure maple syrup
2 tablespoons lime juice
80g (2½oz) pineapple, coconut and lime sorbet

**1** Heat a grill plate (or grill pan) over high heat. Cut cheeks from mangoes using a sharp knife. Cut each cheek into three wedges. Sprinkle each piece evenly with brown sugar.

**2** Grill mango, flesh-side down, for 1 minute or until caramelised and grill lines appear.

**3** Chop half the lime leaves finely; shred remaining lime leaves. Combine maple syrup, lime juice and chopped lime leaves in a small jug.

**4** Spoon lime drizzle over mango cheeks and sprinkle with shredded lime leaves; accompany with a quarter of the sorbet per person.

**TIP** Use ripe mangoes in this refreshing, summery dessert for the best flavour.

**DR JO SAYS**
Pure maple syrup is a good choice of sweetener for blood glucose control as it has a low GI. You only need to use about two-thirds of the amount you would of table sugar, so it helps you to keep total sugar levels down.

# GLOSSARY

**agar-agar powder** is a gelatinous substance made from seaweed and used as a setting or thickening agent. It's available from health food stores.

**agave syrup** a sweetener commercially produced from the agave plant in South Africa and Mexico. It is sweeter than sugar, though less viscous, so it dissolves quickly. Agave syrup is sold in light, amber, dark and raw varieties.

**all-bran cereal** a low-fat, high-fibre wheat bran breakfast cereal.

**bacon, shortcut** is a 'half rasher'; the streaky (belly), narrow end of the rasher is removed leaving the larger 'eye' meat (shortcut).

**baking powder** a raising agent consisting mainly of two parts cream of tartar to one part bicarbonate of soda (baking soda).

**barley**
*black* this nutty-tasting wholegrain is dark mahogany in colour with a white interior. Use it as a substitute for rice. Serve on its own or combine with other grains.
*pearl* a nutritious grain used in soups and stews; has had the husk removed then been hulled and polished so only the 'pearl' of the original grain remains, much the same as white rice.

**basil, thai** (also horapa) is different from sweet (common) basil, having smaller leaves, purplish stems and a slight aniseed taste.

**beans**
*black* also known as turtle beans or black kidney beans; has an earthy flavour and is completely different from the better-known chinese black beans (which are fermented soya beans).
*broad* also known as fava, windsor and horse beans. Fresh and frozen forms should be peeled twice (discarding both the outer long green pod and the beige-green tough inner shell).
*cannellini* small white bean similar in appearance and flavour to great northern, navy and haricot beans – all of which can be substituted for the other.
*kidney* a red bean with a slightly floury texture and sweet flavour.
*sprouts* also known as 'shoots'; tender new growths of assorted beans and seeds grown for consumption as sprouts.

**bicarbonate of soda** also known as baking or carb soda; is used as a leavening (raising) agent in baking.

**bread**
*mountain* a thin, soft-textured bread, that is either filled then rolled up or served flat alongside soups and dips. Available from supermarkets and health food stores.
*pitta* also known as lebanese bread. A wheat-flour pocket bread sold in large, flat pieces that separate into two thin rounds. Also available in small thick pieces called pocket pitta.
*pumpernickel* a form of german bread characterised by its dark brown, almost black, colour, virtually no crust and strong rye taste.
*rye* may be made from 100% rye flour or as a white/rye flour blend.

*sourdough* has been around since the Middle Ages. It is made using a starter dough, a blend of flour and water, which has been left for many days to ferment. A small amount of starter is kept to use in the next batch. These days, sourdough may be made using a commercial yeast, although traditionalists frown on this process.

*tortillas* thin, round unleavened bread originating in Mexico. Two types are available, made either from wheat flour or corn (maize).

**buk choy, baby** also known as pak kat farang or shanghai buk choy, is much smaller and more tender than mature buk choy.

**burghul** is made from whole wheat kernels, which are steamed, dried and toasted before cracking into several distinct sizes, so they develop a rich, nutty flavour. Because it's already partially cooked, burghul only requires minimal cooking. Cracked wheat, which is raw whole wheat, requires much longer cooking.

**buttermilk** originally the term given to the slightly sour liquid left after butter was churned from cream, these days it's made similarly to yoghurt. Despite the implication of its name, it is low in fat.

**capers** grey-green buds of a warm climate (usually Mediterranean) shrub, sold either dried and salted or pickled in a vinegar brine. Baby capers are picked early, and are fuller-flavoured. Whether pickled or salted, capers should be rinsed well before using.

**capsicum** also known as bell pepper or, simply, pepper.
*vine sweet mini caps* can be orange, red or yellow and are about the size of baby red capsicums. They have a very fine skin and few seeds, although still need deseeding.

**cavolo nero** also known as tuscan or tuscan black cabbage. It has long, narrow, wrinkled leaves and a rich, astringent, mild cabbage flavour. It doesn't lose its volume like silver beet or spinach when cooked, but it does need longer cooking.

**celeriac** a tuberous root with a brown skin, soft, white velvety flesh and a celery-like flavour.

**chai tea bags** chai tea usually contains a strong black tea mixed with various spices and herbs; the mix and proportions of flavours vary, but often contains cardamom, cinnamon, cloves and ginger.

**cheese**
*labne* is a yoghurt cheese made by draining yoghurt through muslin to remove the liquid.
*paneer* (panir) is a fresh unripened cows'-milk cheese similar to pressed ricotta. It is available in Indian food stores, health food stores and some supermarkets (near the fetta and haloumi).

**chilli** available in many types and sizes. Use rubber gloves when seeding and chopping fresh chillies as they can burn your skin. Removing seeds and membranes lessens the heat level.
*flakes* dried, deep-red, dehydrated chilli slices and whole seeds.
*long, green or red* available both fresh and dried; a generic term used for moderately hot, long (about 6cm to 8cm), thin chillies.

**234**

**mexican chilli powder** a blend of chilli, paprika, cumin and garlic. **powder** the Asian variety, made from dried ground thai chillies, is the hottest; use as a substitute for fresh chillies in the proportion of $\frac{1}{2}$ teaspoon chilli powder to 1 medium chopped fresh chilli.

**coriander** also known as pak chee, cilantro or chinese parsley; bright-green leafy herb with a pungent flavour. Both the stems and roots of coriander are used; wash well before using. Is also available ground or as seeds; these should not be substituted for fresh as the tastes are completely different.

**cornflour** also known as cornstarch; used as a thickening agent in cooking. If gluten intolerant, buy 100% corn (maize) cornflour, as wheaten cornflour contains some gluten.

**couscous** a fine, grain-like cereal product made from semolina. A semolina dough is dehydrated to produce minuscule pellets, which are rehydrated by steaming, causing them to swell to three or four times their original size.

**pearl** couscous is made from baked wheat rather than semolina. Its granules are larger (its size and shape is similar to a pearl) and it maintains its texture and firmness without sticking.

**cream** we used fresh cream, also known as pouring or pure cream, unless otherwise stated. Minimum fat content 35%.

**sour** a thick, cultured, soured cream. Minimum fat content 35%.

**cucumbers**

**baby** a miniature variety of lebanese cucumber, may also be sold as 'qukes'; are small and crunchy.

**lebanese** short, slender and thin-skinned. Very popular due to its tender, edible skin, tiny, yielding seeds and sweet, fresh taste.

**telegraph** also known as the european or burpless cucumber; slender and quite long, its thin dark-green skin has shallow ridges running down its length.

**curly endive** also known as frisée, a curly-leafed green vegetable with a slightly bitter flavour.

**dashi** is the basic fish and seaweed stock used to flavour many Japanese dishes. It is made from dried bonito (fish) flakes and kelp (kombu). *Dashi miso paste* is simply miso (see also 'miso') with added dashi stock or powder.

**dried bonito flakes** simply flakes of dried, smoked bonito fish, a type of tuna.

**dried seaweed** sold as kelp, nori or yaki nori (toasted seaweed). These are the dark green wrappings around sushi rolls.

**dutch-processed cocoa** processed to neutralize its acids, it has a reddish-brown colour, mild flavour, and is easy to dissolve.

**eggplant** purple-skinned vegetable also known as aubergine.

**farro** a variety of wheat with a nutty flavour and chewy texture; may be substituted for rice, lentils, couscous and pasta in recipes.

**fennel** also known as finocchio; has as slightly anise-like flavour.

**flat-leaf parsley** also known as continental or italian parsley.

**flour**

**buckwheat** a herb in the same plant family as rhubarb; not a cereal so it is gluten-free.

**lupin** these are part of the legume family. Lupin flour is created by discarding the hull then grinding the lupins into a fine flour.

**plain** an all-purpose flour made from wheat.

**self-raising** (self-rising) plain flour sifted with baking powder in the proportion of 1 cup flour to 2 teaspoons baking powder.

**spelt** very similar to wheat, but has a slightly nuttier, sweeter flavour; it contains gluten.

**wholemeal** nothing is discarded, uses the whole wheat grain.

**freekah** a highly nutritious grain made from roasted green grains, including wheat, barley, triticale and others. Because the grains are harvested young, freekeh contains more protein, vitamins and minerals than the mature grain. It's low GI, low carb and high fibre.

**garam masala** a blend of spices based on varying proportions of cardamom, cinnamon, cloves, coriander, fennel and cumin. Black pepper and chilli can be added for a hotter version.

**harissa** a hot Moroccan sauce or paste made from dried chillies. The paste, available in a tube, is very hot and should not be used in large amounts; bottled harissa sauce is milder, but is still hot. If you have a low heat-level tolerance, you may find any recipe with harissa too hot to tolerate. It is available from supermarkets and Middle-Eastern grocery stores.

**kaffir lime leaves** also known as bai magrood, look like two glossy dark green leaves joined end to end, forming a rounded hourglass shape. A strip of fresh lime peel may be substituted for each leaf.

**kale** a leafy vegetable of the brassica family (cauliflower, broccoli). However, as with cavolo nero, it doesn't form a head. It has very firm green or purple leaves and is available in both flat-leaf and curly-leaf varieties.

**maple syrup, pure** a thin syrup distilled from the sap of the maple tree. Maple-flavoured or pancake syrup is not an adequate substitute for the real thing.

**matcha powder** (green tea powder) green tea that has been milled into a very fine powder. Is available from Asian food stores.

**millet** is a small-seeded cereal grain, which has a slightly nutty, corn-like flavour. *Puffed millet* are grains that have been processed under high pressure with steam, causing them to expand and puff. It is available from health food stores and the health food section of larger supermarkets.

**miso** Japan's famous bean paste made from fermented soya beans and rice, rye or barley. *White (shiro) miso* tends to have a sweeter and somewhat less salty flavour than the darker red miso. Dissolve miso in a little water before using. Keeps well refrigerated.

**mung bean noodles** made from mung bean paste; also known as bean thread noodles, and cellophane or glass noodles because they are transparent when cooked.

**mushroom**

*button* small, white mushrooms having a delicate, subtle flavour.

*flat* large and flat with a rich, earthy flavour. They are sometimes misnamed field mushrooms, which are wild mushrooms.

*portobello* mature swiss browns. Large, dark brown mushrooms with a full-bodied flavour.

*shiitake* when fresh are also known as chinese black, forest or golden oak mushrooms; although cultivated, they have the earthiness and taste of wild mushrooms. Are large and meaty. Also available dried from larger supermarkets and Asian food stores.

*swiss brown* also called roman or cremini; are light-to-dark brown in colour with a full-bodied flavour.

**nashi pear** a member of the pear family but resembling an apple with its pale-yellow-green, tennis-ball-sized appearance; more commonly known as the 'asian pear'.

**onion**

*green* also known as scallion or, incorrectly, shallot; an immature onion picked before the bulb has formed. Has a long, bright-green edible stalk.

*spring* have small white bulbs and long, narrow green-leafed tops.

**polenta** coarsely or finely ground yellow or white corn (maize). Also the name of the dish made from it.

**pomegranate** the large fruit is filled with many seeds, each wrapped in an edible crimson pulp having a tangy sweet-sour flavour. To remove the pulp, cut the fruit in half, then hit the skin of the halves with a wooden spoon – the seeds usually fall out easily.

*molasses* thick, tangy syrup made by boiling pomegranate juice into a sticky, syrupy consistency. Available from Middle-Eastern food stores and some delis.

**quinoa** (keen-wa) the seeds of a leafy plant similar to spinach. It has a delicate, slightly nutty taste and chewy texture. The seeds should be washed before cooking as they contain a bitter coating, known as saponins, which requires rinsing. Simply wash until the water runs clear. It spoils easily, so keep sealed in a jar in the fridge.

**rhubarb** has thick, celery-like stalks that can reach up to 60cm (24in) in length; the stalks are the only edible portion of the plant as the leaves contain a toxic substance.

**rice**

*brown basmati* has more fibre and a stronger flavour than white basmati, but takes twice as long to cook.

*Doongara* is an uniquely Australian grown rice, first commercially harvested in 1989. It has two main benefits: a lower GI, so it is digested more slowly, and is hard to overcook, so it remains fluffy.

*microwave* this pre-cooked rice is more porous, so steam can penetrate the grain and rehydrate it in a short time.

**rice paper rounds** made from rice flour and water then stamped into rounds; are quite brittle and break easily. Dipped briefly in water, they become pliable wrappers for food.

**rocket** also known as arugula, rugula and rucola; a peppery-tasting green leaf used similarly to baby spinach. Baby rocket leaves, also known as wild rocket, are both smaller and less peppery.

**rolled oats** oat groats (oats that have been husked) that are steam-softened, flattened with rollers, then dried and packaged.

**rosewater** an extract made from crushed rose petals, called gulab in India; used for its aromatic quality in many desserts.

**seafood**

*blue-eye* also known as deep sea trevalla or trevally and blue-eye cod; a thick, moist, white-fleshed fish.

*firm white fish fillet* blue eye, bream, flathead, swordfish, ling, whiting, jewfish, snapper or sea perch are all good choices. Check for small pieces of bone and use tweezers to remove them.

*mussels, black* must be tightly closed when bought, indicating they are alive. Some mussels might not open after cooking. These might need prompting with a knife or might not have cooked as quickly as the others. Farmed mussels will not all open up during cooking – you do not have to discard these, just open with a knife and cook a little more if you wish.

*prawns* are available as uncooked (green) or cooked, with or without shells.

**shallot** also french or golden shallots or eschalots; small, elongated, brown-skinned members of the onion family.

*red* also known as thai purple shallots, asian shallots, pink shallots or homm. A member of the onion family, they resemble garlic in that they are multiple-cloved bulbs and are intensely flavoured.

**soba noodles** are thin Japanese noodles made of buckwheat flour (soba-ko) and wheat flour (komugi-ko).

**stevia** a natural sugar substitute that comes from the stevia plant. It is about 300 times sweeter than sugar, but free of calories and with no impact on blood sugar levels.

*granules and powder* are suitable to sprinkle on desserts, muesli and fruit, or mixed into dishes when cooking and baking.

*stevia liquid with agave* dissolves readily into liquids.

**sugar-free natural icing mix** a 100% natural sweetener made with a blend of stevia and erythritol (a sugar alcohol); erythritol looks and tastes like sugar, yet has almost no calories.

**sumac** a purple-red, astringent spice that is ground from berries grown on shrubs that flourish around the Mediterranean; adds a tart, lemony flavour to foods.

**tahini** sesame seed paste. *Unhulled tahini* retains the outer kernel, so has a slightly bitter taste. Available from supermarkets.

**tzatziki** a greek sauce made from yoghurt and diced cucumber.

**vinegar**

*apple cider* made from crushed fermented apples.

*balsamic* originally from Modena, Italy, and made from a regional wine of white Trebbiano grapes, specially processed then aged in antique wooden casks, which gives it a deep rich brown colour and a sweet/sour pungent flavour.

*red wine* based on fermented red wine.

*rice* a colourless vinegar made from fermented rice and flavoured with sugar and salt. Also known as seasoned rice vinegar.

*rice wine* made from rice wine lees (the sediment left after fermentation), salt and alcohol.

*white wine* made from a blend of white wines.

**Weet-Bix** oven-roasted whole-wheat grains combined with sugar, salt and barley malt extract – a wheat-based breakfast biscuit.

# CONVERSION CHART

## MEASURES

One Australian metric measuring cup holds approximately 250ml; one Australian metric tablespoon holds 20ml; one Australian metric teaspoon holds 5ml.

The difference between one country's measuring cups and another's is within a two- or three-teaspoon variance, and will not affect your cooking results. North America, New Zealand and the United Kingdom use a 15ml tablespoon.

All cup and spoon measurements are level. The most accurate way of measuring dry ingredients is to weigh them. When measuring liquids, use a clear glass or plastic jug with the metric markings.

The imperial measurements used in these recipes are approximate only. Measurements for cake pans are approximate only. Using same-shaped cake pans of a similar size should not affect your baking. We measure the inside top of the cake pan to determine sizes.

We use large eggs with an average weight of 60g.

## DRY MEASURES

| METRIC | IMPERIAL |
|---|---|
| 15G | ½OZ |
| 30G | 1OZ |
| 60G | 2OZ |
| 90G | 3OZ |
| 125G | 4OZ (¼LB) |
| 155G | 5OZ |
| 185G | 6OZ |
| 220G | 7OZ |
| 250G | 8OZ (½LB) |
| 280G | 9OZ |
| 315G | 10OZ |
| 345G | 11OZ |
| 375G | 12OZ (¾LB) |
| 410G | 13OZ |
| 440G | 14OZ |
| 470G | 15OZ |
| 500G | 16OZ (1LB) |
| 750G | 24OZ (1½LB) |
| 1KG | 32OZ (2LB) |

## LIQUID MEASURES

| METRIC | IMPERIAL |
|---|---|
| 30ML | 1 FLUID OZ |
| 60ML | 2 FLUID OZ |
| 100ML | 3 FLUID OZ |
| 125ML | 4 FLUID OZ |
| 150ML | 5 FLUID OZ |
| 190ML | 6 FLUID OZ |
| 250ML | 8 FLUID OZ |
| 300ML | 10 FLUID OZ |
| 500ML | 16 FLUID OZ |
| 600ML | 20 FLUID OZ |
| 1000ML (1 LITRE) | 1¾ PINTS |

## LENGTH MEASURES

| METRIC | IMPERIAL |
|---|---|
| 3MM | ⅛IN |
| 6MM | ¼IN |
| 1CM | ½IN |
| 2CM | ¾IN |
| 2.5CM | 1IN |
| 5CM | 2IN |
| 6CM | 2½IN |
| 8CM | 3IN |
| 10CM | 4IN |
| 13CM | 5IN |
| 15CM | 6IN |
| 18CM | 7IN |
| 20CM | 8IN |
| 22CM | 9IN |
| 25CM | 10IN |
| 28CM | 11IN |
| 30CM | 12IN (1FT) |

## OVEN TEMPERATURES

The oven temperatures in this book are for conventional ovens; if you have a fan-forced oven, decrease the temperature by 10-20 degrees.

| | °C (CELSIUS) | °F (FAHRENHEIT) |
|---|---|---|
| VERY SLOW | 120 | 250 |
| SLOW | 150 | 300 |
| MODERATELY SLOW | 160 | 325 |
| MODERATE | 180 | 350 |
| MODERATELY HOT | 200 | 400 |
| HOT | 220 | 425 |
| VERY HOT | 240 | 475 |